# Facial features
# of neurologic syndromes

# Facial features
# of neurologic syndromes

**PAUL R. DYKEN, M.D.**

Professor of Pediatric Neurology,
Departments of Neurology and Pediatrics,
School of Medicine, Medical College of Georgia, Augusta, Georgia

**MAX D. MILLER, Ed.D.**

Associate Professor, Department of Family Practice and
Division of Educational Research and Development,
Medical College of Georgia, Augusta, Georgia

*with illustrations by*

**KAREN WALDO, M.S.**

Medical Illustration Services,
Medical College of Georgia, Augusta, Georgia

*and*

**JOHN HAGAN, M.S.**

Medical Illustration Services,
Medical College of Georgia, Augusta, Georgia

# The C. V. Mosby Company

ST. LOUIS · TORONTO · LONDON    1980

Copyright © 1980 by The C. V. Mosby Company

All rights reserved. No part of this book may be reproduced in any manner without written permission of the publisher.

Printed in the United States of America

The C. V. Mosby Company
11830 Westline Industrial Drive, St. Louis, Missouri 63141


Library of Congress Cataloging in Publication Data

Dyken, Paul R
     Facial features of neurologic syndromes.

     Bibliography: p.
     Includes index.
     1. Nervous system – Diseases – Diagnosis. 2. Facial
manifestations of general diseases. 3. Syndromes.
I. Miller, Max D., 1940-      joint author. II. Title.
[DNLM: 1. Face. 2. Nervous system diseases – Diagnosis.
WL100.3 D996f]
RC348.D93      616.8′04′72      79-17012
ISBN 0-8016-1485-6


C/CB/B  9  8  7  6  5  4  3  2  1      01/D/030

# Prologue

## THE JOHN ARTHUR SLADE STORY

During a recent clinical investigation of a large, interbred, black family that had an unusual inherited disease, I encountered a strikingly alert and intelligent 70-year-old member of the family. The lady, Mrs. Slade, was a maternal great aunt of an infant who had Tay-Sachs disease. Through various laboratory investigations, the diagnosis in her grandniece was confirmed as the type of gangliosidosis that results from the total absence of the enzyme hexosaminidase A. In an effort to trace this defect, which is unusual in blacks, a full family investigation was performed. Mrs. Slade seemed to realize the potential benefits of such a study, especially for those young members of her family who were of reproductive age. She therefore consented to furnish information about past generations of the family that she represented as matriarch. It was through this investigation that I became familiar with the life of Mrs. Slade's son John Arthur.

Mrs. Slade had given birth to 11 children during the depression period. The depression in the South brought hard times for even the most affluent persons, and more so for blacks. Although of low socioeconomic status and undereducated in relationship to her intelligence, Mrs. Slade and her husband had chiseled out a relatively comfortable life for themselves and their children in the face of many hardships. Even to give birth in that period and in that place was an accomplishment. Poor blacks did not always have available to them the modern conveniences — or the everyday necessities of life — that we in the more modern South take for granted. Southern black women in that era spent their maternity confinements at home. If they were aided by anyone in the labor and birth process, they were helped by friends or relatives or occasionally by a midwife but rarely by physicians or trained professionals. Thus all of Mrs. Slade's children were born at home without modern conveniences to aid her in labor; expert medical or nursing supervision was not available.

One might speculate that the trying circumstances associated with even the simplest and most basic of human functions must have tended to solidify the maternal-child bond. In the instance of Mrs. Slade and her children and other family members, this was certain. The first-born son was the pride and joy of both Mrs. Slade and her husband. When compared to his older sisters, he was never strong or precocious. Yet until he was 7 months old, he was, for all intents and purposes, normal. He was a plump, healthy baby until that time, when he began to become irritable and fussy and to lose weight. His motor skills began to deteriorate, and he seemed "loose" and "floppy," according to Mrs. Slade's clear descriptions.

Although medical care was expensive in those hard times, Mrs. Slade's son was taken to local medical practitioners to be examined and, it was hoped, treated—regardless of the medical debts to be incurred. Yet the examinations were of little diagnostic value. Continued deterioration occurred in spite of all attempted treatments. The boy became progressively more dull, developed excessive "jumpiness," and finally died at 21 months of age after an illness of 14 months.

The loss of her son was a great sadness to Mrs. Slade and her family, but life had to continue. Several females, all of them normal, were born. Then a daughter was born who developed in a way very much like that of the son. She was at first a robust infant, but, to the horror of the family, a clinical course similar to the son's began at about 7 months of age. Again physicians were consulted, but mysteries persisted as to the proper diagnosis and treatment of the condition. The physicians were far from oblivious of Mrs. Slade's grief. The pitiful sorrow mapped eloquently upon her pleading face must have driven them to make maximum use of their abilities. Great effort was expended to be able to tell her something—to make a diagnosis at least, if not to cure her child's unrelenting disorder. Any knowledge would have been helpful to assure the family that this second tragedy was not a punishment for some imagined sinful act of this God-fearing, kindly woman. One physician even asked a consultant from Atlanta to drive to the rural community in which Mrs. Slade lived to examine her daughter. Since the consultant was related to the practitioner, this additional examination was accomplished at no expense. In the simple home of Mrs. Slade, the two physicians performed detailed examinations in an almost frantic attempt to elucidate the cause of the disease.

Unfortunately, they were unsuccessful. The second child died in a fashion similar to the first. Mrs. Slade bravely existed after this second tragedy. Other members of her family needed her attention and strength, and she returned to her previous activities as devoted mother and wife. She bore other children, all of whom were female, all of whom were strong and healthy. Finally another son was born. He was the apple of his parents' eye and a pet of the many older sisters, some of whom by this time had grown to adolescence. What a fine specimen he was, a well-formed and handsome lad, male heir to the family name. The birth occurred in the height of the depression in 1936, and times were indeed hard. Even the next meal was uncertain because of failing businesses and finances. Still, the Slades, remembering the kindly physician who had unsuccessfully but energetically tried to help them years before, sought this man out for reassurance that their son, named John Arthur, did not have the "disease."

Examinations in early infancy were normal, but familiar symptoms later began, again at about 7 months of age. The experience of many years before had not been forgotten by the physician, an honest, hard-working, and intelligent general practitioner who himself was overworked and underpaid. No modern medical library was available to him, but continued search through his textbooks allowed him to categorize John Arthur's disease in the best fashion possible, considering then prevailing medical views. A diagnosis was finally suggested, the accomplishment of which was only a small comfort. An illustration in a new medical book showed a child with Werdnig-Hoffman disease. The similarities to John Arthur's condition were noted, and Mrs. Slade was told that John had "spinal muscular atrophy."

The initial joy of achieving the diagnosis was soon dampened by the realization that nothing could be done to stop the progressively downhill course of the disease. "Spinal" was all that Mrs. Slade could remember about the diagnosis when relating the story to an interested physician some 40 years later. "The doctor said my son had 'spinal' and that nothing could be done to help him."

This blow, the third tragedy, was almost too much for Mrs. Slade to bear, but she knew things that we who are perhaps more affluent often never know. She knew that life was hard, that life is hard. It was not in the nature of this strong woman of the South, a personification of her race and time, to give up on life. But for her especially, life was difficult at that time. Meals were scarce, but enough money was saved to pay a last tribute to the male child Mrs. Slade had hoped beyond hope would be the inheritor of her husband's name. Tragically, another child would not survive infancy. The others had small graves, but they were forgotten— their faces would never be viewed by persons who had not seen them in life.

John Arthur would be different. Mrs. Slade made a decision to keep his memory alive—regardless of the sacrifice to herself or her family. The small amount of money saved would serve as the down payment for his photograph. A traveling photographer was contacted and asked to come to the small house where the Slades lived. John Arthur was already very weak and debilitated. It was feared that he might succumb to infection if taken out in the winter air. One photograph was all the photographer could take at the price the Slades could afford to pay him. Therefore, detailed preparations were made prior to the scheduled appointment. John Arthur was dressed in his finest. He was already so weak that he could not sit unsupported. Pillows were needed to support him. They were borrowed, and he was propped on the one household couch. He was a small child, and Mrs. Slade believed that she could hold her rather large and wrinkled hand behind him to keep his arms to his sides. One feature of John's disease was sudden jerkiness of the arms, which occurred both spontaneously and when he was startled by any tactile, visual, or auditory stimulus. When the photographer rustled his equipment immediately before he snapped the one picture allowed, John Arthur's left hand jerked upward in a typical manner. This "startle" reaction seemed to characterize the disease, which had been mistakenly diagnosed as "spinal."

Through this posture, caught so dramatically in the one photograph the family had sacrificed so much to take as a memorial to the young son and brother who everyone knew would be dead in a few weeks, a specific neurologic diagnosis can be made. To this photograph and to this story, but most importantly to Mrs. Slade and to John Arthur, this book is dedicated. For John Arthur's story, culminating in a single photograph, represents the most eloquent argument possible for the facial diagnosis of neurologic disease.

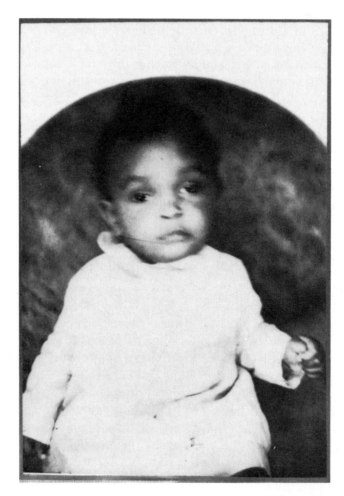

John Arthur Slade—born September 17, 1936, died June 12, 1938. In 1937, he was mistakenly diagnosed as having spinal muscular atrophy. He was the son of a carrier for hexosaminidase A deficiency and the cousin of a patient who 40 years after John Arthur's death was proved to have classical Tay-Sachs disease, or hexosaminidase A deficiency. Observe the dull facial expression, the exotropia of the left eye, the cortical thumb posture of the clenched left fist, and the excessive abduction of the left upper extremity, which resulted from John Arthur's being startled by a noise when the photograph was taken.

# Preface

For several years we have been interested in the facial diagnosis of neurologic disease. One of us, a clinical pediatric neurologist, has collected thousands of photographs of patients seen in his practice. The other, an educational specialist and curriculum planner, realized the potential for a unique approach to teaching a complex subject. To both of us it was apparent that collaboration on a book on facial diagnosis might be of benefit both for the student of neurologic disease and for the practicing physician. The first collaborative efforts were attempts to blend our sometimes divergent philosophies and training to produce a book that was both scientifically and medically accurate and educationally sound.

Our objective was soon found to be more difficult than we had expected. The rapid growth of knowledge in the fields of birth defects, metabolic diseases, and neurologic processes, as well as in medicine in general, made us realize that our registry of thousands of patient photographs was deficient if we sought, even in the most superficial fashion possible, to cover the entire field of the face as it relates to neurologic disease. We found that our knowledge and expertise in studying the face were also deficient, and we learned that covering the field comprehensively was an impossibility. It was with this background that we approached what turned out to be an extremely interesting project.

In order not to seem too amateurish to our peers and to the true giants in the field of facial diagnosis, including our personal teachers William DeMyer, Arthur Drew, Douglas Buchanan, Alexander Ross, Philip White, Wolfgang Zeman, Jans Miller, Peter Harper, and others, we soon began to supplement not only our meager knowledge about the face but also our understanding of the structural and metabolic bases of many diseases whose presence may be suspected as a result of simple facial viewing. In the process we borrowed photographs from our co-workers and friends, including Dr. William DeMyer, Dr. Arthur Drew, Dr. Douglas Buchanan, Dr. Alexander Ross, and Dr. Ray Chun. These borrowed photographs were few in number, however, and we had personally examined most of the patients involved.

In the final agonies of our endeavor, we supplemented our collection of photographs with additional photographs borrowed from our current co-workers at the Medical College of Georgia. These helpful physicians include Dr. Thomas Swift, Dr. Charles Linder, Dr. Patricia Hartlage, Dr. Theo Thevaos, Dr. Farivar Yaghmai, Dr. John Bigger, and Dr. Floyd Haar. With few exceptions the patients in these photographs were also personally examined. In addition, Dr. Taher El Gammal supplied many pertinent roentgenograms, and Dr. Farivar Yaghmai supplied several photographs showing pertinent pathology. Dr. John Bigger allowed the use of several photographs of the eye from his personal collection and was most helpful in reading part of the text.

The institutions at which we have worked must be lauded. The patients whose conditions are discussed in this book were seen at these institutions, and many of the photographs were taken by staff members of their illustration and photography departments. The institutions include Indiana University School of Medicine, the Milwaukee Children's Hospital, the Milwaukee County Hospital, Washington University School of Medicine, the University of Chicago Hospitals and Clinics, the Muscatatuck State School and Training Center of Indiana, the Southern Wisconsin School and Training Center, the Gracewood State School and Training Center of Georgia, and the hospitals of the Medical College of Georgia, with which we are currently affiliated.

Much praise must be given to others in the formation of the book. Highest on the list perhaps are our families, who sacrificed much to enable us to find the time in our busy schedules to compose the text. Special thanks must be given to our wives, Mrs. Linda Dyken and Mrs. Melva Miller, for their patience and understanding. Our friends also were of great help. Mrs. Frances Powell not only did most of the typing and retyping of the manuscript but also helped in the organization and did much of the never-fully-appreciated leg work involved in coordinating the project. Help was also given by the secretarial services of our institution. Mrs. Margaret Holtam and Mrs. Andrea Swift contributed expert editing. Dr. John Bigger contributed greatly as an ophthalmologic consultant. The contributions of Dr. Joseph Green, Chairman of the Department of Neurology, Dr. Alex Robertson, Chairman of the Department of Pediatrics, and Dr. Jon Calvert, Chairman of the Department of Family Practice also must be acknowledged. These men allowed us to devote to the preparation of this book much time that otherwise would have been spent in performing more tedious tasks.

Early in the process of developing this book it became apparent that supplemental art work had to be prepared. Mrs. Karen Waldo and John Hagan, of the Department of Medical Illustration of the Medical College of Georgia, performed this task expertly and cheerfully. Other artists involved in the project included David Mascaro, Kristina Walters, Robert Margulies, and Thomas Waldrop.

Most importantly, the authors thank the patients for their cooperation in helping us to complete this project.

Paul R. Dyken
Max D. Miller

# Contents

1  **The normal face,** 1

Facial observation, 2
Embryogenesis of the face and cranium, 5
Facial lines, 13
Facial segments, 18
General facial features, 29
Facial growth, 30

2  **Upper facial and cranial segment abnormalities,** 33

Primary suture abnormalities, 36
Secondary suture abnormalities, 43
Topographic abnormalities, 51

3  **Middle facial segment abnormalities,** 58

The eyes, 59
Nasal base and midface proper, 72
Nasal bridge and tip, 76
Zygomata and lateral bony orbits, 77
The ears, 79

4  **Lower facial segment and neck abnormalities,** 82

External lower face, 83
Internal lower face, 92
The neck, 97

5  **Syndromes of the upper facial and cranial segment,** 102

Syndromes characterized by premature closures of cranial sutures, 104
Syndromes characterized by other suture disturbances, 123
Syndromes characterized by simple macrocephaly, 130
Syndromes characterized by microcephaly, 156
Syndromes characterized by abnormalities of the hair, 166
Cranial neurocutaneopathies, 172

6  **Syndromes of the middle facial segment,** 181

Syndromes of the central middle face, 182
Syndromes of the lateral middle face, 277

7  **Syndromes of the lower facial segment and neck,** 295

Syndromes of the central lower face, 296
Syndromes of the peripheral lower face, 325
Syndromes of the oral cavity, 333
Syndromes of the neck, 344

8  **Syndromes of the total face,** 359

Syndromes of multisegmental involvement, 360
Syndromes of abnormal facial expression, 397

**References,** 423

I that am curtailed of this fair proportion, cheated of feature by dissembling nature, deformed, unfinished, sent before my time into this breathing world, scarce half made up and that so lamely and unfashionable that dogs bark at me as I halt by them.

King Richard III, Act 1, Scene 1

# CHAPTER ONE

# The normal face

Your face, my thane, is a book where men may read strange matters.
*Macbeth*, Act 1, Scene 5

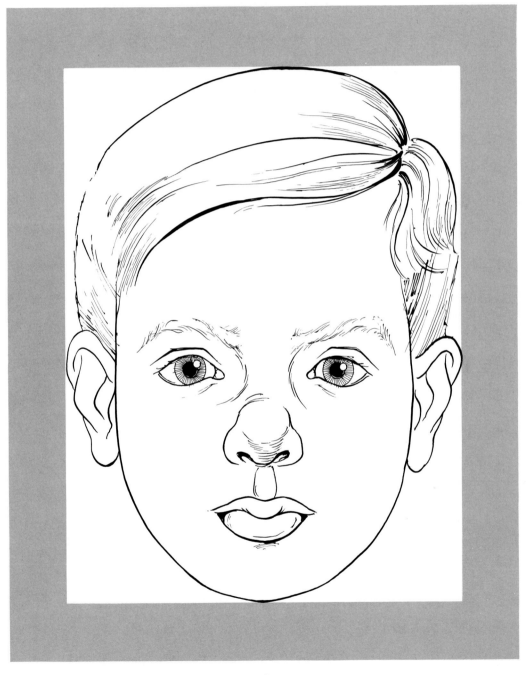

In this world there are many commonplace things of which people take little note but which can give much useful information if properly observed. Most people do not notice in detail the facial characteristics of others. They believe they can glance at a person's face and quickly determine whether it looks different from normal or, in some instances, that it appears unequivocally abnormal. A glance, a quick analysis of the parts, and the development of an *impression* of normality or abnormality comprise an intrinsic skill that is characteristic of all intelligent human behavior.

One of the most important indications of the state of health of a human being is how he appears. The face, of all parts of the human body, provides much information to the astute observer. Close observation of the facial features of many individuals reveals wide variation in the relationships of the features to each other and in proportion, shape, symmetry, and size. Thus there is great variation in what might be considered normal. The "normal" human face may be elongated, round, square, or triangular but is not necessarily symmetrical. In fact, most faces are not symmetrical at all. How, then, does one determine whether a lack of symmetry is a normal variation or a sign of an abnormality that needs investigation? When should a variation in proportion or size or shape be considered abnormal? In order to answer these important questions, it is necessary—despite the difficulty of the task—to determine what constitutes normal shape, size, proportion, and position for various features of the human face. For only in being able to recognize normal features can one begin to identify unusual or abnormal characteristics.

## FACIAL OBSERVATION

Physicians frequently encounter mothers who are certain their children are "sick" even though standard, early medical evaluations "prove" that they are normal in every known way. The clever physician learns to make use of these maternal observations and often because of them is able to make early medical diagnoses and to establish treatments before more abnormalities develop. Although the physician may receive credit for the ultimate diagnosis in such a case, the mother should receive much of the credit. Her observation may not be explained in medical terms, and her analysis of the observation may be faulty. However, in some unknown fashion, such a mother is able to observe an abnormality.

While a mother's impression of "sickness" may not be explained medically, her observation is often so accurate that it supersedes a physician's observation of normality. But many people do not have these natural observational abilities, and some who do have them need to cultivate their skills further. Development of skill in facial diagnosis starts with improvement in observational ability.

One of the physician's most important tools is the power of observation. The skillful physician has perfected the ability to look, to see, and to perceive. He or she accurately uses perceptual stimuli—auditory, tactile, olfactory, or visual—to better understand a patient's problems. In facial observation, however, the physician relies primarily on his or her power of visual perception.

The process of meaningful facial observation and perception is based upon three physiologic mechanisms: (1) adequate input (stimulus) being carried by visual sensory pathways to the observers' brain, (2) associative brain pathways (central processing) being activated to allow proper analysis of the input and conscious recognition of the impression, and (3) an output (response) being originated by the brain. The brain functions very much like a complex and sophisticated computer. Like a computer, the brain must have properly furnished, accurate input for meaningful recognition and output to occur. Also like a high-speed computer, the human brain is unlimited in its ability to handle a large volume of input without distortion. Furthermore, through selective attention, the mind is able to increase its ability to deal with this large volume. Thus a person may be able to perceive that a face is not normal without being able to state exactly why until further, more intensive observation is made.

Even if one is unable to state in accurate, scientific terms why a face appears abnormal, he may be able to say that it is "out of proportion," "strange," or "odd." Close observation may reveal disproportion from the top of the head to the chin or from one side of the face to the other. While facial distances—that is, distances between various facial features—can be accurately measured and exact proportions mathematically determined, the major goal of this chapter is to establish an overall concept of normal. We are concerned with a *facial gestalt*—in other words, with looking first at the whole. Yet we are also concerned with the precise characteristics of the parts. Examination of each facial element, in a systematic way and in relation to other facial elements, can reveal patterns of normality or abnormality. It has been stated by DeMyer (1975) that once a clinician decides that a patient's face looks unusual, he must then decide whether the problem is one of the face as a whole or solely of a region or segment of the face. Localization of the abnormality to one region of the face greatly reduces the number of syndromes that need to be considered and suggests a pathogenesis and in some cases the cause. Therefore, we agree with DeMyer that a rational division of the face and an analytic approach become the first tasks in developing skill in facial diagnosis.

One obvious place to start in facial diagnosis is to develop a common, consistent, and proper nomenclature in describing facial features. We could begin by describing the overall shape and structure of the face. Common terms that have been applied to the face as a whole include "expressionless," "coarse," "fine," "dull," "pinched," "distressed," and "elfin-like." Individual features also have been described in various ways. Noses have been described as "pug," "large," "small," "long," "short," "fat," "wide," or "pursed"; ears have been termed "flat," "elephantine," "cauliflower," and "jug." Terms that describe the shape or position of the eyes—"squinted," "wide-eyed," "pig-eyed"—have been used in a similar fashion. However, few of these terms are scientific or even wholly accurate (Feingold, 1975).

One purpose of this chapter is to develop a system that may be helpful in improving skills in facial observation. For persons already skilled in observing facial details, the following exercises may provide a better understanding of the analysis of facial abnormalities.

The face may be divided into separate parts, each of which has special features that can be used for detailed observation. In Fig. 1-1, a drawing of the child, you see the cranium and face and some of its individual parts. Your initial impression is that this child appears normal, and this "gestalt" impression is correct. Yet the drawing shows much more. Look at the face and study its features in more detail. You see cranial hair, a forehead, temples, ears, eyes, eyelids, eyebrows, a nose, a

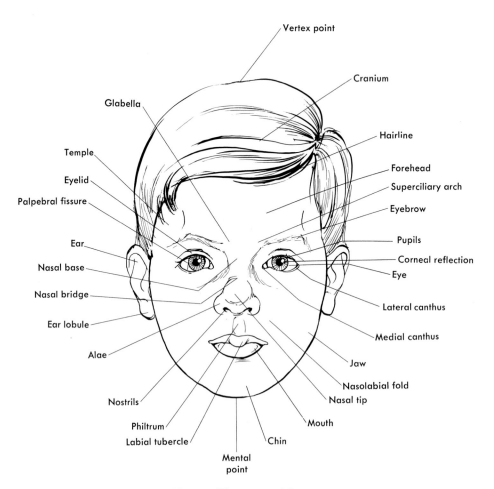

**Fig. 1-1.** The normal face.

mouth, nares, lips, a chin. In this instance of obvious normality, analyses of parts and details make little difference in the final impression. It is simple enough to identify parts of the face, the cranium, and the neck in general terms; but in order to understand deviations from normal, you must analyze more fully *why* this face is normal. Observe the shape of the head, the size of the face, the position of the eyes, the ears, the nose, the mouth, and the chin. Observe the distances between the various structures, and note proportionality—especially as it relates to the cranium, the forehead, the middle of the face, and the lower part of the face. Look along the vertical planes and along the horizontal planes. Try to determine what constitutes normal proportion and normal placement of features. Try also to imagine what would constitute abnormality or disproportion, remembering that there is enormous variety in what might be considered normal.

## EMBRYOGENESIS OF THE FACE AND CRANIUM

Understanding abnormal or disproportionate faces is enhanced by understanding the embryogenesis of the face and cranium.

Early in gestational life the human organism consists of a simple plate composed of three types of tissues: endoderm, from which the gut is derived; mesoderm, from which bone and muscle are derived; and ectoderm, from which skin is derived. Soon after these tissues form, they become specialized. The ectoderm thickens along the median raphe to form neuroectoderm and a neural plate. Soon after neuroectoderm has formed, specialized junctional tissues between the ectoderm (which will become skin) and the neuroectoderm (which will become the brain and spinal cord) develop. These specialized tissues, called neural crest, are induced to differentiate and migrate, possibly by underlying mesenchyma: the notochord in the caudal end of the embryo and the mesenchymal frontonasal plate in the rostral end. The rostral segments of the neural crest tissue migrate extensively to give rise partially or totally to most of the derivatives of the face (Patten, 1968). The only major components of the face not of neural crest origin appear to be the retina and lens, epithelial tissues, vascular endothelia, and skeletal muscle (Remnick, 1970). Crest tissue contributes extensively to cartilage, connective tissue, teeth, and bone. The migration of crest tissue and the tissues of the frontonasal plate occurs concomitantly with dramatic changes in the rostral end of the neural tube as the early brain develops. These changes include marked increases in all types of tissue growth and many flexions of the primitive brain and its early diverticula, the eyes (optic stalk), the ears (ear placode or vesicle), and the nose (nasal placode). (See Fig. 1-2.)

The face has a dual embryologic origin. Median face structures arise from a frontal prominence that will be referred to as the frontonasal process. Lateral facial structures, on the other hand, arise from the branchial arches. The frontonasal segment of the fetal face (see Fig. 1-2) produces the forehead, the glabella, the interorbital region, the nose, the

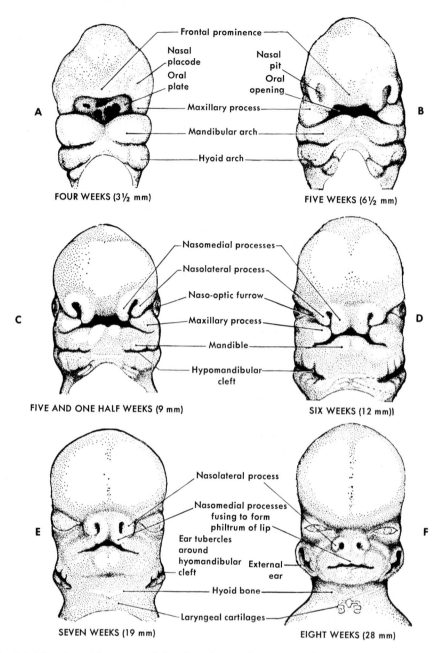

Fig. 1-2. The frontal aspect of the developing human embryo at various stages of embryonic life. (From Patten, B.: Human embryology, ed. 3, New York, 1968, McGraw-Hill Book Co. Used with permission.)

prolabium (extending laterally from the midline on both sides to the middle third of the upper lip, rostrally to the lower level of the nose, and caudally to the stomodeum or mouth), and the underlying midline structures. The branchial clefts are paired and produce many adult facial analogues. The first branchial arch forms the maxillary and mandibular

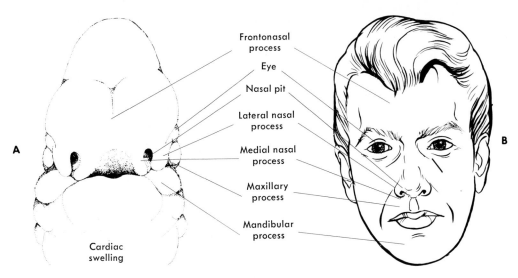

Fig. 1-3. Adult analogues of the embryonic face. Note especially the lateral to central movement of the parts, which is also evident in Fig. 1-2. (A, From Sperber, G. H.: Craniofacial embryology, Baltimore, 1973, The Williams and Wilkins Co. Used with permission.)

Table 1. Facial derivatives of embryonic parts

| Embryonic part | Skeletal derivative | Fleshy derivative |
|---|---|---|
| Frontal process | Frontal bones | Forehead |
| Prolabium | Nasal base | Dorsum and apex of nose |
| Median nasal process | Ethmoid and vomer | Nasal septum, medial portion of upper lip, and upper gum |
| Junction of median nasal processes | | Philtrum, frenulum |
| Lateral nasal process | | Alae |
| Junction of lateral nasal and maxillary processes | | Nasolabial fold |
| Maxillary process (first branchial arch) | Maxilla | Upper lip and gum, upper cheek region |
| Mandibular process (first branchial arch) | Mandible | Lower lip and gum, chin, lower cheek region |

processes. The second branchial arch contributes to the hyoid bone in the adult. As the embryo develops, the first branchial arch is of vital importance to the formation of the face, and the other arches are of less importance. (See Table 1 and Fig. 1-3.)

The frontonasal process and the structures derived from the branchial arches provide a convenient embryologic means of viewing and describing facial features. As the neural crest mesodermal mass of the frontonasal process grows (primarily outward and downward in symphony with the flexing nervous system), the eventual contour of the face becomes noticeable. A large frontal prominence forms epithelial placodes that thicken and later form the nasal pit. The globular process eventually helps form the contour of the nose and the naso-optic furrow. Caudally, two subdivisions occur, forming the nasomedial process and the lateral process (Fig. 1-2). The former contributes to the nose, the latter to the medial aspect of the orbit and to the palpebral fissure and conjunctival sac. In general, the frontonasal prominence forms the major midline structures of the face, including the philtrum, nostrils, alae, nasal bridge, nasal base, glabella, forehead, and orbits. The frontonasal prominence also contributes to the latter portion of the eye, the temporal fossa, and the cranium proper. The first branchial arch contributes to the primitive stomodeum, as outlined by the maxillary and mandibular processes. As these processes grow and merge, they extend to the chondrocranium superiorly from the developing floor of the mouth (Arey, 1974). The nasomedial process and the maxillary process continue to grow and merge to form the developed upper lip. The nasomedial portion of the frontonasal process develops vertical and horizontal extensions into the oral chamber, thus forming the nasal septum and primitive palate (Patten, 1961).

The branchial arches form various facial structures, including the maxillary and mandibular processes and their subdivisions, the zygomatic arch, parts of the temporal bone, parts of the lips, the chin, and parts of the ear, as shown in Fig. 1-3 and Table 1. It is important to note that the first branchial arch also contributes to many midline facial structures.

The cranial base, as well as the bones of the face, is derived from cartilaginous precursors. By the twelfth week, chondrification is at its height, and the limits of the future bones are set. Precursors of the sphenoid bone and capsules of the otic and nasal sense organs begin to form cartilage. The ethmoid cartilage gives rise to the nasal base and bridge, and its terminal portion becomes the cartilaginous nasal septum. The otic capsule is derived from multiple centers of ossification in the temporal cartilage, with the mastoid process being formed from the petrous portion of the temporal bone. The bones of the middle face originate primarily in the cranial base, the two most important being the orbitosphenoidal bone (which encapsulates the eye) and the ethmoid bone (which forms the nasal base and the nasal bridge).

DeMyer (1975) uses the embryologic development of the face as a convenient basis for standard facial diagnosis. Fig. 1-4, A, shows the cranioface divided into three segments — upper, middle, lower. This simple, time-honored, but arbitrary classification was originated by clinicians and artists, who were concerned with artistic symmetry and the estab-

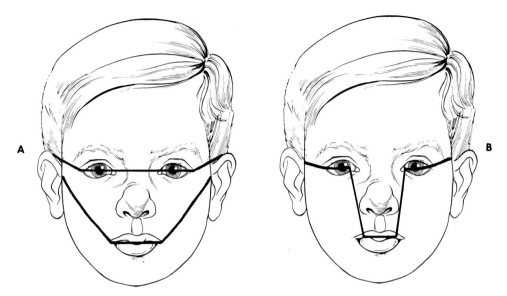

**Fig. 1-4.** Two ways of dividing the face. **A,** Traditional division of the face into upper, middle, and lower segments. The cranium is considered to be part of the upper facial segment, and the neck is considered to be part of the lower facial segment. **B,** Embryologic division of the face into a central or medial portion, which is derived from the frontonasal process, and a lateral portion, derived from the branchial clefts.

lishment of roughly equal parts. We have maintained much of this non-functional system of facial division in this book. However, an embryologically and anatomically more functional way of dividing the face is shown in Fig. 1-4, *B*. This later illustration shows the facial structures derived from the frontonasal process and the first branchial arch. The frontonasal process contributes to the cranial and midline portions of the middle and lower face at least to the level of the mouth. The first branchial arch contributes to most of the lower face and the lateral aspects of the middle face.

The two ways of dividing the face are not incompatible with each other. It is logical to think of the face as consisting of three horizontal divisions. The upper facial segment and cranium are derived primarily from the frontonasal process. The lower face, with the exception of a small but important midline wedge called the prolabium, which extends from the nose to the mouth, is derived from the first branchial arch. The middle face is derived from both the frontonasal process and the first branchial arch, with the more medial structures (including the nose and the eyes) primarily of frontonasal process derivation and most of the more lateral structures (including the zygomatic arches and the ears) primarily of first branchial arch derivation.

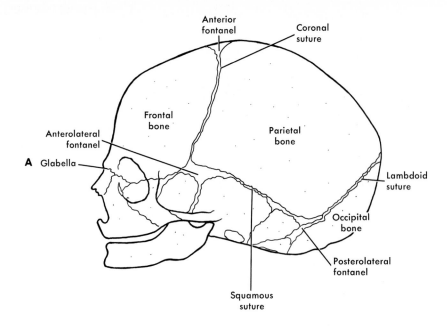

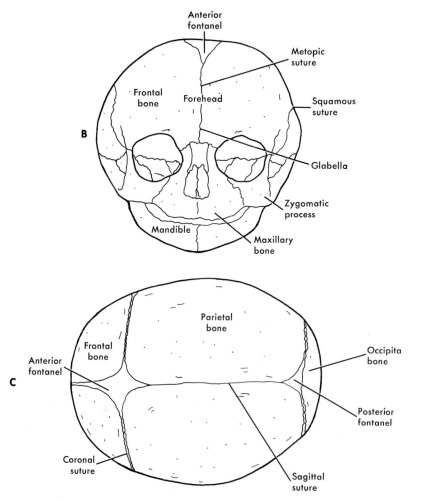

Fig. 1-5. Major bones, sutures, and fontanels of the newborn skull. Note especially the major sutures—the sagittal and the coronal. A, Lateral view. B, Frontal view. C, Top view.

## Embryologic formation of the cranium

Embryologically, the cranium is formed from both the membranous cranial vault and the cartilaginous cranial base (Sperber, 1973). During embryologic development and through differential growth patterns, the frontal mesenchyma, the extension of the notochord, envelops the cranial end of the primitive neural tube to form a capsule around the developing brain. Through bifurcation the mesenchymal membrane divides. The inner portion becomes the exomeningeal covering of the brain, giving rise to the dura mater, which remains unossified. The outer superficial membrane gives rise, through ossification, to cranial bone. The vault of the skull is thus formed of membranous bone that grows from several ossification centers to form the individual cranial bones found in the postnatal human. Ossification of the cranial vault begins early in the third month of gestational life and is not completed until well after birth. The union of individual bones, however, is not completed until well into childhood. The separations are called sutures. At birth the individual cranial bones are separated—apparently to accommodate rapid growth of the brain. To fuse, bones grow in breadth at their margins. Progressive decreasing of suture spaces takes place through the deposit of matrix unequally on the external surface while the internal surface experiences resorption. Fontanels are formed in certain areas along the unclosed margins between bones. The paired frontal, parietal, occipital, and squamosal parts of the temporal bones compose the cranial vault. (See Fig. 1-5.)

The ultimate shape and size of the cranial vault depend largely upon the internal forces that result from the expanding brain. The brain, as it grows, exerts pressure upon the cranial bones, thereby stimulating bone growth and determining the ultimate cranial size.

## Embryologic formation of the middle face

As noted previously, the middle face is of two embryologic origins—the frontonasal process and the first branchial arch. The middle face contains structures important to facial development and ultimate facial appearance and also, therefore, to subsequent facial observation by a physician. Each major structure—the eyes, the nose, the external ears—will be discussed separately. (See Figs. 1-2 and 1-3.)

**Embryologic formation of the eye.** Developing from the primary optic primordial process, the eye becomes one of the most complex of the sense organs. The various structures of the eyes originate embryologically from three sources: (1) the retina and optic fibers, the sensory portions of the eye, develop from the embryonic diencephalon; (2) the lens and cornea develop from the ectoderm; and (3) the sclera, parts of the cornea and iris, and the muscles of the eye develop from the mesoderm.

A pair of sac-like depressions form the lateral walls of the developing diencephalon, the proximal portions being connected to the brain proper through the optic stalk. With growth and further developing and thickening of the exterior wall, the retina proper develops. The retina of the eye is thus an organ of the brain that contains light-sensitive cells. These cells send stimuli through the optic nerve to the occipital lobe for processing.

The lens is formed as a local thickening, known as the lens placode, on the superficial ectoderm. The lens placode becomes invaginated as the cavity in the optic cup deepens; the number of cells in the inner wall increases greatly, bringing an overall thickening of the lens, which eventually breaks away to form an epithelial body lying in the optic cup. A thin overlapping part of the cup forms the iris from the mesenchyma. The eyelids form as a fold of skin growing back over the cornea.

**Embryologic formation of the nose.** The nose is formed from the bilateral nasal placodes and changes the appearance of the frontal prominence at about 5 weeks of embryologic age. The nasal placodes eventually form the olfactory sense organs as the placodes become surrounded by the growing, horseshoe-shaped lateral and median nasal processes. The "sinking" nasal placodes deepen, form the olfactory epithelium, and subsequently form the nasal pits—the precursors of the anterior nares. The lateral nasal processes form the alae of the nose; the median processes form the tip of the nose, the philtrum, and the frenulum. The median nasal processes merge to form the philtrum of the lip. The lower edge of the nasal septum fuses with the upper surface of the palate, thus forming the two nasal fossae. The fusing of the lateral nasal processes with the maxillary processes forms the nasolabial folds. The bridge of the nose results from the fusing of the median nasal processes in the midline or median plane. The merging of the bilateral median nasal processes thus forms a single median nasal bridge, with the elevation of the bridge being the result of the predominant anterior-to-posterior growth at the nasomaxillary junction.

**Embryologic formation of the external ear.** The earliest embryologic sign of an external ear is local thickening of the ectoderm otic placodes at about the third week of embryologic life. Continued expansion and growth elevates the otic placode, which takes on the appearance of an auditory pit. The external ear makes its appearance at about the fifth week. The various structures of the external ear are derived from the first and second branchial arches, with surface irregularities appearing on the borders of the arches and specific structures such as the tragus beginning to be noticeable. By the seventh week of embryologic life, these ridges start to take on the shape of an external ear. The tragus and the anterior crus of the helix margin are derived from the mandibular arch, while the helix, the anthelix, the scapha, the antitragus, and the lobule are derived from the hyoid arch (Haines, 1965).

## Embryologic formation of the lower face

Ectomesenchymal migration of neural crest tissue forms five ectodermally lined mesenchymal elevations or processes that correspond to growth centers in the underlying mesenchyma. These growth centers are, as previously noted, the frontonasal process and the paired maxillary and mandibular processes.

The ectodermal grooves or furrows between these processes form the various features of the postnatal face and provide a convenient basis for describing the precursors and developing structures of the lower face.

The primitive mouth or stomodeum begins as a depression in the early facial region and is bound laterally by the first pair of branchial arches (the mandibular). (See Figs. 1-2 and 1-3.) The maxillary process of the first branchial arch is the precursor of the maxilla and forms the maxillary structures of dentition—two lateral palatal shelves, various ossification centers including those for the bilateral sphenoid wings and the vomers, and various muscles of mastication. Continued growth and merging with the frontonasal process and the mandibular process provide continuity of the facial structures.

The mandible is also a derivative of the first branchial arch and is first formed as Meckel's cartilage, which serves as a template for later mandibular bone growth and development. Portions of Meckel's cartilage develop into the bones of the middle ear (malleus, stapes, and incus) and parts of the sphenoid bone. The mandibular arch is also the precursor of various muscles of the lower face.

Embryologic development of the face and subsequent growth produce typical symmetries and proportions that are slightly different in childhood, adolescence, and adulthood. At each stage of development a series of artificially but logically drawn facial lines can be used for systematic study of the face and cranium.

## FACIAL LINES

Since a primary objective of this book is to teach the early detection of abnormalities in facial features, which in many instances leads to early diagnosis of neurologic syndromes especially prevalent in children, emphasis will be placed on viewing the faces of children directly—that is, from the front.

The face can and should be studied systematically. In order to understand the whole, one must develop certain concepts about individual parts of the face. In addition to the embryologic (or central-to-peripheral) approach, we have found it useful to devise a system of key vertical and horizontal lines that divide the frontally viewed face into several horizontal and vertical segments. These segments have been developed for the beginner in facial viewing and can aid in forming a gestalt impression of normality or abnormality, which in turn may help in diagnosing disorders. Fig. 1-6 shows the same "normal" face of the child shown in Fig. 1-1, but this face is now divided into an initially confusing grid of vertical, horizontal, and oblique lines. We have found the subdivisions of the face based upon these lines to be useful.

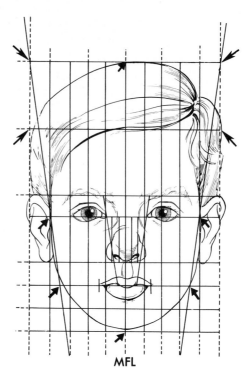

MFL

**Fig. 1-6.** Facial lines, points, and segments used in this book. This complex arrangement of horizontal, vertical, and oblique lines divides the face into subdivisions that are useful in describing facial abnormalities.

## Horizontal facial lines

The most important horizontal facial lines are shown in Fig. 1-7; the vertical limits of the cranioface are set by the *horizontal vertex line* (HVL) and the *horizontal mental line* (HML). The point where the HVL touches the cranium is called the *vertex point* (VP), and the point where the HML crosses the chin is called the *mental point* (MP). In the child, the *browline* (BL), which is also called the horizontal midfacial line, divides the cranioface into approximately equal portions. On the other hand, in the adult the cranioface is bisected approximately by the *intercanthal line* (ICL). Embryologically, the browline roughly approximates the juncture of the frontonasal process and the cranial base. The upper half of the cranioface is itself divided into halves (or quarters of the entire cranioface) by the *hairline* (HL). The lower half of the face is bisected by the *nasal line* (NL), which crosses the lower limit of the nose and approximates the embryologic juncture of the maxillary process and the prolabium. The lower facial segment is divided into approximate thirds by the *horizontal oral line* (HOL) and the *upper mental line* (UML). Under normal conditions the HOL connects the *jaw angle points* (JAP$_1$ and JAP$_2$) and both *mouth corners* (MC$_1$ and MC$_2$). The HOL coincides with

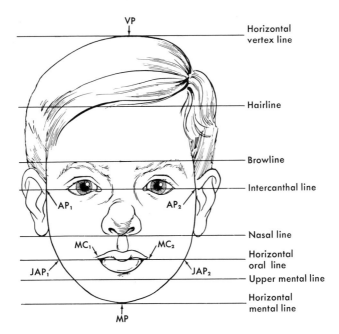

**Fig. 1-7.** Major horizontal lines. In children the cranioface is divided into halves by the browline. These halves are further divided (into equal quarters) by the hairline and the nasal line. The lower facial segment (or that segment below the nasal line) is divided into approximate thirds by the oral line and by the upper mental line. The middle facial segment, or that part of the face between the browline and the nasal line, contains another important horizontal line—the intercanthal line. This line connects the four canthi and, in adults, tends to divide the cranioface into halves. *VP*, Vertex point. *MP*, Mental point. *AP*, Aural points. *MC*, Mouth corners. *JAP*, Jaw angle points. Subscripts in abbreviations indicate sidedness. Odd number means right side of patient (left side of examiner); even number means the opposite.

the mouth or stomodeum. The jaw angle points are those points where the angle of the jaw is greatest. When the face is viewed from the front, these points fall at approximately the HOL. The UML delineates the upper limit of the chin and the lower limit of the lower lip and has no useful embryologic analogue.

One of the most useful horizontal lines is the *intercanthal line* (ICL), which also could be called the horizontal pupillary line. This line is drawn between the four canthi—lateral and medial on both sides. The ICL is extremely important in facial diagnosis, for in the normal Caucasian face it (1) touches all four canthi and thus sets the normal "tilt" of the eyelid and palpebral fissures, (2) delineates the most anterior part of the upper ear as it connects to the face (at the aural points), (3) crosses the narrowest part of the base of the nose, (4) usually passes through both pupils, and (5) represents, in the normal adult, a more equal division of the entire cranioface into halves than the browline, which performs this function in the child. Anatomically, the ICL is the most important horizontal line of the middle facial segment. In the child, the ICL is located one third of the distance from the browline to the nasal line.

### Vertical facial lines

The most important vertical facial lines are shown in Fig. 1-8. These lines divide the face into roughly equal segments and are useful in determining symmetry. The horizontal extent of the cranium is established by drawing a vertical line on each side of the head to delineate the maximum width. These two lines, which are the basis for further division and subsequent determination of symmetry, are designated the *vertical cranial lines* (VCL$_1$ and VCL$_2$, from the viewer's left to right).

Once the maximum horizontal extent of the cranium has been established, drawing the *vertical midfacial line* (VMFL) is important. This

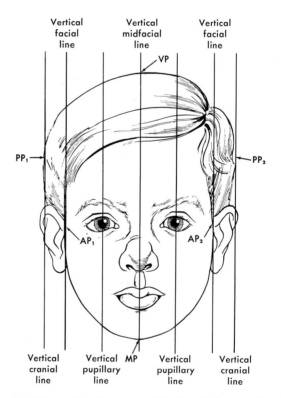

Fig. 1-8. Major vertical lines. The horizontal limits of the cranium are the vertical cranial lines. The most important vertical line is probably the vertical midfacial line, which touches the VP, the MP, the tip of the nose, and the philtrum and divides the face into halves. The lateral limits of the face are the vertical lines drawn at the junctions of the ears with the face at the aural points (AP$_1$ and AP$_2$). The face is further divided (into equal quarters) by the vertical pupillary lines, which are equidistant from the vertical midfacial line and the vertical facial lines. *VP*, Vertex point. *MP*, Mental point. *AP*, Aural points. *PP*, Parietal points.

line, which runs parallel to the vertical cranial lines, divides the normal cranium and face in half. The VMFL delineates the embryologically derived median plane and is extremely important in determining the degree of symmetry. The roughly equal vertical divisions of the cranioface are themselves bisected by the *vertical pupillary lines* (VPL), which are designated from the viewer's left to right as $VPL_1$ and $VPL_2$.

In addition to the major vertical lines, several other vertical lines are important in the construction of the normal face in its proper proportions. From a pathologic viewpoint, these lines are important only in the middle and lower facial segments. The *lateral canthal lines* ($LCL_1$ and $LCL_2$) are important in the middle facial segment and mark the lateral borders of the palpebral fissures. The *medial canthal lines* ($MCL_1$ and $MCL_2$) are important because they delineate the medial borders of the palpebral fissures. When extended downward, the medial canthal lines also touch the lateral extent of the soft tissue of the nose and come close to the mouth corners.

The maximum extent of the face proper is marked by the *vertical facial lines* ($VFL_1$ and $VFL_2$). The distance from the VMFL to the VPL is equal to the distance from the VPL to the VFL.

## Oblique facial lines

Since the cranium is larger horizontally than the face proper, it is useful to draw two oblique lines, which become important when examining the face for asymmetry (Fig. 1-9). Many obliquely drawn lines could be used. However, we have found that the two *oblique facial lines* (OFL), each of which is drawn between three points, are most useful. These lines connect (1) the *upper cranial points*, $UCP_1$ and $UCP_2$, where the horizontal vertex line intersects the vertical cranial lines; (2) the *aural points*, $AP_1$ and $AP_2$, located at the junctions of the intercanthal line and the vertical facial lines; and (3) the *jaw angle points*, $JAP_1$ and $JAP_2$. The OFL are important in establishing normal facial contour and proportion in comparison to the cranium. When normal faces are viewed frontally, they ususally have a rounded rather than a severely angular, square, or rectangular appearance.

In understanding the relationship between the fetal development of the face and certain facial defects, it is important to consider one other oblique line. This line extends from the medial canthus to the lateral aspect of the labial tubercle on the same side. This line also falls on the lateral aspect of the nares and is thus called the *canthal labial line* (CLL). The CLL represents the junction of the frontonasal process and branchial arch–derivative structures.

## Normal facial proportion

It is important to remember two general factors when analyzing the "normal" face. First, as mentioned before, the face is generally rounded, although minor variations occur. Second, the width of the normal face is

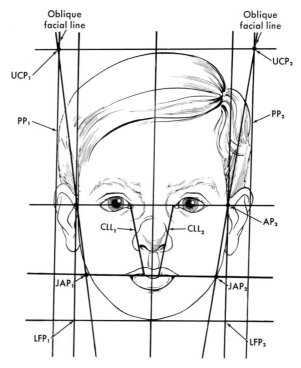

**Fig. 1-9.** Major oblique lines. Many lines can be drawn obliquely in relation to facial features. On logical, embryonic, and anatomic grounds, only two are shown here—the oblique facial line (OFL) and the canthal labial line (CLL). The OFL connects the upper cranial point, the aural point, and the jaw angle point on the same side. The CLL connects the medial canthus, the lateral aspect of the nares, and the lateral aspect of the labial tubercle on the same side. The CLL represents the junction of the paramedian-frontal process and the first branchial arch derivatives. *UCP*, Upper cranial points. *PP*, Parietal points. *AP*, Aural points. *JAP*, Jaw angle points. *LFP*, Lower facial points.

approximately two thirds its length. A person whose face is unusually broad is said to be brachyfacial ("wide-faced"), whereas a person whose face is much longer than it is wide is considered dolichofacial ("long-faced"). A person with a long and narrow face is said to be dolichostenofacial. There are mildly angular, square, rectangular, and triangular variations of normal, but severe deviations from roundness are considered abnormal.

## FACIAL SEGMENTS

In facial observation, it is convenient to separate the face and cranium into three major horizontal segments. Whereas the vertical midfacial line separates the face into left and right halves, the horizontal facial lines form the borders of the horizontal divisions, designations of which will be used extensively in this chapter and subsequent chapters. The horizontal segments are (1) the upper facial and cranial segment,

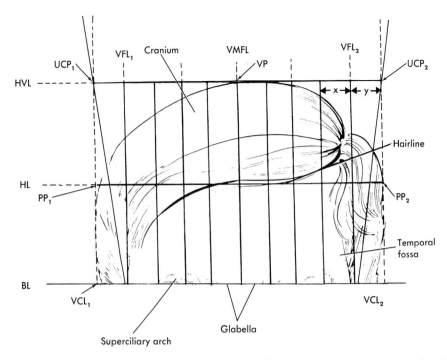

**Fig. 1-10.** Upper facial and cranial segment. This segment is bordered by the browline, the vertical cranial lines, and the horizontal vertex line. *HVL,* Horizontal vertex line. *VMFL,* Vertical midfacial line. *HL,* Hairline. *BL,* Browline. *VCL,* Vertical cranial lines. *VFL,* Vertical facial lines. *VP,* Vertex point. *UCP,* Upper cranial points. *PP,* Parietal points. $x = y$.

which includes all the area above the browline; (2) the middle facial segment, which includes the area between the browline and the nasal line; and (3) the lower facial segment, which is the area below the nasal line. The neck is considered part of this segment.

## Upper facial and cranial segment

The upper facial and cranial segment (Fig. 1-10) consists of the upper half of the cranioface in the child. This segment is limited by the browline inferiorly, by the horizontal vertex line superiorly, and by the two vertical cranial lines laterally. The actual maximum lateral extent of the cranium is designated by what we call the *parietal points* (PP$_1$ and PP$_2$, from the viewer's left to right). Included in the upper facial and cranial segment is the entire cranium, the hairline, the forehead, the temples, the superciliary arches, the temporal fossae, the eyebrows, and the area between the brows (the glabella). In the normal upper facial and cranial segment, the most prominent characteristics important in facial observation relate to the proportion evident in Fig. 1-10. The segment is more or less symmetrical, and this symmetry should be closely observed. The distances between the VMFL and each vertical cranial line, respectively, are roughly equal, as are the distances from the brow line to the hairline and from the hairline to the horizontal vertex line. Deviations from these proportions should be noted and more precise measurements taken. Specific abnormalities in these distances will be more fully discussed in Chapter 2.

## Middle facial segment

Included in the middle facial segment (Fig. 1-11) are the eyes, the ears, and the nose. Because of the importance of this segment of the face, especially in syndrome diagnosis, individual features will be described in detail.

**The eye.** The structures of the eye that are helpful in establishing a concept of normal are shown in Fig. 1-12. The palpebral fissure is the dis-

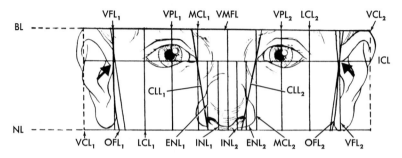

Fig. 1-11. Middle facial segment. This segment of the face is bordered by the browline, the nasal line, and the vertical cranial lines. *BL*, Browline. *NL*, Nasal line. *VCL*, Vertical cranial lines. *LCL*, Lateral canthal lines. *VFL*, Vertical facial lines. *VPL*, Vertical pupillary lines. *MCL*, Medial canthal lines. *VMFL*, Vertical midfacial line. *CLL*, Canthal labial lines. *ICL*, Intercanthal line. *OFL*, Oblique facial lines. *ENL*, External nares lines. *INL*, Internal nares lines. Arrows indicate aural points.

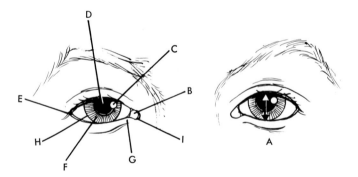

Fig. 1-12. Normal eyes. Each of the structures shown may be helpful in facial viewing. Special note should be taken of the relationships between the various parts, especially the limbus and the lacrimal papilla, since these structures, considered in combination with the corneal light reflection sign, can indicate the placement of the eye in the orbit. *A*, Palpebral fissures. *B*, Caruncle. *C*, Corneal light reflex. *D*, Pupil. *E*, Lateral canthus. *F*, Iris. *G*, Lacrimal papilla. *H*, Limbus. *I*, Medial canthus.

tance between the upper and lower eyelids when the eyes are in a relaxed and open position. The canthi represent the points of the angles between the upper and lower eyelids, both medially (the medial canthus) and laterally (the lateral canthus). The lacrimal papilla, which surrounds the lacrimal duct, is a small elevation of the lower lid close to the medial canthus. Other structures that are important in later descriptions of abnormalities of the eye are the pupil and the iris. The pupil is the small opening of the iris through which light passes on its way to the retina. A "negative" structure, the pupil is delineated by the inner termination of the circular iris. The constriction or dilation of the muscles of the iris determines pupillary size and is influenced by many physiologic and pathologic events. The iris, of course, is pigmented, and its appearance varies from individual to individual.

In ordinary facial viewing of eye structures, especially in photographic study, it is important to be aware of the corneal reflection sign. A reflection of light from the cornea is seen in photographs taken with a flash or in normal clinical examination of the eyes with a flashlight. This reflection and its clinical uses will be explained in detail. The cornea itself is usually not seen in normal situations but is delineated in ordinary frontal eye observation by the outer limits of the circular iris. The junction of the outer iris and the transparent conjunctiva overlying the white sclera of the eye is called the limbus. The limbus in general delineates the cornea from the sclera and the conjunctiva.

Measurement of the distances between the eyes is made using the medial canthal distance, the lateral canthal distance, and the interpupillary distance, as shown in Fig. 1-13. Pryor (1969) and Laestadius et al.

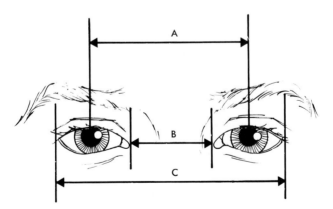

Fig. 1-13. Normal proportions of the eyes. The distance between the eyes can be useful in determining the condition of the midface proper. Normally, the medial canthal distance (B) is equal to approximately one third of the lateral canthal distance (C). In fact, an artist's trick is to imagine a "third eye" located in this space. If the "third eye" overlaps the actual eyes, the eyes are too close together (hypotelorism). If there is space between the third eye and the actual eyes, the eyes are too far apart (hypertelorism). A, Interpupillary distance.

(1969) have discussed the importance of the accurate measurement of distances between the eyes as a means of substantiating or denying visual impressions of abnormal spacing. Pryor states that

> A clinical impression of ocular hypertelorism may be misleading because of the fat tissue surrounding the eye. There may be narrow palpebral slits, epicanthal folds, a flat nasal bridge or widely spaced eyebrows any of which could influence the observer.

An unusual appearance in this region of the middle facial segment should alert the physician to observe more closely and to distinguish between ocular hypertelorism, relative lateral displacement of the inner canthi (as is present in children generally in true dystopia canthorum), and "short" palpebral fissures, since each of these conditions may have distinctive diagnostic implications. Other conditions that may be confused with true hypertelorism include blepharophimosis, microphthalmia, small faces, and small noses (DeMyer, 1975). Any deviation from the normal proportions should be noted, and more precise measurements should be taken and compared to those in normal tables (Laestadius, 1969; Pryor, 1969). The medial and lateral intercanthal and interpupillary distances should be measured. The interorbital distance, taken from posterior/anterior skull x-ray film, is roughly equal to the medial intercanthal distance and is believed to offer the most accurate and reliable means of recording abnormally wide-set eyes (DeMyer, 1975).

In the normal eye, the distances between the medial limbus and the medial canthus and between the lateral limbus and the lateral canthus are about equal. A normal exception is in early childhood, when the iris is relatively large in relation to the palpebral fissure. The medial limbus then falls closer to the medial canthus and the lacrimal papilla. Whereas in adults the lacrimal papilla is medial to the innermost border of the limbus, in children the medial limbus is at the papilla or even closer to the midline than the papilla. The normal iris-canthus relationships in the child and the adult, as well as the condition dystopia canthorum, are shown in Fig. 1-14.

Dystopia canthorum (literally, "displaced canthus") is the condition characterized by an abnormally laterally placed medial canthus. A "closer" relationship exists between the medial limbus and the lacrimal papilla than is normal. This condition, which is related to no functional deficit, may be mistakenly diagnosed as esotropia or hypertelorism, two much more significant abnormalities of the middle face.

Sometimes a fold of skin covers the inner or medial canthus. Such a fold is called an epicanthal fold. Like dystopia canthorum, epicanthal folds are not associated with functional deficits. In certain situations they are variations of normal. For example, epicanthal folds are not uncommon in Orientals, especially Japanese. Epicanthal folds are important to recognize, for they may give the false impression, as does dystopia canthorum, of esotropia or hypertelorism.

*Corneal reflection sign.* Under ordinary situations, the eyes or eye-

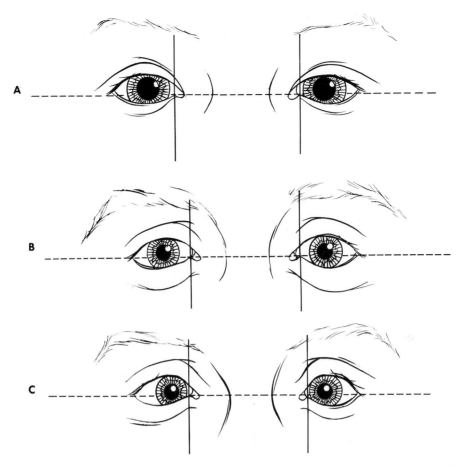

**Fig. 1-14.** Iris-canthus relationships. The normal iris, **B**, is equidistant from the canthi—that is, the iris is set in the exact center of the orbit. An exception to this rule is in infancy, **A**, in which the eyes are displaced medially and may, in fact, touch a line drawn through the lacrimal papillae. An abnormal condition, dystopia canthorum, **C**, exists if the iril limbus is near or touches this imaginary line as a person looks straight ahead.

balls are exactly aligned in order to keep us from having diplopia, or double vision. The corneal reflection sign offers a useful way of evaluating subtle malalignments of the eyes. The cornea is a reflecting surface, and when a light is placed in front of a person in a semidarkened room, a reflection can be observed on the cornea. When a person with normally aligned eyeballs looks at a light held before his eyes, a small reflection can be seen slightly laterally from the midpoint of the pupil. The reflection is seen at the same point in each cornea (Fig. 1-15). If a person is looking at a distant object and a light is held only a few feet from his eyes, the corneal reflection falls slightly to the medial aspect of the center of each pupil but in exactly the same position in each eye, if there is no malalignment. If one of a person's eyeballs is deviated, or if malalign-

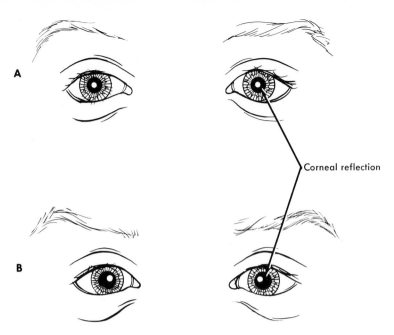

Fig. 1-15. The corneal reflection sign. The reflection of light off the cornea changes position as a person shifts his point of focus from a nearby object, **A**, to a distant object, **B**. As the eyes diverge to gaze at a distant object, the corneal reflections appear to move medially even though the eyes themselves move laterally.

ment is present, the corneal reflections in the two eyes will be asymmetrical. One reflection might be in the middle of the pupil of the eye that is fixating, and the other reflection could be in an asymmetrical location. Thus, in this book — and especially in later chapters dealing with photographic study — the reader will find the corneal reflection sign a useful detector of ocular malalignment.

**The nose.** The nose is a prominent feature that is often neglected or ignored in a close examination of the face. The shape, size, and position of the nostrils or alae, the relation of the nose to other facial features, and the characteristics of the bridge and base of the nose are very important in facial diagnosis (see Fig. 1-16). The nose can be divided into distal, middle, and proximal portions. The proximal part consists of the bony base and can be defined as that portion of the nose that rests mainly between the eyebrows and medial canthi. This portion of the nose is primarily osseous. The base of the nose of a normal face, when seen in profile, forms an angle with the forehead. A flat nasal base (hypoplasia of the base of the nose) forms no angle with the face and may create an illusion of wide-set eyes when the face is viewed frontally. The intermediate, or middle, portion of the nose consists of the narrow bridge of carti-

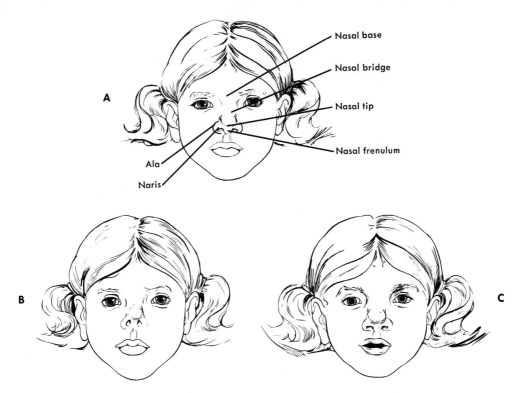

Fig. 1-16. Normal variations of the nose. A, Normal nose. B, Anteverted nares. C, Flat nasal base. The flat nasal base may give the illusion of wide-set eyes.

lage that contributes to much of the shape of what is commonly called the nose when seen in profile. Finally, the distal part of the nose consists of the fleshy tip and the lateral, more flared, fleshy parts called the alae. The external openings of the nose are called the nares, and the fleshy area that separates the nares is called the nasal frenulum. Each of these divisions of the nose is important in facial diagnosis but contributes in a different fashion depending on whether the face is observed from the front (as is the case in the vast majority of the clinical examples in this book) or in profile. The fact that many combinations of proximal, middle, and distal nasal characteristics are possible accounts for the many variations in human noses.

The ears. Although the ears are not seen ideally when a patient is viewed face-to-face, one can still observe certain ear features that are of importance in facial diagnosis. The anatomy and terminology of the ear are presented in Fig. 1-17. The normal shape, size, and position of the ears when seen from the front should be noted, and the fact that the rostral-caudal limits of a typical ear cover the entire vertical extent of the middle facial segment should be particularly observed. The caudal limit of the ear, the lobule, when viewed directly from the front, rests upon the

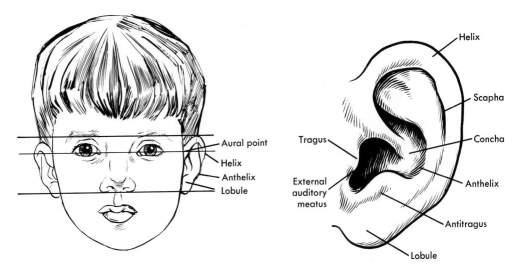

Fig. 1-17. Normal ear. The top of the ear is approximately at the level of the nasal line. Thus about a third of the ear is situated above the intercanthal line.

nasal line, with the rostral limit resting on the browline. These lines also set the rostral-caudal limits of the middle facial segment. As mentioned before, it is important to note that the point where the ear is attached to the temple (the aural point) falls on the intercanthal line.

The extent of protrusion of the ears when viewed from the front is important cosmetically, if not so much medically. Exceptions to this statement will be discussed in Chapter 3. An illusion that the ears are large and protuberant is seen frequently in persons with small craniums.

Much importance is given to the "set" of the ears. When the rostral limit of an ear falls below the browline, the ear is said to be "low-set," a phenomenon of questionable use in clinical diagnosis. It should be stressed that, when a person tips up his face or when the viewer is not on the same plane as the person viewed, a natural distortion gives the impression that the ears are low set.

Since anatomic details of the ear are not fully appreciated during frontal facial viewing, it is important to observe the ears directly as well. The normal anatomic features that are best appreciated by direct ear viewing are important but will not not be emphasized here or in future chapters (see Fig. 1-17).

• • •

The "midface proper" is an important concept in facial diagnosis. Although the eyes, the nose, and the ears may be unremarkable when considered by themselves, the "gestalt" of the middle face is extremely important. The midface proper is often considered to include the total area or volume of the middle facial segment as viewed from the front. It

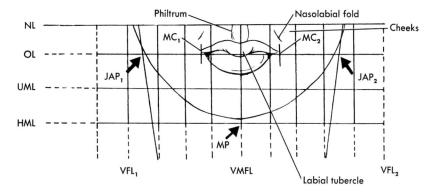

**Fig. 1-18.** Lower facial segment. This segment includes the area below the nasal line. The neck is considered to be part of this segment. *NL,* Nasal line. *OL,* Oral line. *UML,* Upper mental line. *HML,* Horizontal mental line. *VFL,* Vertical facial lines. *VMFL,* Vertical midfacial lines. *MC,* Mouth corners. *JAP,* Jaw angle points. *MP,* Mental point.

is more accurate, however, to say that the midface proper is the central portion of the middle facial segment—the portion that develops from the embryologic frontonasal process. The midface proper has been called the central part of the middle face because, technically, it excludes the more laterally placed structures of the middle facial segment (as defined previously), which are derived from the first branchial arch.

## Lower facial segment

In the lower facial segment (Fig. 1-18), there are several important landmarks that are useful in facial diagnosis. We have included the upper neck in this segment because this nonfacial structure is easily seen in ordinary frontal facial viewing. For convenience it is best to think of the lower face as composed of two major parts: the external part, which can be viewed easily, and the internal part, which generally cannot be properly appreciated unless the patient opens his mouth. The external features of the lower facial segment will be discussed first and in more detail. Basically, the external lower face consists of the mouth proper, the cheeks, the nasolabial folds, the chin, and the jaws. The internal lower face consists of the buccal mucous membranes, the gums, the tongue, and the teeth. The palate is also visible when the mouth is held widely open. (See Fig. 1-19.)

**The mouth and cheeks.** The anatomic limits of the mouth are difficult to establish because we use this term both scientifically and in ordinary conversation. In its most restricted use, the term refers only to the oral opening, which is bounded by lips. In this sense, the mouth is a "negative" structure that is more or less comparable to the other negative

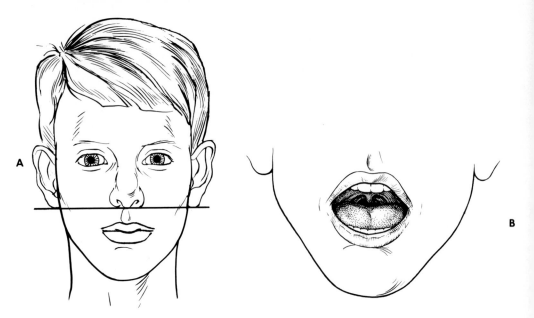

Fig. 1-19. The external lower face, **A**, consists of the area below the nasal line and includes those structures derived from the branchial arches. The external lower face also includes the neck. The internal lower face, **B**, includes the teeth, the gums, the buccal surfaces, the palate, and the tongue.

structures we have discussed, the pupil and the nares. In this restricted sense, the mouth is more appropriately referred to as the horizontal oral line (HOL), a term that will be used in this book. There are many less restrictive definitions of the mouth, however. Some include, in addition to the oral opening: both the vermilion border of the upper and lower lips and the fleshy part surrounding it; the midline depressed crease extending from the nose, also called the external frenulum; the median labial tubercle of the upper-lip vermilion border; the corners or angles of the mouth; and the lower part of the lip, which extends to the upper mental line. The areas included in these definitions can also be referred to as the "mouth proper." The normal HOL extends from one corner of the mouth to the other. It is a straight line that runs parallel to all other horizontal lines of the face but that usually crosses the median labial tubercle. The nasolabial folds divide the mouth proper from the cheeks. The cheeks, in turn, extend to the zygomata and the temporomandibular joints.

Close observation of the symmetry and proportionality of the mouth and cheeks is paramount in facial diagnosis. It should be noted that, except during animation and relaxation, the lips and mouth are usually closed. A mouth that is habitually held open suggests an abnormality. Asymmetry of the mouth and unusual elevation or depression of one mouth corner or both corners usually represents an abnormality. An unusually long or short HOL, an unusually angled mouth, or a peculiarity in the size or proportion of one of the mouth areas in relation to another may be important in diagnosis. The character of the nasolabial folds is a clue to certain neurologic abnormalities. A subtle flattening of one nasolabial fold, for example, might lead to the diagnosis of a one-sided facial nerve lesion.

**The chin and jaws.** Although wide variation is seen in the size and shape of the normal chin and jaws, this area is also important in facial viewing for syndrome diagnosis. The chin includes the area below the lower lip, which is delineated inferiorly by the UML. The chin blends into the jaws on each side. Unusually large, protruding chins or very small, receding, pointed chins may suggest certain syndromes. The chin area shows marked growth changes as a child progresses to adulthood.

The angle of the jaw, particularly at the JAP, is an important landmark in the frontal facial view and acts as a basis for more detailed facial viewing—not only because the presence of unusually severe angles or the absence of angles suggests abnormalities but also because the angle of the jaw delineates the lateral limits of the lower face. Certain conditions tend to cause overgrowth of the jaw. The shape and size of the jaw thus are important in early facial diagnosis.

**The internal mouth.** Special care should be taken to observe for characteristics of the teeth at variance with a patient's age. A 20-year-old person without teeth may be abnormal, yet a newborn with teeth must also be considered a deviation from normal. Care should be taken to note abnormally large or small, or unusually shaped, teeth. Significant abnormalities may lead to a syndrome diagnosis. The gums should be observed for unusual growth, hypertrophy, edema, or unusual plaques and lesions.

# GENERAL FACIAL FEATURES
## Hair

The characteristics of cranial and facial hair vary considerably among normal individuals of different ages, sexes, races, and social dispositions. Yet normal texture, position, and color are important in the diagnosis of several clinical syndromes. In all normal situations, hair is distributed over the cranium and around the eyes (that is, forming the eyebrows and eyelashes). In the postpubescent adult male, lower facial hair occurs normally, the extent and characteristics of which are partially dependent upon current social mores. Naturally occurring and highly visible facial hair is rare in females and children, and its presence suggests an abnormality. Most persons, regardless of age, have at the most sparse midline hair across the base of the nose; the eyebrows are usually separated by an area nearly devoid of hair. The presence of a heavy midline eyebrow in a younger person is abnormal. Likewise, the presence of universal baldness or an unusually high or low hairline is abnormal, as is the absence of the normal curve of the hairline as it extends from the apex of the forehead, around the frontal bones and temporal areas, to the areas in front of, on top of, and behind the ears.

## Skin

Except for such innocuous skin marks as freckles, occasional nevi, pimples, and wrinkles, the normal skin—especially in older children and adults—is essentially devoid of blemishes. The teenager with acne vulgaris is ubiquitously seen, but one must still consider this condition an abnormality. Not all teenagers have acne, and those who do have hormonal imbalances that may account for the transient and nonserious skin blemishes that result. Thus, although any skin blemish constitutes an abnormality in the context of this book, every abnormality does not lead to the clinical diagnosis of a syndrome.

## FACIAL GROWTH

The previous discussions often have been related to the face of a child. As a child grows, his head and face grow also, and the proportions of the face change. The growth of the face occurs in horizontal, vertical, and anterior/posterior directions. Roentgenographic studies indicate that, by age 10, the skull has reached about 96% of adult length, breadth, and circumference; yet there is remarkable change in facial appearance between preadolescence and postadolescence. The direction of facial growth in the childhood period is primarily forward because of growth in the cranial base. In the preadolescent and adolescent periods, maximum

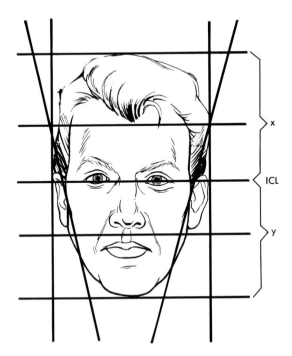

Fig. 1-20. The adult face. (Compare to child's face in Fig. 1-6.) Note that the face is bisected not by the browline, as in the child, but by the intercanthal line (x = y). Observe also that the eyeballs are relatively smaller, the chin is broader and more protruding, the nose is longer and broader, the jaws are wider, the hairline is higher (at the temples especially), the superciliary arches are more pronounced, and the face is more wrinkled.

growth occurs in the vertical direction, primarily in the maxillary region. In the postadolescent period, maximum growth is in the posterior/ anterior and horizontal directions, primarily in the mandibular region. The length and depth of the mandible increase as it grows toward the chin. The jaw therefore becomes thicker, wider, and somewhat more projecting. Maxillary growth at this time is not as pronounced as mandibular growth (Tanney, 1962). Much of the change is in the lower face, with the mandible growing fastest in the latter part of the growth spurt; the mandible lags somewhat behind the rest of the face in its development.

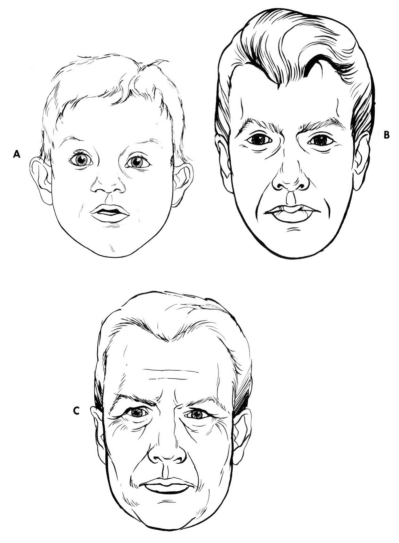

**Fig. 1-21.** The face and the aging process. Changes in the proportions of the face from childhood, **A,** to early adulthood, **B,** are dramatic. The changes from early adulthood to late adulthood are less pronounced but equally important. As cutaneous and subcutaneous changes take place, the character of the face alters and the characterisitcs of old age, **C,** emerge.

In addition to changes in the size and shape of the jaw, there are changes in the middle facial segment. These changes are related primarily to growth before puberty. The growth of the cranial base, the maxillary/mandibular bones, and the upper face (including the pterygopalatine suture) results in changes in proportion during the preadolescent and postadolescent periods. Change is most pronounced in vertical directions. The horizontal midfacial line in the child is represented by the browline, which divides the face into upper and lower parts. In the adult, however, the face is divided into roughly equal parts by the intercanthal line. The growth of the face proceeds in such a way that the eyebrow line moves upward in relationship to the entire face. Other changes in the proportions of the face that occur during adulthood are shown in Fig. 1-20. It should be noted that the lower face changes considerably during adulthood as well as during childhood.

One of the basic facts of human existence is change, and perhaps in no other place is change more evident than the human face. The creases and lines that are faintly observable in youth become pronounced with age (Fig. 1-21). The normal features of the face at various ages deserve special note. Features that are not appropriate to age may be important clues to abnormalities.

In youth there are few lines, creases, or wrinkles other than those associated with the junctions of anatomic areas, such as at the nasolabial folds, on the upper mental crease, between the eyes, and on the external nasal frenulum. During adulthood, these lines become more pronounced, and deep creases develop in other areas.

# CHAPTER TWO

# Upper facial and cranial segment abnormalities

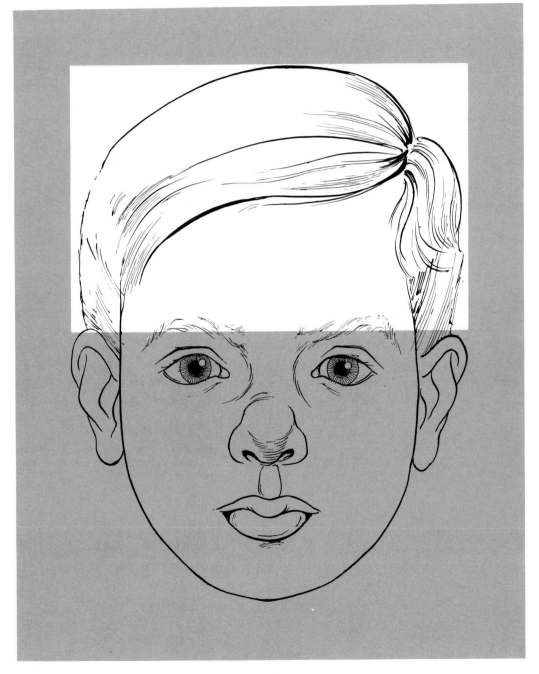

The next three chapters are concerned primarily with abnormalities of the face that do not necessarily represent syndromes, which will be discussed in Chapters 5 through 8. Abnormalities may be either major or minor and may occur alone. Many abnormalities characteristically occur together, however, and when two or more seem to fall into a predictable pattern, the term "syndrome" is appropriate. Nevertheless, attention to the major abnormality of a syndrome is important, and that is the primary concern of this chapter and the next two chapters.

It is pertinent to refer to a major abnormality—one that is predictable because of an anomaly of development in embryogenesis—as an anomalad. Many such abnormalities will be discussed in the immediately following chapters. There are also many minor abnormalities, which result from minor anomalies. Although they are of no serious medical or cosmetic consequence, they will be discussed briefly in these chapters because they serve as indicators of altered morphogenesis and may be valuable clues to the pattern or presence of malformation.

This chapter discusses abnormalities involving primarily the upper facial and cranial segment. Abnormalities in this segment may involve irregularities in size, proportion, shape, and/or alignment. Other abnormalities consist of skin blemishes or involve the hair.

The shape and size of the cranium are largely determined by highly specialized characteristics of bone and bone growth. Most bones of the body, including the bones of the face and the cranial base, are cartilaginous (see Chapter 1). The cranium proper, or vault, however, is formed by membranous bone. The major bones that compose the cranial vault are the paired frontal, temporal, parietal, and occipital bones. Connections between two membranous bones are called sutures, which are necessary for continued, unimpeded growth of the underlying brain. In fetuses and infants the sutures are widely separated to allow for rapid brain growth. Areas where the separation is greatest are called fontanels. The anterior fontanel—the "soft spot" known to every parent—is the largest of the fontanels.

Knowledge of suture physiology and pathology is important in craniofacial viewing. The two most important sutures are the sagittal suture, which divides the cranium into a left half and a right half, and the coronal suture, which divides the cranium into an anterior portion and a posterior portion. Other sutures are of somewhat less importance. The metopic suture separates the forehead into left and right halves and is an extension of the sagittal suture. The paired, semicircular squamous sutures separate the frontal and parietal bones from the temporal bones on both sides of the cranium. Of much less importance to the craniofacial observer is the lambdoid suture, which separates the occipital from the parietal bones. The lambdoid suture is, however, an important determinant of cranial growth (see Chapter 1).

A suture's most important function is to remain open until the brain has slowed its growth rate. The determinant of ultimate cranial contour is essentially unknown. Whether this determinant involves a hormone or represents a mechanical message transmitted purely from the pressure of the growing brain is not absolutely known. The message is relayed to the sutures in some fashion, however, and when it is no longer necessary for them to remain open, they close.

Interestingly, each suture closes at a different time. The closure of the sagittal suture, with some contribution by the metopic suture as well, appears to determine the extent of maximum lateral cranial growth; when the sagittal suture closes, little more lateral expansion of the cranium, and therefore of the brain, is possible. The coronal suture, with some contribution from the lambdoid suture, seems to be the primary determinant of cranial growth in the anterior/posterior direction. The squamous and metopic sutures, although minor sutures, also have significant effects on cranial facial formation. The squamous suture primarily allows for vertical growth of the cranium, while the metopic suture is important in the development of the ultimate shape and configuration of the forehead. The squamous suture becomes particularly important when either or both the sagittal and coronal sutures close prematurely. In such a situation the squamous suture functions as a safety valve to allow continued expansion of the brain in a vertical direction.

When sutures close earlier than usual, the condition called premature suture closure exists. By tradition, there are two types of premature closure of the sutures—primary and secondary. It is important to distinguish between primary and secondary premature suture closure conditions, although at times this can be difficult in clinical practice. Primary suture closure abnormalities are believed to be relatively independent of brain stimulation. Certain factors, some of them undoubtedly inherited and probably mainly osteogenic, cause the sutures to close even though there is adequate stimulation for them to remain open because of pressure from underlying brain growth. These primary suture closures, known as *suture dysostoses* and also as *craniosynostoses,* are of several types. Secondary premature suture closure, on the other hand, results from inadequate stimulation of the sutures to remain open by the underlying brain. In this situation, which can result from a wide variety of brain defects, there is no need for the suture to remain open, and closure passively occurs. It is important to remember that brain growth or lack of growth can be either asymmetrical or symmetrical and either localized or diffuse.

An unusual cranial shape does not necessarily establish that a morbid condition is present. The heads of persons of the Mongoloid race, for example, characteristically are not only smaller than those of Caucasians but also shorter and relatively broader—that is, the anterior/posterior distance is relatively shorter than the horizontal or lateral distance. This is an anthropologic difference that must be taken into account when one defines abnormality. It is not abnormal for an Oriental to have such a relatively shortened cranium, whereas the same extent of shortening may be decidedly abnormal in a Caucasian. The term used to describe this variation, which thus can be either anthropologic or pathologic, is *brachycephaly* ("broadened cephalus"). Likewise, the variation characterized by a cranium that is relatively longer than "normal" is termed *dolichocephaly* (dolich = long). In premature infants, particularly, there is a tendency for the cranium to be relatively much longer than in older infants and children. This tendency results from relative differences in growth activity – probably in response to brain growth – between the sagittal and coronal sutures. This situation in a premature infant also is called dolichocephaly, but the term is used simply as a description rather than as an indicator of a true abnormality. However, an excessively long cranium later in infancy, or in a full-term neonate, would be considered an abnormality, but not necessarily a serious or significant one.

## PRIMARY SUTURE ABNORMALITIES

Suture dysostosis is a nonspecific term referring to any primary disturbance in a suture. The term "craniosynostosis" refers more specifically to premature closing of a suture. Craniosynostoses, particularly in early life, may represent clinical emergencies because of the development of increased intracranial pressure. However, the manifestations of some of the craniosynostoses are delayed, producing clinical symptoms of increased intracranial pressure in late infancy or even in the juvenile or adult periods.

When only one suture is involved in the early closure process, others remain open or even may become wider as a means of compensation to allow for increasing brain growth without acute increased intracranial pressure. Since certain sutures close and others remain open, the cranium is formed into predictable shapes (Gorden, 1959). Individuals with severe variations of these shapes tend to be more prone to developing decompensated, increased intracranial pressure in later life after simple insults that would not otherwise be clinically significant. Minor head trauma, subclinical infections, minor toxins, and excessive stress from almost any source can cause the deterioration of a previously compensated or balanced situation. Observation for such suture dysostotic conditions is of great importance in clinical medical practice, even if at the time of medical evaluation a patient does not show signs of increased intracranial pressure.

### Dolichoscaphocephaly

The term dolichocephaly means a relatively long and narrow cranium, in an anthropologic sense. The term used for the pathologic condition existing when the sagittal suture closes prematurely while other sutures (especially the coronal) remain open is scaphocephaly (scapho = boat-shaped). A preferable term might be *dolichoscaphocephaly*. In such a situation, there are distinct abnormalities in the cranial contour when the face is viewed from the front, as in Fig. 2-1. Although the face proper is of normal proportion, the cranium is obviously abnormal. The cranium in the patient shown is not only much narrower than normal but also slightly higher—that is, towered. Fig. 2-1, *C*, shows the growth characteristics of this cranial abnormality. One can visualize the patho-anatomy of the long, narrow cranium that results if the sagittal suture closes prematurely.

Individuals with dolichoscaphocephaly have a much less efficient defense against noxious stresses, which might produce increased intra-cranial pressure and brain damage, than persons with normal cranial contours. Thus, persons with this abnormality may have a variety of neurologic deficits other than acute increased intracranial pressure, especially in later life.

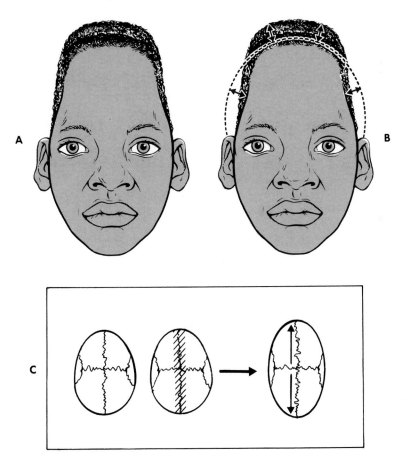

Fig. 2-1. Dolichoscaphocephaly. **A,** Typical frontal view of person with a long, narrow cranium. **B,** Presumed normal contour superimposed. **C,** Top of the normal skull with the major sutures indicated, early closure of the sagittal suture, and resulting cranial growth. *Vertical line,* Sagittal suture. *Horizontal line,* Coronal suture.

## Acrobrachycephaly

The term brachycephaly refers to a broadened cranium and may be an anthropologic designation. The pathologic suture dysostosis characterized by an extremely broad cranium is called *acrobrachycephaly* (acro = extreme). This condition results from premature closure of the coronal suture. In acrobrachycephaly the growth of the cranium is impeded in the longitudinal direction, the reverse of the situation that exists in scaphocephaly. If the sagittal and metopic sutures remain reasonably open, expansion of the brain and the growth of the cranium in width continue. Because of the increased horizontal distance, it is quite obvious that the cranial contour of the patient in Fig. 2-2 is abnormal. Acrobrachycephaly produces several other craniofacial abnormalities:

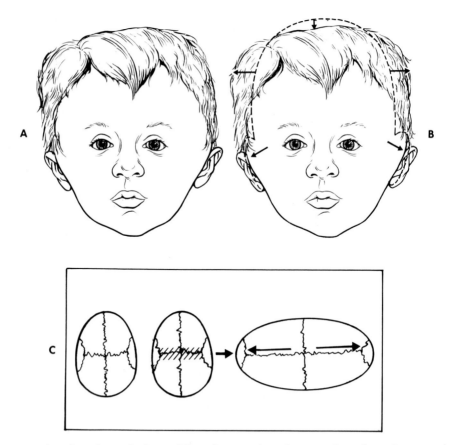

**Fig. 2-2.** Acrobrachycephaly. **A,** The abnormality that results when there is premature closure of the coronal suture, resulting in anterior-posterior growth being impeded. **B,** Normal contour superimposed. **C,** Normal skull, closure of the coronal suture, and the resultant direction of cranial growth. *Vertical line,* Sagittal suture. *Horizontal line,* Coronal suture.

(1) the eyes may be tilted downward laterally, (2) the ears also may be tilted downward, and (3) the temporal area usually appears to be bulging outward and slightly downward.

In acrobrachycephaly the coronal suture closes prematurely while all other sutures—including the sagittal, the squamous, and the metopic—remain relatively open. It is apparent that early closure of the coronal suture is less easily compensated for than early closure of the sagittal suture. Normal brain growth tends to be more in an anterior/posterior direction than in a lateral direction. Thus, when there is early coronal suture closure, compensation from continued opening of the sagittal suture is not as efficient as compensation from early closure of the sagittal suture when the other sutures remain open. The squamous suture, along with other minor sutures, must remain open longer to compensate for continued normal brain growth. Without this "safety valve," brain growth would be inhibited, and increased intracranial pressure could ensue. The growing brain continues to keep the squamous suture open, and the lower part of the temporal bone may be observed to bulge. This development causes the intercanthal line to be tilted downward and the ears to be pushed outward and downward. In addition, the zygomatic processes become prominent and tilted downward. The metopic suture also contributes to this unique cranial and upper facial disturbance. It too must remain open longer to compensate for continued brain growth. Frequently in acrobrachycephaly a prominent metopic suture, clinically seen as a keel or hyperostotic line, may be present in the middle of the forehead.

Acrobrachycephaly is an important cranial abnormality. The risk of decompensated increased intracranial pressure and subsequent signs of brain damage is greater than with scaphocephaly. In addition, more facial abnormalities are possible with this defect than with scaphocephaly. Acrobrachycephaly is also associated with many general physical abnormalities, including other dysplastic defects such as syndactyly and polydactyly (Apert, 1923; Book and Hesselvik, 1953; Kahn and Fulmer, 1955). These abnormalities and the syndromes associated with them will be discussed in more detail in Chapter 5.

## Oxyturricephaly

Turricephaly means "tower skull." When the major determinants of anterior/posterior and lateral growth are impeded, the cranial vault grows vertically rather than in its normal longitudinal and horizontal directions. Since such a cranium occasionally comes to a sharp point at the vertex, the term oxycephaly is also used to designate this condition (oxy = sharp or pointed). A combined term, oxyturricephaly, will be used here. Fig. 2-3 shows such a cranial configuration. The skull is much higher and somewhat narrower than normal. In this cranial abnormality, most (if not all) major sutures appear to be dysostotic and prematurely closed. Because of persistent opening of the basilar synostosis and synchondrosis (connections between cartilaginous bones or between

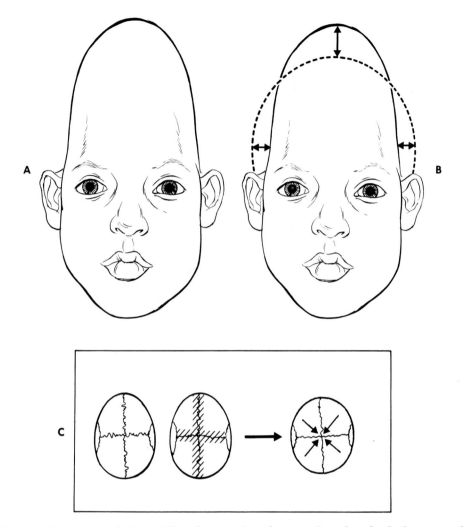

**Fig. 2-3.** Oxyturricephaly. **A,** The abnormality that results when both the coronal and the sagittal sutures close prematurely. **B,** Normal contour superimposed. **C,** Directions of forces of skull growth when both the major sutures close prematurely. *Vertical line,* Sagittal suture. *Horizontal line,* Coronal suture.

cartilaginous and membranous bones), the brain is allowed to grow only in a vertical direction, and the cranium thus becomes towered. Since the base of the cranium is usually wider than the most rostral parts, the cranium also appears sharp or pointed. From the front, a person with oxyturricephaly resembles the scaphocephalic child in Fig. 2-1 except that the skull has a greater vertical distance. In oxyturricephaly, other abnormalities (like proptosis) are so common that they fit into a fairly distinct syndrome. Further discussion of oxyturricephaly will appear in subsequent chapters, especially Chapter 5.

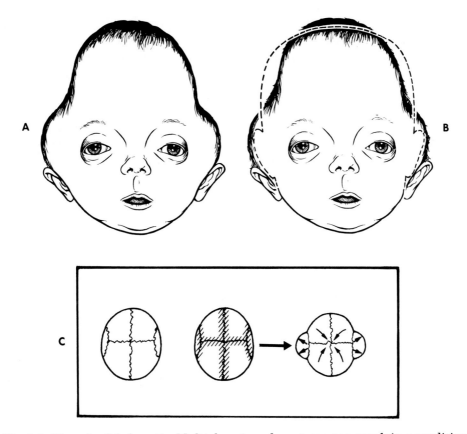

Fig. 2-4. Cloverleaf deformity. Multiple suture dysostoses can result in a condition A, in which there are upward and lateral growth pressures. B, Normal contour superimposed. Note especially the downward displacement of the features of the middle facial segment, with the ears being pushed into an extremely low position. C, Presumed directions of pressures when several major sutures close prematurely. *Vertical line,* Sagittal suture. *Horizontal line,* Coronal suture.

## The cloverleaf deformity

The cloverleaf deformity, which is also considered to be a multiple-suture dysostosis, is caused by a persistent opening of the squamous sutures. In this regard the abnormality is very similar to acrobrachycephaly. In the cloverleaf deformity, however, it would seem either that the entire temporal bone is dysplastic and extra-pliable or that there is such extensive skull growth impediment in utero that the brain pushes on the temporal bone strongly enough almost to destroy it. As Fig. 2-4 shows, the expanding brain grows into the temporal fossae. Thus, from both the front and the top, a cloverleaf configuration develops (Angle and others, 1967; Feingold and others, 1969).

• • •

In clinical practice multiple suture dysostoses are rare because suture defects usually produce immediate secondary symptoms; for example, acute increased intracranial pressure is common and develops very early because there is less opportunity for compensation for brain growth. Thus it is more common to encounter such defects in infants than in older children or adults. One must remember that there are other directions of brain growth possible even when multiple suture closure occurs. In the infantile period brain growth may be directed anteriorly and downward on the still-soft and pliable bony orbits and pituitary sellae. This direct pressure on the bony orbits and retroorbital soft tissues exerts an effect upon the eyeballs. Exostosis or proptosis, therefore, occurs in conditions characterized by multiple suture dysostoses.

### Other suture dysostoses

The term *plagiocephaly* refers to an unusual slanting or tilting of the cranium (plagio = slanting). This condition occurs when there is premature and asymmetrical closure of one suture or a part of one suture. Examples would be the premature closure of one squamous suture or half of the coronal suture or the lambdoid suture. Plagiocephaly is often associated with an underlying brain defect and thus is frequently a secondary rather than a primary craniosynostotic abnormality. Plagiocephaly should be distinguished from the less specific term *cranioscoliosis*. Cranioscoliosis, or abnormal turning of the cranium, which is best appreciated when viewing the cranium from the top, may be a product of positional restraints in infancy. However, restraining an infant's head in order to mold it is itself an abnormal situation. Certain primitive cultures engage in infant skull binding for cosmetic purposes, but such a practice encountered in Western society would lead one to suspect child abuse. Thus, unusually molded crania in infants result not from faulty positioning on the part of parents but rather from abnormal inactivity on the part of the child. An infant who is so immobile that asymmetrical molding of the head occurs probably has severe motor handicaps.

The metopic suture is very important in facial viewing, since ultimate forehead size and shape are greatly dependent upon it. When there is premature closure of the metopic suture, *trigonocephaly* occurs. This condition is characterized by a narrow and frequently "keeled" forehead, as shown in Fig. 2-5. Trigonocephaly is often associated with a small forehead, a low hairline, and ridging or hyperostosis along the edges of the metopic suture. The reverse of the trigonocephalic abnormality is seen in conditions characterized by persistent opening of the sutures. These conditions will be discussed in Chapter 5. In a person with *persis-*

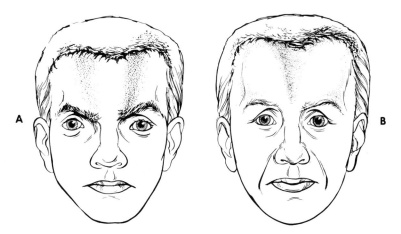

Fig. 2-5. Metopic suture dysostosis. Premature closure of the metopic suture results in a frontal keel and often a very narrow forehead, while persistent opening results in a "funnel" appearance. **A**, Persistent suture opening. **B**, Frontal keel.

*tent metopic openings*, a V-like funnel is seen in the forehead. This funnel is almost always associated with a large cranium as well.

It is important to remember that suture dysostoses commonly produce continuing variations in cranial and facial appearance and that, although simple abnormalities have heretofore been discussed, in practical clinical practice suture dysostoses usually appear in combination with other abnormalities (Opitz and others, 1969).

## SECONDARY SUTURE ABNORMALITIES

We have discussed cranial abnormalities that result from defects of the sutures or cranial bones themselves. These were named primary suture abnormalities. There are also secondary suture abnormalities, which result from primary brain abnormalities. The distinction between primary and secondary suture abnormalities has important clinical implications but may be diagnostically difficult. Therefore special attention must be given these secondary abnormalities.

The secondary suture abnormalities, usually resulting from major brain defects, are of several types, but the most frequently encountered are abnormalities in cranial size. The size of the cranium is extremely important in clinical medical practice and can be readily determined. It then can be compared to standards for age, sex, and race. This book will not dwell upon aspects of physical diagnosis other than simple facial and cranial viewing, but head measurement must be discussed briefly. The standard procedure is to determine the maximum occipital-frontal circumference (OFC). See Table 2 for normal OFCs at

**Table 2.** Composite graphs of head circumference in boys and girls from birth to 18 years of age*

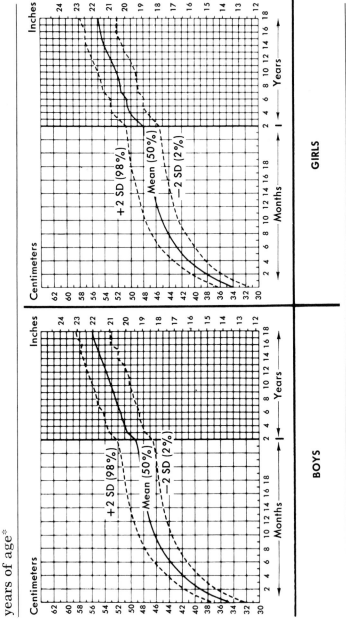

*From Nellhaus, G.: Pediatrics 41:106, 1968. Copyright American Academy of Pediatrics, 1968.

various ages. Age obviously is the greatest influencer of head size, but sex and race are also important. Heads of females are smaller than those of males, and heads of Orientals are smaller than those of Caucasians and Negroes. The measurements shown in Table 2 are those found in Caucasians. For total accuracy, all head measurements should be compared to standards for the sex, race, and exact age of the individual being measured. Since in clinical practice it is inconvenient to carry a set of tables, a simple rule for determining whether a head size is clearly abnormal has been devised. This is the *rule of five*.

## The rule of five

Study of the figures in Table 2 allows one to recognize clear abnormalities in head size. One simply remembers the following ages: birth (newborn at term), 3 months, 9 months, 30 months, and 15 years. A newborn male at term has a mean OFC of 35 cm, as shown by several repeated measurements. One standard deviation at this age is about 1 to 1.2 cm; two standard deviations is about 2 to 2.4 cm. Thus a newborn term male with an OFC of 32 cm, which is more than two standard deviations below the mean, is clearly abnormal, as is a newborn with a head size of 38 cm, which is more than two standard deviations above the mean. A full-term female newborn usually has an OFC about 1 cm less than that of a male. Thus the mean for a newborn term female is about 34 cm. The rule of five adds 5 cm to the mean OFC for each additional age level mentioned. Thus for a male infant, the mean OFC at 3 months is about 40 cm, at 9 months about 45 cm, and at 2 ½ years about 50 cm. A male juvenile of about 15 years has an OFC of about 55 cm. Females are usually about 1 cm smaller. The standard deviation at each age level is usually 1 to 1.2 cm, regardless of sex.

The size of the cranial vault correlates only slightly with intelligence. Yet head measurement should be a standard physical diagnostic test for any patient—young or old, but especially in the pediatric age group—in whom mental retardation, learning disability, dementia, or degenerative disease is suspected.

Although actual head measurement is the best method of determining whether the head is too small or too large, certain features suggesting these conditions can be detected through frontal viewing of a person's cranium and face.

## Microcephaly

The term microcephaly means "small cephalus." This condition exists statistically when the maximum occipital-frontal circumference falls two standard deviations or more below the mean for the age, sex, and race when, of course, the other body measurements are relatively normal. Several of the conditions described in later chapters are characterized by microcephaly in addition to other more specific abnormalities, and some of the contour abnormalities already discussed are accompanied by microcephaly. A prime example is oxyturricephaly (see Fig. 2-3), in which the maximum OFC obviously is deficient because the major volume of the brain is displaced vertically to cause the tower deformity.*

It is obvious, even on initial inspection, that the person shown in Fig. 2-6 has a diminished cranial volume. His cranium is both narrow and short. (Compare this cranium with the turricephalic cranium in Fig. 2-3. In oxyturricephaly the cranium is narrow but towered.) When the face in Fig. 2-6 is viewed from the front only, one must speculate about the condition of the posterior cranium, but one would assume it to be equally small. This person has an abnormality called simple microcephaly, which usually does not involve suture dysostosis. Although small, the cranium is symmetrical. Such an abnormality is almost always associated with deficient growth of the brain. The cranium is small because the brain is small. Although such a situation may follow many types of brain lesions, such as those resulting from birth trauma, congenital infections, metabolic disturbances, and cytogenic abnormalities, simple microcephaly occasionally runs in families and is not associated with severe mental deficiency (Book and others, 1953; Crome, 1952; Pryor and Thelander, 1968).

Distinguishing between microcephaly associated with suture dysostosis and simple microcephaly is not as easy as one would like, especially in young infants who may have small heads but have not had the opportunity to develop characteristic cranial stigmata. Skull roentgenograms are useful in making the distinction because they show hyperostotic suture changes and even suture "ridging" in instances of actual suture dysostosis.

*Anencephaly* is the ultimate and most severe form of microcephaly.

---

*One must remember that the OFC is not necessarily a measure of the brain volume or even the surface area of the head. For example, four squares measuring 1 cm are arranged to form a large square as follows,

the total circumference is 8 cm. If, however, the 1 cm squares are placed end-to-end,

the circumference totals 10 cm. In this arrangement, even though the total area remains the same, the circumference is greater. Thus in dolichocephaly, as an example, the OFC may be greater than normal, even though the area and the volume are the same in both situations.

To visualize oxyturricephaly, the squares can be thought of as a three-dimensional block,

and the OFC is represented by the circumference of one block—that is, 4 cm. Thus, although a small OFC suggests severe microcephaly, the brain volume may not be different.

Such simple mathematics show why the correlation between head circumference and mental retardation is weak. One would expect a more positive correlation between brain volume and intelligence.

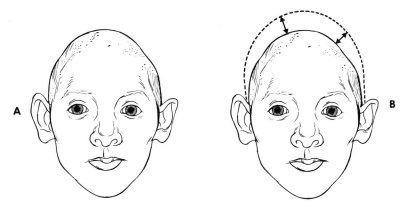

Fig. 2-6. Microcephaly. **A,** An abnormally small cranium. **B,** Normal contour superimposed.

Although the term literally means "without brain," in most cases some rudiments of brain are found. This defect is believed to represent, in some instances, a failure of the rostral neural tube to close. In many other instances, it is likely that a destructive insult takes place after closure has occurred or that an inducer of brain proliferation is missing. An *Encephalocele* (a herniated brain) is another defect resulting from incomplete closure of the rostral neural tube. Since this defect is partial, the condition is not necessarily incompatible with life. Frontal encephalocele is particularly important in relation to the upper facial and cranial segment. Both encephalocele and anencephaly potentially can be associated with macrocephaly if hydrocephalus occurs as a complication. *Hydranencephaly* may be an example of anencephaly complicated by hydrocephalus.

## Macrocephaly

Macrocephaly (literally, "large cephalus") is a nonspecific abnormality as well. This condition occurs statistically when the OFC is more than two standard deviations greater than the mean measurement for age, sex, and race (see previous exceptions). It is important to emphasize that a large cephalus does not necessarily indicate a large brain or, an even more common mistake, a hydrocephalic condition. The cephalus may be large for various reasons, including enlargement of (1) the scalp (cranial subcutaneous hematoma, leprosy, acromegaly), (2) the subperiosteum (cephalohematoma), (3) the skull (Paget's disease, cranial neurofibromatosis), (4) the meningeal spaces (subdural hematoma), (5) the brain (megalencephaly), and (6) the ventricles of the brain (hydrocephalus). (Refer to Table 3.) The major causes of macrocephaly range from life-threatening conditions (like subdural hematoma and hydrocephalus) to benign conditions (like familial megalencephaly). Although life-threat-

Table 3. Type, source, and differential diagnosis in macrocephaly*

| Type | Source | Differential diagnosis |
|---|---|---|
| Hydrocephalus | Communicating hydrocephalus | Meningeal fibrosis<br>Vascular malformation<br>Neurocutaneous malformation<br>Destructive lesions |
| | Noncommunicating hydrocephalus | Arnold-Chiari malformation<br>Aqueductal stenosis<br>Neoplasms |
| Brain edema | Toxins | Lead<br>Vitamin A<br>Tetracycline |
| | Endocrine | Hypoparathyroidism<br>Hypoadrenocorticism |
| | Galactosemia<br>Idiopathic edema | |
| Subdural effusion | Hematoma<br>Hygroma<br>Empyema | Head trauma<br>Child abuse<br>Nutritional disturbance |
| Thickened skull | Cranioskeletal dysplasia | Osteopetrosis<br>Osteomyelitis<br>Osteogenesis imperfecta<br>Craniofacial dysostosis<br>Cleidocranial dysostosis<br>Epiphyseal dysplasia |
| Megalencephaly | Anatomic megalencephaly | Neurocutaneous diseases<br>Familial ganglioneuroma |
| | Metabolic megalencephaly | Aminoacidurias<br>Leukodystrophy<br>Lysosomal diseases |

*Adapted from DeMyer, W.: Megalencephaly in children, Neurology 22:634-643, 1972.

ening conditions are more common than benign conditions and more important to recognize early, a large head does not always mean that a serious problem exists. Since the major causes of macrocephaly are important to the neurologist, most of them will be discussed further in subsequent chapters.

It is not always possible to distinguish between different types of macrocephaly through simple craniofacial inspection, although certain clues are important. Persons who suffer from hydrocephalus often, but not always, have increased intracranial pressure. In infants and young children, chronic increased intracranial pressure exerts an effect on the overlying soft pliable skull. Thus one might expect to see certain concomitant features in hydrocephalus in infants, including (1) engorged superficial cutaneous cranial veins (because the increased pressure causes a relative stagnation of intracranial circulation), (2) a bulging

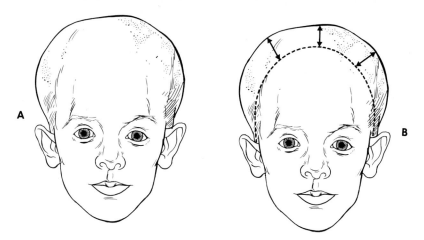

Fig. 2-7. Macrocephaly. **A,** The middle and lower facial segments can be relatively normal, with most of the enlargement occurring in the upper facial and cranial segment. **B,** Normal contour superimposed.

and tense anterior fontanel (a safety valve peculiar to young infants that allows them to tolerate increased intracranial pressure better than older infants, juveniles, and adults), (3) proptosis (resulting from pressure on the still soft and pliable bony orbits of the eyes, which in turn push the eyes outward), which accounts for the so-called setting sun sign (a feature to be discussed in more detail in subsequent chapters), and (4) cranial nerve palsies, especially those of the extraocular muscles and pupils. None of these coexistent abnormalities, however, is always present in infants with hydrocephalus.

Young children and infants who have macrocephaly secondary to chronic subdural effusion often have a peculiar configuration of the cranium. Such crania have been described by some as "square-shaped" because of the tendency of the subdural fluid (especially if it is blood, for example, secondary to trauma) to fill the subdural space rather equally in anterior-to-posterior cranial compartments. In such infants there is a greater propensity for cranial nerve palsies and other signs of increased intracranial pressure, but seldom to the extent or severity that they occur in patients with hydrocephalus.

The patient in Fig. 2-7 has an obviously large, though symmetrical, cranium. No other abnormalities are evident. Although one could not be certain, considering his pleasant countenance and his presumed age, one might conclude that his macrocephaly probably has a benign cause. Distinctions of this type will be discussed further in subsequent chapters.

It should be emphasized that a large head could result from a combination of factors. For example, a person with familial megalencephaly could fall, develop a subdural hematoma, and then develop obstructive hydrocephalus as a result of clotted blood being spilled into the cerebro-spinal fluid pathways and obstructing them.

A traumatic condition that has little clinical significance either at the time of injury or later is frequently encountered in newborns. This condition, called cephalohematoma, results from hemorrhage in the periosteum of the skull caused by the trauma of birth. When large enough, cephalohematomas may produce moderate enlargement of the cephalus. One can recognize the condition by the asymmetry it produces in the cephalus. Although cephalohematoma can be quite disfiguring and alarming, it seldom produces problems itself and usually disappears in time with no treatment. Cephalohematomas are differentiated from subcutaneous hemotamas by the fact that they are confined to the compartments of the cranial bones, while subcutaneous hemorrhages are not.

### Asymmetries

Cranial asymmetries can result either from primary brain lesions or from abnormalities of the scalp, bone, periosteum, meninges, or ventricles. Included in the many possible abnormalities are localized growths or atrophies of skin, subcutaneous tissue, and bone. Most of these will be discussed in the section on topographic abnormalities, which follows. Subdural hematomas may be purely unilateral and, when long standing, may have an effect upon the growth of the cranium and the upper face. When the brain is also involved, the residual effects may be far more extensive and can influence other parts of the face and soma as well. Localized atrophy of the brain, as is seen in birth trauma, acquired trauma, and asymmetrical brain malformations, may be obvious by its effects upon the cranioface. Localized ventricular enlargements result not only from trauma but also from vascular neoplastic and malformation processes.

Asymmetrical abnormalities of the cranioface include atrophic and hypertrophic or hyperplastic features. Fig. 2-8 shows how facial observation can be important in properly assessing such situations. It is obvious that the cranial vault on the patient's right is much smaller than the more normal corresponding segment on the patient's left. The right cranium in this patient is obviously abnormally shaped. When one superimposes the major facial lines (as is done in Fig. 2-8), this initial impression is dramatically confirmed.

Such an obvious abnormality in cranial symmetry represents a defect that is seldom limited to the cranium. Such an abnormality is usually seen when there is an underlying defect involving asymmetry of the brain. This defect in turn often has far-reaching somatic and neurologic consequences, usually even more obvious than the facial abnormalities.

Many asymmetries of the cranioface have been discussed in the section on primary suture abnormalities. Plagiocephaly, for example, in some situations truly represents a suture dysostosis, but it can result

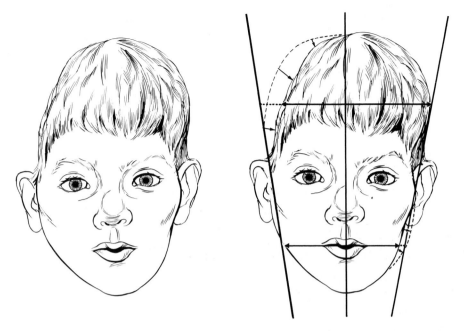

Fig. 2-8. Asymmetry in cranial contour. The major facial lines can be used to confirm an impression of asymmetry.

from a localized underlying brain disturbance. (Refer also to the discussion on cranioscoliosis in the same section.)

## TOPOGRAPHIC ABNORMALITIES

The upper facial and cranial segment represents over half of the entire face and cranium. In this segment there is thus more total skin surface in which various topographic abnormalities can occur than in the other segments. These abnormalities include simple blemishes, birthmarks, abnormalities of hair (too much or too little or abnormal distribution), and other deformities. Most topographic disturbances tend to cross facial segments or to be associated with other abnormalities that would more appropriately be discussed in subsequent chapters. Yet many are limited to the upper facial and cranial segment and need to be mentioned in this chapter.

### Abnormalities of the skin

**Depigmentation abnormalities.** The definition of *Leukoderma*, literally "white skin," has not been clearly established by clinicians. The most acceptable definition suggests that it is a congenital nonprogressive skin blemish—in other words, a birthmark. The lesion is common among blacks, although it has been reported in persons of all races. Although leukoderma may be distributed over the entire body, it has been suggested that the condition has particular significance when located on the cranium and other parts of the face. Leukoderma tends to be found on the forehead but may extend past the hairline, thus producing white hair (Dyken and others, 1972). Several syndromes characterized by such localized congenital depigmentation will be discussed in later chapters. (See Fig. 2-9, A.)

*The white forelock* is another topographic abnormality of the upper facial and cranial segment. This lesion is an example of simple leukoderma except that it is confined to the area behind the hairline. Rather than being asymmetrical, the white forelock tends to occur closer to the midline of the forehead. There is usually no other feature of skin depigmentation either on the face or on the rest of the body, although heterochromia may occasionally occur. A white forelock seems to have more specificity for Waardenburg's syndrome (to be discussed in later chapters). The white forelock, as opposed to plain congenital leukoderma, is more common in Caucasians than in persons of other races. (Campbell, 1962; DiGeorge and others, 1960). (See Fig. 2-9, B.)

*Poliosis* is a condition of white hair that is associated with leukoderma when the poliosis is congenital. There are, however, examples of acquired poliosis. Poliosis is distinguished from white forelock by its distribution, which usually is generalized over the cranium. Poliosis, in fact, tends to occur posteriorly.

Smaller depigmented lesions also may be observed over the forehead and behind the hairline. When present over the cranium, such lesions are associated with poliosis. These depigmented lesions are called *nevus anemicus* or *ash-leaf spots* (because of their shape) and usually vary

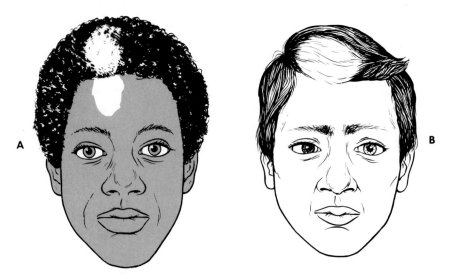

Fig. 2-9. Topographic abnormalities. **A,** Typical situation of a white patch of skin (leukoderma) accompanied by a white lock of hair. **B,** A less typical constellation of signs, one of which is a white lock of hair.

from 0.5 to 1 cm in size. They are usually smaller than the lesions seen in leukoderma and are more likely to be distributed over the body.

**Hyperpigmentation abnormalities.** There are many cutaneous lesions that, although not confined to the upper facial and cranial segment, or even to the face, may and frequently do affect this area. The most well known but certainly not the most common is the *café-au-lait spot* or *coffee-with-milk spot.* This lesion is of variable size and is the color of coffee mixed with cream. It is flat and has a shaply demarcated but irregular border. In blacks this lesion may be darker. More deeply colored (and rarer) hyperpigmented skin lesions occur in association with other cutaneous abnormalities. The *Albright type of café-au-lait spot* has a much more irregular border than the typical cafe-au-lait spot. The rough *sharkskin lesion* or *shagreen patch* is usually observed on the back, in the flank, and has a dermatome distribution. When it appears in this location, it has great significance in the diagnosis of tuberous sclerosis. This lesion may also occur over the cranium and the upper face. The sharkskin patch often appears more bronzed when pigmented, and the overlying epidermis is usually hypertrophied. *Chocolate spots* also may occur over the cranioface, especially in blacks. These spots may have diagnostic meaning when they appear in certain areas. *Freckles* or *lentigines* are of several varieties. They may be distributed over the forehead but are especially meaningful when seen around the lips and in the central middle face. Sometimes they are blue-gray vertical bands limited to the epidermis. *Giant hyperpigmented skin lesions* are seen in several neurocutaneous diseases. Such lesions usually have the same characteristics as the cafe-au-lait spots but are darker and larger and are distributed over the body rather than the cranioface. Usually this lesion is distributed over the sacrum, buttocks, or upper spine. *Poikiloderma congenita* is a unique skin lesion that involves both pigmentation and depigmentation and that usually changes over a period of time. First, irregular erythema develops, which progresses to telangiectasia, scarring, and atrophy. This lesion has universal distribution in most cases and thus may affect the cranium and upper face.

**Vascular nevi.** The precise medical meanings of vascular birthmarks are highly debatable. General knowledge of their form, shape, color, location, and consistency—especially in the craniofacial area—may be of extreme importance in diagnostic classification, management, and prognosis. There are three major types of persistent vascular nevi or hemangiomas: (1) *cavernous hemangiomas,* (2) *capillary hemangiomas;* and (3) *mixed hemangiomas,* which are combinations of cavernous and capillary hemangiomas. Capillary hemangiomas are of three subtypes, the so-called *nevus vasculosus,* the *nevus flammeus,* and the *nevus telangiectasis.* All vascular nevi are distinguished by size, form, location, and border demarcation, among other minor criteria.

The cavernous hemangioma is often extensive and bluish because it is usually located in the deeper layers of the skin and subcutaneous tissues. This hemangioma can involve much of the face and large parts of the body. Cavernous hemangiomas are primarily subdermal or subcutaneous and seldom involve the epidermis. They may be associated with hypertrophy of the underlying tissues and organs.

Capillary hemangiomas generally are located in the superficial areas of the skin. The nevus vasculosus is also called a strawberry mark. It is usually slightly elevated, has a sharp demarcation but an irregular border, and tends to occur over the body rather than on the face. There are, of course, exceptions to this rule. The nevus flammeus consists of two subtypes. The more clinically significant subtype resembles a port wine stain in color. This "port wine" nevus flammeus is contrasted to the lighter, more irregular, flat, pink, "rose wine," nevus flammeus that occurs quite commonly, but transiently, in the neonatal period. The nevus telangiectasis or spider nevus represents a dilation of the end point of an arteriole. This hemangioma usually occurs singly rather than in clusters and does not cover a large area of skin, as in both nevus vasculosus and nevus flammeus.

Mixed hemangiomas usually do not represent simply a miscellaneous category. Most often the combination is between a typical cavernous hemangioma and the capillary hemangioma that has a "strawberry" appearance—the nevus vasculosus. The mixed hemangioma is, of course, important to the dermatologist, but it also has diagnostic importance for the general physician. Such a birthmark may occur in the gastrointestinal tract, the respiratory tree, and other areas. In the central nervous system such lesions may produce subarachnoid hemorrhage.

The distribution of vascular nevi may have as much importance as the type of lesion. The port wine nevus flammeus commonly is distributed predominantly on one side and sometimes does not extend much past the midline, if at all. This lesion often involves other facial segments on the same side of the face. Rarely, however, the port wine mark, which is usually associated with mild hypertrophy of the overlying epidermis, will be distributed almost exactly in the midline in the upper facial and cranial segment. The rose wine nevus flammeus is so commonly seen in the infantile period that it is usually believed not to have much importance. An exception to this statement is the purely midline forehead rose wine nevus flammeus, which has been associated with other cranial defects. In such instances, the vascular lesions have persisted into adult life, whereas in the more common varieties (including those in which the lesions are distributed more widely on the forehead), they usually disappear by the second year of life. (See Fig. 2-10.)

**Hypertrophic and hypotrophic lesions.** *Fibrous dysplasia* (Fig. 2-11, *A*) with associated cutaneous hypertrophy and hyperpigmentation occasionally involves the upper face and cranium. This condition affects the bone and subcutaneous tissues especially and often the skin as well. When it involves the face, lesions are usually distributed on the forehead

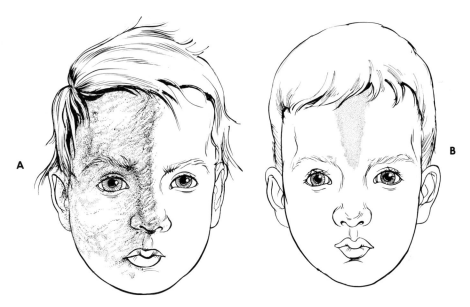

Fig. 2-10. Topographic abnormalities: vascular nevi. There are several types of vascular nevi or hemangiomas. The two depicted here are perhaps the most common—the port wine stain, **A**, and the "pink" nevus flammeus, **B**.

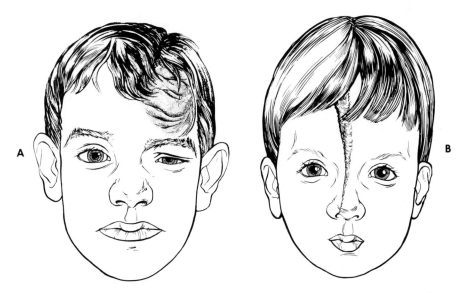

Fig. 2-11. Topographic abnormalities. **A**, Fibrous Dysplasia. **B**, Coup de sabre.

in an asymmetrical fashion. Fibrous dysplasia may be associated with other cutaneous and systemic abnormalities, especially tuberous sclerosis (see Chapter 5). It is important to remember that this condition involves hypertrophic rather than atrophic lesions.

*The coup de sabre* (Fig. 2-11, *B*) is a linear, hypotrophic lesion, primarily of the skin, that gets its name from its resemblance to the scar left after the slash of a sabre. This lesion is progressive and may involve skin, subcutaneous tissue, bone, and even brain if the lesion covers the cranium. Coup de sabre is closely related to the hemifacial atrophy (Parry-Romberg) syndrome (Rogers, 1977).

Usually the coup de sabre lesion can be distinguished from a similarly progressing skin lesion called a *linear organoid nevus* or *sebaceous nevus of Jaddasohn*. This slowly progressing birthmark is raised and has a dirty, waxy appearance. The nevus is not confined to the cranioface, but it has particular diagnostic significance when it appears there (Swaiman, 1975, p. 749).

Small punched-out lesions sometimes are seen, especially behind the hairline, this *congenital absence of the skin* is significant only in that it may indicate abnormalities in underlying tissues and their formation. Usually there is no hair growing in the area of the lesion.

### Abnormalities of the hair

**Baldness.** Although a newborn child may be bald, baldness in an older child or a woman is considered abnormal under any circumstances. In an adult male, it may not be an absolute abnormality. Yet certain types of baldness are always abnormal. Frontal baldness (Fig. 2-12, *A*) begins in the midline area of the forehead and extends backward, sparing the temporal areas. Temporal baldness is a more common type of baldness in adult men and is not an absolute abnormality. The significance of frontal baldness in male (or female) members of families in which one or more members have the disease dystrophia myotonica cannot be denied. (Refer to the discussions of dystrophia myotonica in subsequent chapters.)

*Alopecia* is an abnormal dropping out or absence of hair. This condition may be patchy (*alopecia areata* or *partialis*) or universal (*alopecia universalis*).

**Hirsutism.** Abnormal amounts and distribution of facial hair, especially in children, may have important diagnostic implications. Eyebrows that meet in the midline of the face and facial hirsutism may be seen in normal persons, especially adults. Marked hyperplasia, on the other hand, especially in a child, suggests an abnormality. When a midline brow occurs with other abnormal facial and somatic features, it may have great diagnostic meaning, as in de Lange's syndrome, which will be discussed in more detail later. (See Fig. 2-12, *C*.)

One should also take note of excessive hairiness of the eyebrows, especially of the medial aspects.

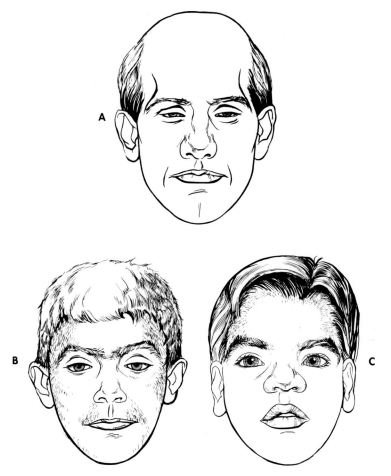

**Fig. 2-12.** Topographic abnormalities. The absence or abundance of hair may be a sign of a serious abnormality. Furthermore, the distribution of the hair about the head and face is important. **A,** Frontal baldness. **B,** Synophrys (midline brow) and hyperplasia of the superciliary arch. **C,** Frontal hirsutism.

Even without other abnormal facial or somatic features, hyperplasia of the superciliary arches, from which the eyebrows originate, is also of significance. This deformity occurs more often in certain mentally retarded, chronically hospitalized patients than in normal persons and is almost always associated with hirsutism of the forehead. Superciliary arch hyperplasia is commonly associated with mental retardation or related disorders. For example, excessive cranial and upper facial hair and superciliary hyperplasia occur in the mucopolysaccharidoses and related diseases, which will be discussed in later chapters. (See Fig. 2-12, *B.*)

# CHAPTER THREE
# Middle facial segment abnormalities

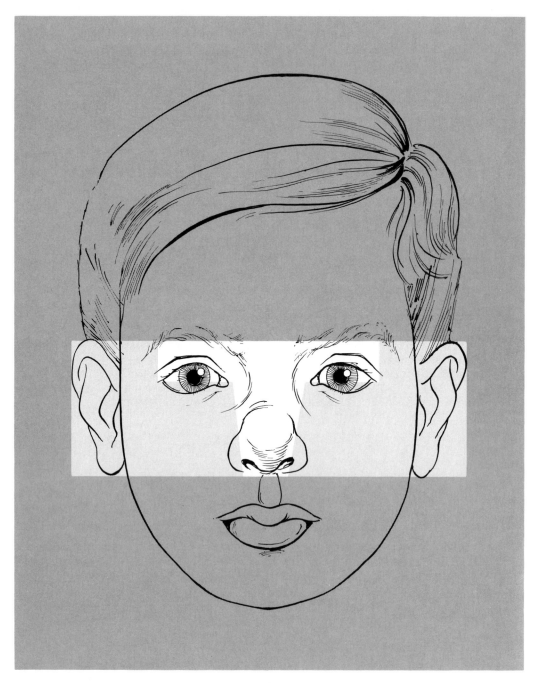

The middle face is an important segment of the cranioface because it includes the eyes, the nose, the ears, and midface proper, the maxilla, and the particularly important zygomatic processes. The middle facial segment is the focus of most casual facial viewing. The eyes, the nose, and the ears are ubiquitously dwelled upon in romantic literature and are the features that remain in our memories longest when we try to recall the uniqueness of the face of a person we have met. Yet, from a purely medical viewpoint, the middle face is often relatively ignored—partly because guidelines for absolute abnormality and normality have never been commonly accepted and partly because, until recently, the medical profession has not been as prone to study this area with as much vigor as other disciplines (for example, anthropology) have shown. If we include for discussion all deviations from normal of the eyes, the ears, and the nose, we include perhaps the largest aspects of two traditional medical specialties—ophthalmology and otolaryngology.

As discussed in Chapter 1, the middle facial segment can be divided into parts according to embryologic origin. The central portion of the developed face is supplied by the embryonic frontonasal process, which is induced to develop by the rostral extension of the notochord. The lateral portions of the mature face are derived primarily from the first branchial arch, although the second branchial arch also contributes in a small way to formation of portions of the ear. The dividing lines between these parts of the middle face are important and may be seen in the illustration with which this chapter begins. These borders drop from the eyebrow line along the vertical lateral canthal lines and then follow the horizontal intercanthal line until they reach the canthal labial lines, along which they travel to the nasal line, which marks the termination of the middle facial segment. This division of the middle facial segment allows discussion of the following central middle face structures: (1) the eyes and the eyelids; (2) the nose, including the tip, base, and bridge; and (3) some of the maxilla. The term "central middle face," or "midface proper," refers to the bony nasal base, the middle eyebrow, the cartilaginous nasal bridge, and the immediately surrounding maxillary bone. The "lateral middle face," on the other hand, consists of the ears, the zygomatic processes, and the lateral bony orbits of the eyes, in addition to contiguous maxillary structures.

## THE EYES

The eyes are amazingly complex organs whose main function is to allow the three-dimensional viewing of objects in the environment. Since this book is not concerned with ophthalmology per se, details about basic function or dysfunction will not be dwelled upon in length. Rather, some deviations in the structure and expression of the eyes that are useful in neurologic diagnosis will be stressed. The eyes are an important clue in the diagnosis of neurologic conditions.

## Abnormalities involving size and protrusion

The size of the eyeball depends upon a wide range of factors including age, sex, race, and various individual characteristics (see Chapter 1). Thus, when a size discrepancy does not involve asymmetry, an abnormality might not be recognized. It is important to emphasize again that, relatively speaking, the eyeball is larger in childhood than in adulthood (see Fig. 1-14, *A*). Thus, relatively, the eyeballs in a child may appear to be closer together or to be deviated inward. Still, the relative position of the eyeball in the orbit remains fairly constant at any age.

Dystopia canthorum (see Fig. 1-14, *C*) is a condition in which the position of the eyeball in relation the the eyelid is abnormal. Relative dystopia canthorum exists in childhood normally. The child's eye appears to be situated more toward the medial part of the palpebral fissure than the adult's eye. This condition will be discussed more fully in the section of the eyelids later in this chapter.

The term *macrophthalmia* refers to an absolute increase in the volume of the eyeball when compared to the average size in a known population. The term does not refer to the size in comparison to the space available within the bony orbit. This distinction is important. One therefore must consider two possibilities when confronted with an individual who appears to have a larger eye—(1) true macrophthalmia (that is, a truly large eyeball) or (2) pseudomacrophthalmia (an eyeball that is large in comparison to the space available in the bony orbit). True macrophthalmia (Fig. 3-1, *A*) is also called *buphthalmos* (bous = ox, or large). The most common cause of buphthalmos is congenital glaucoma, as is seen in the Sturge-Weber syndrome (Chou, 1959) (See Chapter 6). In

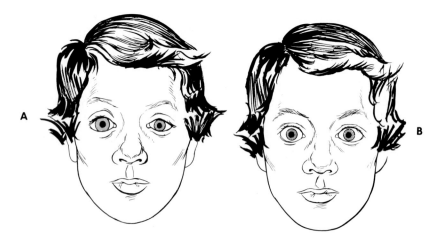

**Fig. 3-1.** Abnormalities in ocular size and protrusion. **A,** True macrophthalmia (buphthalmos) or enlargment of the eye. In this unilateral example the patient's right eye is larger than the left. Compare this condition to that in **B,** in which there is an abnormal protrusion of the globe (exophthalmos or proptosis) with a resulting retraction of the eyelids.

true macrophthalmia there is usually no distortion of the surrounding soft tissues of the orbit because the bony orbit and soft tissues also are larger than normal. There is little retraction of the eyelid over the enlarged eye.

While macrophthalmia involves a true enlargement of the eyeball, pseudomacrophthalmia involves an illusion of eyeball enlargement as might be seen in exophthalmos or proptosis. We usually use the term *exophthalmos*, literally meaning "condition in which the eyes are placed or pushed outward," to refer to a condition in which the eye is fairly symmetrical. We use the term *proptosis*, meaning to "fall out" or to "fall forward," to refer to a more severe, usually unilateral, condition. Many authors of medical textbooks, including ourselves on occasion, use these terms interchangeably.

From a clinical viewpoint, the distinction between exophthalmos and proptosis is not completely clear and perhaps is of only minor significance. The distinction between true macrophthalmia and pseudomacrophthalmia, however, is of utmost importance because entirely different mechanisms and associated diseases are involved. Fig. 3-1, *B* shows mild exophthalmos, an example of pseudomacrophthalmia. The eyeball protrudes anteriorly in this condition because of lack of space in the bony orbit. The lack of space results from the protrusion of the brain or intracranial contents into the back of the orbit (a condition seen in infants who have increased intracranial pressure), from the presence of a mass (such as a tumor) in the back of the orbit, or from edema of the soft tissues in the back of the orbit. Exophthalmos in adults is often related to thyroid dysfunction. In fact, it has been stated that the most common cause of exophthalmos is probably hyperthyroidism (Guyton, 1971; Werner and others, 1974).

A useful clinical distinction between pseudomacrophthalmia and true macrophthalmia can be made by observing the relationship of the eyeball to the surrounding soft tissue of the eyelids. In exophthalmos and proptosis the eyelid is often actually retracted from the eyeball. The white of the eye or the rostral conjunctiva is often seen in proptosis, but usually is not seen in true macrophthalmia. In addition, associated megalocornea is seldom seen in proptosis but is usually seen in macrophthalmia (Flippen, 1950).

The term *megalocornea* refers to an enlargement of the cornea or, in frontal viewing, that area within the limbus that separates the cornea from the surrounding conjunctiva. In a practical sense this demarcation line also falls at the junction of the pigmented iris and the white sclera. The cornea, of course, may be enlarged along with the rest of the eyeball, and megalocornea would be expected in any macrophthalmic condition. Occasionally, however, selective or relative enlargement of the cornea occurs. This selective megalocornea is seen in several syndromes that will be mentioned further in Chapter 6. It is important to remember that young children have not only eyeballs that are large in relation to their faces and their bony orbits but also corneas that are large in relation to their eyeballs.

*Microphthalmia,* like macrophthalmia, involves the comparison of the size of an eyeball to what has been established as normal. The extreme of microphthalmia is no eyeball at all, or *anophthalmia.* The distinctions between a small eyeball that produces an eyelid alteration and the various primary eyelid abnormalities will be mentioned later in the chapter in the discussion of ptosis and pseudoptosis (Warburg, 1960; Warkany and others, 1966). (See Fig. 3-5, *A*.)

The term *enophthalmos* means a retraction of the eyeball. This condition is the opposite of exophthalmos and thus constitutes a "pseudomicrophthalmia." Enophthalmos is less frequently encountered clinically than exophthalmos. Enophthalmos, or an abnormal retraction within the depths of the bony orbit of a normal-sized eyeball, occurs after lesions of sympathetic pathways. It also is reported to be due to necrosis of the soft tissue in the back of the orbit. Apparent enophthalmos may occur in cases of microphthalmia in which the entire eyeball is small or atrophic. Apparent enophthalmos is seen especially in acquired types of microphthalmia, such as those that are secondary to trauma or infections.

### Pupillary abnormalities

The pupil, an important part of the eye, is very useful in facial diagnosis. The pupil's reaction to light and accommodation is important in ophthalmologic and neurologic assessments. Light striking the pigmentary absorptive substance of the retina produces a reaction that ultimately ends in constriction of the pupil of the eye originally stimulated by light (direct response) and in constriction of the opposite pupil (indirect or consensual response). Since facial viewing is performed in light and many of the photographs illustrating the examples in following chapters were taken with an artificial light source (a flash), it is pertinent to know these fundamental details of the pupillary light reaction.

The pupillary accommodative reaction occurs when a person attempts to adjust the convexity of the optic lens in order to focus light directly on the retina. Usually the accommodative reaction occurs with convergence of both eyes, but not necessarily. Both pupils constrict. During facial viewing, the physician must be aware of the current accommodation of a patient's pupils. Since most facial observation is at close range—eyeball to eyeball, so to speak—and most of the photographs taken are also at close range, a patient's pupils will usually be relatively accommodated. In addition, the eyeballs of a patient are usually in a state of relative convergence.

The size of a person's pupil depends upon two opposite actions. The pupillary constrictor muscle is under the influence of parasympathetic nerves. When a parasympathetic stimulation occurs, the pupil constricts. The pupillary dilator muscle, conversely, is under the influence of sympathetic nerves. When a sympathetic stimulation occurs, the pupil dilates. Pupillary dilation in response to alarm results from the liberation of epinephrine into the bloodstream and the consequent stimulation of the pupillary dilator muscles of the iris. The sympathetic and parasympathetic actions on the pupil during both wakefulness and sleep are in tone. Which action is dominant at any given time depends on the prevailing circumstances.

The resting pupillary size and shape are particularly important in facial diagnosis. Pupil size varies under ordinary conditions because the amount of light let into the inner eye varies. In order for a person to see in different environmental circumstances, the need for pupillary size variation is essential. Hormones and the autonomic nervous system have great and almost immediate effects on pupillary size. It should be noted that there is symmetry to the pupil whether it is small or large; the pupil is usually a perfect circle located in the exact center of the iris. Thus variations seen in a patient's pupils during standard facial viewing are reasonably balanced.

The terms *miosis* and *mydriasis* (or *corectasis*) are conditions characterized by small and large pupils, respectively. Certain refraction abnormalities have an effect upon pupillary size. The myopic or near-sighted eye is often associated with relative mydriasis or dilated pupils. Certain local eye diseases such as glaucoma may be associated with mydriasis, while cataracts are usually associated with miosis. Inflammatory conditions of the iris may cause unusually small pupils. An alarmed or highly anxious person may have larger pupils than the normal relaxed person because of the effect of epinephrine on the pupil. Narcotics may produce miosis. In general, however, if the pupil is symmetrical, pupillary size alone can seldom be used to diagnose a medical condition. For the purposes of this book it is important to point out that an illusion of both abnormal miosis and abnormal mydriasis may be given. Miosis may occur during photography because both an accommodation reflex (from the eyes converging at near) and a light reflex (from the flash) take place. Occasionally the patient is startled, resulting in an alarm reaction characterized by mydriasis. An attempt has been made to standardize the drawings and photographs to balance these effects.

An asymmetry of pupils is always abnormal, although the clinical significance of the abnormality varies. Usually, pupillary asymmetry or *anisocoria* (without equal pupils) results from a disturbance either locally in the eye (for example, in an active child who plays in the woods, ragweed may be rubbed into the eye, producing sympathomimetic effects and transient anisocoria from the atropine contained in this plant) or in the neural pathways. (See Fig. 3-2, A.) The most worrisome neurologic cause of anisocoria is a structural disruption of the third cranial nerve, parasympathetic fibers of which innervate the pupil. Oculomotor disturbances are quite common in neurologic diseases (see Chapter 6), especially those associated with asymmetrical brain masses, increased

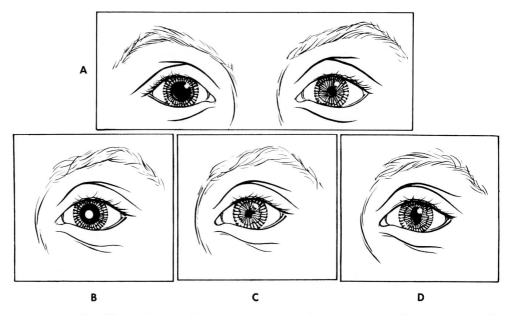

**Fig. 3-2.** Pupillary abnormalities. **A,** anisocoria (aniso = unequal; coria = pupil). Note difference in size of pupils. **B,** Mydriasis, or extreme dilation of the pupils. **C,** Irregularly shaped pupils, as might be found in some syndromes. **D,** Elliptical pupil, which may be a normal variation.

intracranial pressure, and herniation syndromes. A common location for brain herniation is at the incisura of the tentorium. At the incisura, the oculomotor nerve lies freely within the subarachnoid space in its path from the midbrain, where it exits the brain, to the superior orbital fissure, where it enters the bony orbit of the eye. In the bony orbit, the preganglionic parasympathetic fibers that are destined to innervate the pupil are particularly susceptible to injury from masses and herniated brain.

It is quite common to see irregularly shaped pupils in a variety of old ocular infectious states usually resulting from an iridocyclitis (inflammation of the iris), which may be due to syphilis, sarcoidosis, or other infectious or parainfectious disorders. (See Fig. 3-2, *C.*) The Argyll Robertson pupil is a specific example of an old infectious disease that affects the pupil. This pupil is miotic, irregular, and nonreactive to light but reactive with accommodation. The Argyll Robertson pupil is considered very suggestive, if not pathognomonic, of tertiary syphilis. Tertiary syphilis also frequently, but not necessarily, produces anisocoria (Adie, 1931; Merritt and Moore, 1933).

Elliptically shaped pupils are seen in a wide variety of disorders but are far more nonspecific in identifying the site of neural involvement. The so-called wilsonian pupil, which is eccentrically located in the iris, reportedly is seen in midbrain lesions (Walshe, 1967). (See Fig. 3-2, *D.*)

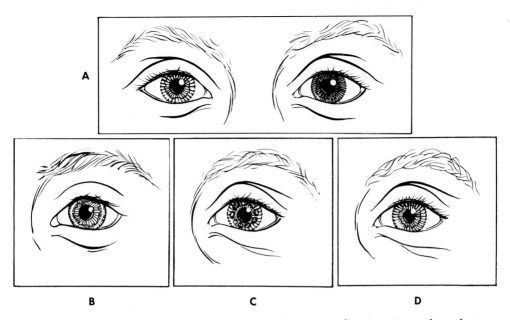

Fig. 3-3. Abnormalities of the iris. Heterochromia iridis, **A**, exists when the two irides are not the same color (hetero = other; chromia = color). The Kayser-Fleischer ring, **B**, which results from the deposit of copper in the membrane of Descemet, gives an illusion of color changes in the iris. Brushfield spots, **C**, often seen in chromosomal abnormalities, are depigmented patches that surround the iris. Arcus senilis, **D**, which is believed to be a sign of the atherosclerotic process, is a pale ring around the margin of the cornea.

*Heterochromia* and other unusual iris patterns are encountered in many dysgenetic syndromes. Most of these syndromes are characterized by a defect in migration of melanocytes from the neural crest early in embryogenesis. In heterochromia (Fig. 3-3, *A*), there is a difference in pigmentation in the irides—usually one eye is colored differently from the other. The term has also been used to refer to the condition in which different colors exist within the same iris. However, we will use the term in the former sense and not in the latter. Heterochromia may be associated with other defects in pigmentation, some of which may involve other parts of the cranioface. (See Chapter 6.) Heterochromia may be associated with a white forelock, auditory problems, and other abnormal facial features such as those seen in Waardenburg's syndrome (DiGeorge and others, 1960). (See Chapters 5 and 6.)

The pattern of the iris also is of some diagnostic importance. *Brushfield spots* (Fig. 3-3, *C*) are an irregular pattern of depigmented chains or patches that surround the iris. This "lumpy" pattern is highly characteristic of trisomy 21 and was once considered pathognomonic for it. Brushfield spots are seen only in light-complexioned individuals and are certainly not specific for trisomy 21 because these spots are seen in other conditions as well (Warkany and others, 1966). When Brushfield spots are not highly developed, they are said to produce a "mosaic" pattern in the iris. Although this mosaic pattern does not always point to a specific syndrome, such a pattern is seen much more commonly in persons with "dysplastic" syndromes (Solomons and others, 1965).

Various color changes in addition to pattern disturbances of the iris are helpful to the diagnostician and, in fact, may themselves be abnormalities of importance. One such iris sign in the *Kayser-Fleischer ring* (Fig. 3-3, *B*), which is believed to be pathognomonic for Wilson's hepatolenticular degeneration (Walshe, 1967). The ring actually is not in the iris at all. It results from deposits of free cooper in Descemet's membrane and only gives the illusion of being in the iris. The Kayser-Fleischer ring is a homogeneous, fairly wide ring that appears to involve the outer third of the iris, extending to the limbus.

Another ring commonly encountered in facial viewing is the *arcus senilis* (Fig. 3-3, *D*). This ring, which occurs in older persons, is itself not diagnostic of any particular disease. It is believed to result in some fashion from atherosclerotic changes associated with aging. Rarely, younger people develop the condition. Arcus senilis is seen more often in blacks than in persons of other races.

## Eyeball malalignment

Eyeball malalignment is one of the most important abnormalities of the eye. In order for a person to see normally binocularly, the eyeballs must be exactly aligned. Otherwise diplopia or double vision occurs—a distracting situation that drastically interferes with normal existence. A simple clinical test can be performed to determine whether the eyeballs are properly aligned.

**Corneal reflection sign.** When a flash is used in direct facial photography, the cornea, which is able to reflect light, reflects the flash. The center of each cornea, if the eyeballs are reasonably well aligned, will show a tiny dot of light when the photograph is studied. These dots can give a clue to the alignment of the eyes at the time the photograph is taken and are also important as a clue to the abnormalities seen in the patients who will be shown both in the drawings and in later more detailed photographs.

The principle of the corneal reflection sign is also of great use in clinical examination for ocular malalignment. An essential physical examination tool is a flashlight, but a penlight flashlight is of particular use. In a normally ocularly aligned person, the eyeballs fixate together on an object in such a way that light beams from the object radiate to a corresponding point on the retina of each eye—the fovea centralis, which represents the most central point of the macular region. Neural relays are thereafter activated to allow the brain to receive the stimulus so that a visual image may be produced in three dimensions. Precise alignment of the eyeballs is necessary and is accomplished by fine adjustments of the extraocular muscles, which move the eyeball.

The corneal reflection sign allows a simple test of ocular alignment. (See Fig. 1-15.) One procedure is to ask a patient to look at a penlight that is held several feet away. If the eyeballs are aligned properly, a small reflection of the light on the cornea can be observed when the patient fixates on the light. Since the eyeballs are slightly converged (deviated inward) when the patient looks at an object only a few feet away, the reflection will be in the center or located slightly to the lateral aspect of the exact center of each pupil (Fig. 1-15, A). When the eyeballs are not aligned properly, one reflection is deviated asymetrically—that is, to one side or above or below the center of the pupil. The deviantly reflected light usually is in the malaligned eye.

To further characterize the suspected abnormality suggested by observation of the corneal reflection sign, it is wise to perform an additional procedure. The patient should be asked to look into the distance, thus eliminating convergence as much as possible. The penlight then is held at the same distance as before—a few feet away. The corneal reflection will still be close to the center of the pupil on both sides, but instead of being on the outer side, it will be closer to the actual center or on the inner side (Fig. 1-15, B). Again, if the eyeballs are malaligned, one corneal reflection will be elsewhere than expected.

After performing the corneal reflection sign tests, a physician can next do what is called the cover-uncover test. The patient's eye is alternately covered and uncovered. This procedure is done with the examiner's thumb while the rest of the hand is steadied on the patient's forehead. (The patient is still looking at a distant object.) When an ocular malalignment is present, a subtle movement of the eye is seen when it is uncovered. When a suitable rate of covering and uncovering is established in a cooperative individual, the examiner sees a rhythm developing that is characterized by movement of first one and then the other eyeball. Young children sometimes have difficulty in fixating on a distant object, and it may be better to perform this cover-uncover test while they are looking at the light source with their eyes converged (DeMyer, 1975).

There are, of course, other means of recognizing malalignment of the eyeballs. The simplest but not the most accurate is ordinary observation, the success of which depends largely on the skill of the examiner. The accuracy of conclusions drawn from observing the corneal reflection sign also depends to a great extent upon the skill of the examiner. When the corneal reflection sign is further studied by photography, however, as has been done in this book, more objective data are accumulated.

Regardless of the method of detecting abnormal ocular alignment, certain definitions of the abnormality are of great importance in diagnosis. Malalignment of the eyes can be designated in several fashions. In layman's terms malalignments are referred to as "squints" or as "strabismus." These terms are frowned upon for medical use because of their scientific inexactness.* The preferred general term for a manifestly

---

*Using "squint" to refer to malalignment is confusing because the word also means "to partially close the eyes." Strabismus is an ancient medical term. Reportedly Strabo, a famous Roman nobleman who was examined by Galen, had a deviated eye. Galen called the condition strabismus—literally, "the condition of Strabo."

malaligned eyeball is *heterotropia* (hetero = different; trop = turn; ia = condition of).

Heterotropias may be defined more specifically according to the direction in which the eye is deviated. In the usual instance of heterotropia, the fixating eyeball is normal and the nonfixating eyeball is turned. If the nonfixating eye is deviated inward in relationship to the fixating normal eye, the condition of malalignment is called *esotropia* (eso = inward). If the deviation is outward, the condition is called *exotropia* (exo = outward). Likewise, if the abnormal deviation is upward, the condition is called *hypertropia* (hyper = excessive — that is, upward) and if downward, *hypotropia* (hypo = deficient — that is, downward). These simple heterotropias are shown in Fig. 3-4.

These definitions are useful in everyday medical practice. Yet the conditions they refer to are only the simplest and not necessarily the most common. There are combinations of heterotropias that affect one eye and combinations that affect both eyes. Especially in some highly complex neuro-ophthalmologic conditions, one may see almost any combination of heterotropias possible. Such a clinical condition might be congenital toxoplasmosis involving mild to severe lesions of the brainstem and supratentorial brain that are complicated by bilateral chorioretinitis. More common, however, are transient ocular malalignments and heterotropias that alternate with other heterotropias. Other adjectives, such as "bilateral," are also often used to describe heterotropias, and combinations of heterotropias are given names such as hyperesotropia, hypoexotropia, and the like.

Although "nonmanifest" ocular alignment disturbances are very important to the ophthalmologist, they are less important for the purposes of this book and will not be dwelled upon at length. Nonmanifest "squints" are brought out by procedures, such as the alternating cover-uncover test, and are not obvious in simple facial viewing. Nonmanifest eyeball deviations are called *heterophorias.* Since many of the photographs in this book have been taken with a flash, in a sense we have introduced an artifact that may bring out some heterophorias. Nevertheless, most of the ocular malalignments shown are heterotropias.

## Abnormal eye movements

Abnormal eye movements, which are important in facial diagnosis, are difficult to illustrate with still photographs and drawings. Yet some discussion of these movements is necessary. *Nystagmus* means simply ocular nodding. Some types of nystagmus represent not abnormalities but rather physiologic actions important for normal eyeball movement. An example is *opticokinetic nystagmus*, a phenomenon of which any train or automobile traveler is well aware. Opticokinetic nystagmus occurs when the eyeballs look at a series of moving objects. For example, a row of telephone poles might be outside the window of a person seated in a moving vehicle. The eyeball of the individual slowly follows a "mov-

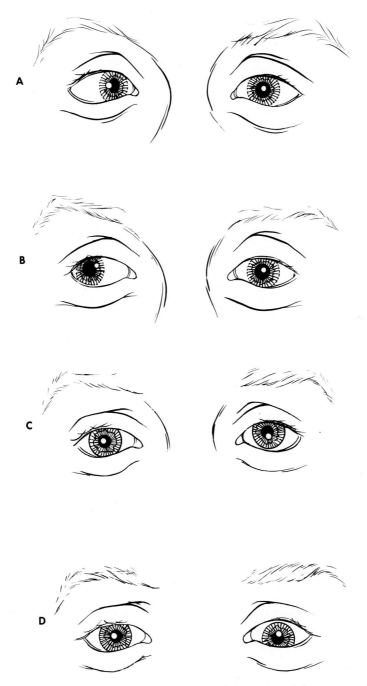

Fig. 3-4. The heterotropias. Several abnormal alignments of the eyes, as indicated by the corneal reflection sign, are possible. A, Eyes deviated inward (esotropia). B, Eyes deviated outward (exotropia). C, Eyes deviated upward (hypertropia). D, Eyes deviated downward (hypotropia).

ing" pole until it is past the window and then jerks (or nods) back to fol-low the newly approaching pole. Opticokinetic nystagmus is an impor-tant neurologic physical diagnostic sign and may even help in assessing vision in newborns. *End-position nystagmus* is an example of an abnor-mal eyeball movement that is of little clinical significance. End-position nystagmus is elicited during a neurologic or ocular examination when the patient is asked to follow an object to the extremes of gaze (most commonly horizontally). Normally, this is accomplished, but when the patient is asked to hold this extreme position, a fast-slow jerking move-ment of both the abducted eyeball and the adducted eyeball eventually is seen. Mild end-position nystagmus, however, is not considered abnor-mal. Other forms of physiologic nystagmus are elicited by head or body rotation (rotational nystagmus) or by stimulation of the semicircular canals with warm or cold water placed in the external auditory canal (caloric nystagmus). These types of eyeball nodding are normally pres-ent, and their absence after stimulation represents an abnormality. They are not of importance, therefore, in standard facial viewing.

Other spontaneous eyeball movements that are definitely abnormal may be observed. Some of them are ocular dysmetria, ocular flutter, op-soclonia, abnormal saccadic movements, cogwheel nystagmus, all forms of pendular or ocular nystagmus, see-saw nystagmus, ocular bobbing, and many other spontaneous or elicted ocular movements. Since the movement of the eyeball cannot be seen in simple facial viewing as it is illustrated in this book, further details of these phenomena will not be discussed.

### Eyelid abnormalities

Another condition that affects the appearance of the eyes is *ptosis* or drooping of the upper eyelid. When this drooping occurs while a person is looking straight ahead, it is considered an abnormal condition; drooping of the lid when a person is looking downward is not considered abnor-mal. Ptosis should be considered when the upper lid covers more than half of the iris (Fig. 3-5, *B*).

When true ptosis occurs, one should suspect a lesion of the nerve that goes to the levator palpebri, the function of which is to hold the upper eyelid up. This is not the only reason for a drooping eyelid, however. In-trinsic muscles around the palpebral fissure are in tone and are innervat-ed by sympathetic nerves. When lesions occur in the sympathetic nerves, as in Horner's syndrome, these intrinsic muscles are affected, and there is a relative asymmetry of the palpebral fissures. This type of lesion sel-dom causes the drooping eyelid to cover more than one third of the iris (see Fig. 3-5, *C*). It is common clinical practice to distinguish between true ptosis, which suggests an oculomotor lesion, and *pseudoptosis*, which suggests sympathetic involvement or another type of lesion (Hanson and Rowland, 1971).

As previously mentioned, an illusion of pseudoptosis can be observed

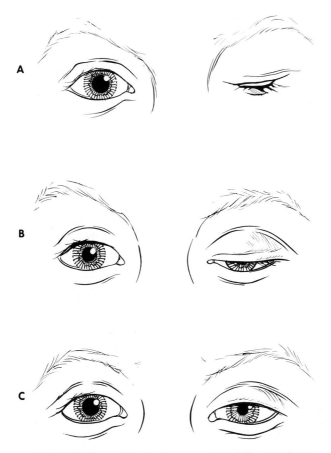

**Fig. 3-5.** Abnormalities of the eyelid. **A,** In a condition in which the eye is absent (anophthalmia) the eyelid may be completely closed. **B,** In the condition called ptosis, which generally involves the levator palpebrae muscle, the eyelid droops and covers more than half the iris. **C,** If the eyelid covers only about one third of the iris, the condition is called pseudoptosis if the levator palpebrae nerve is not involved.

when the eyeball is relatively small or is retracted into the orbit. In order for the palpebral fissure to be of normal width, the eyeball also must be normal in size and intraorbital placement. When the eyeball is retracted into the bony orbit, the palpebral fissures normally become smaller because there is no mechanical force to keep them open. Such posterior retraction is usually not designated as either ptosis or pseudoptosis but rather as *enophthalmos* (the eyeball is "in"). When the eyeball is absent, we designate the condition anophthalmia (an = without), and when the eyeball is smaller in size than the limits of normal variation, the condition is called microphthalmia (micro = small). These conditions may resemble each other and should be differentiated. (See Fig. 3-5.)

The medial and lateral canthi have been defined in Chapter 1. An *epi-*

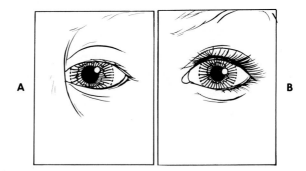

**Fig. 3-6.** Other abnormalities involving the lids. Epicanthal folds, **A**, sometimes cover the medial canthi. This condition may be a normal, familial, or racial variation, or it may be one sign of a syndrome. Long eyelashes, **B**, while sometimes quite fashionable, may be associated with some congenital neurologic syndromes.

*canthal fold* (Fig. 3-6, *A*) is merely a fold of redundant skin and tissue that overrides the medial canthus. This fold is seen most often in persons with dysgenetic disorders, particularly trisomy 21. An epicanthal fold, however, is neither specific nor necessarily always abnormal. It may be seen in a wide range of normal children and adults and it is quite common in Orientals, especially Japanese.

*Dystopia canthorum* has been mentioned in the section on ocular size and protrusion (see Fig. 1-12, *A*). This condition must be considered abnormal, although its significance is not always great. Dystopia canthorum, or displaced medial canthi, is a condition in which the relationship between the medial limbus of the eyeball and the lacrimal papilla of the lower eyelid is altered. This condition may be seen in the normal young child, who has a relatively large eyeball in comparison to the surrounding eyelids and soft tissues. As a child grows, the "displacement" disappears. Thus it is perhaps best to reserve the term dystopia canthorum for permanent conditions. An example is seen in Waardenburg's syndrome (see Chapter 6), in which the altered relationship does not change with age. It is important to distinguish dystopia canthorum from two conditions it may resemble—hypertelorism and esotropia, which are abnormalities of entirely different clinical significance.

Abnormalities of the eyelashes may occur in certain syndromes. These abnormalities range from absent eyelashes to excessively long and sometimes curled eyelashes. Lateral eyelash hyperplasia also may be significant (Smith, 1970).

## NASAL BASE AND MIDFACE PROPER

The central portion of the middle face includes that part of the face located between the eyes, below the eyebrows, and at the base of the nose. The nasal bridge and tip are also derived from the embryonic structures that supply this area in the adult, but they will be discussed in a separate section.

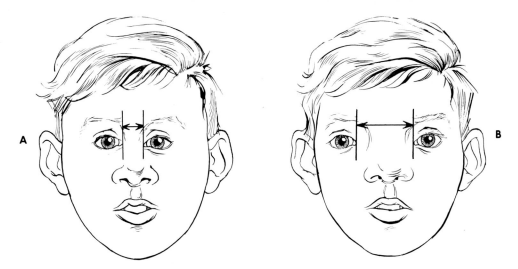

**Fig. 3-7.** Abnormalities in distance between the eyes. In hypotelorism, **A,** the eyes are too close together (hypo = under or deficient; telouros = distance). The condition in which the eyes are too far apart is designated hypertelorism (hyper = over), **B.**

## Hypotelorism and hypertelorism

The terms hypotelorism and hypertelorism are best used to refer to the positions of the bony orbits in relationship to each other. As pointed out by DeMyer (1975), much confusion exists concerning the derivation and precise meaning of these terms. Hypotelorism refers to less-than-normal distance between the medial aspects of the bony orbits, whereas hypertelorism refers to an excessive distance. These measurements have been standardized (Pryor, 1969). In Fig. 3-7, the two conditions are contrasted.

## Midface hypoplasia and hyperplasia

Being able to recognize hypertelorism and hypotelorism is extremely important, but of even greater importance may be whether the entire central portion of the middle face is hyperplastic or hypoplastic, concepts that are not absolutely dependent upon the positions of the bony orbits in relation to each other. Fig. 3-8 shows the relationships of the central portion of the middle face and how the area should be assessed. Several dysgenic disorders, particularly, are characterized by disturbances in this area. Recently recognized cytogenic syndromes especially, such as the short-arm-18-deletion syndromes, involve abnormalities in the central middle face.

## Birthmarks and other skin blemishes

Since the middle face is a focal part of the total face and represents at least one fourth of the total area, many skin lesions characteristically involve this segment. Although almost any skin blemish may involve the

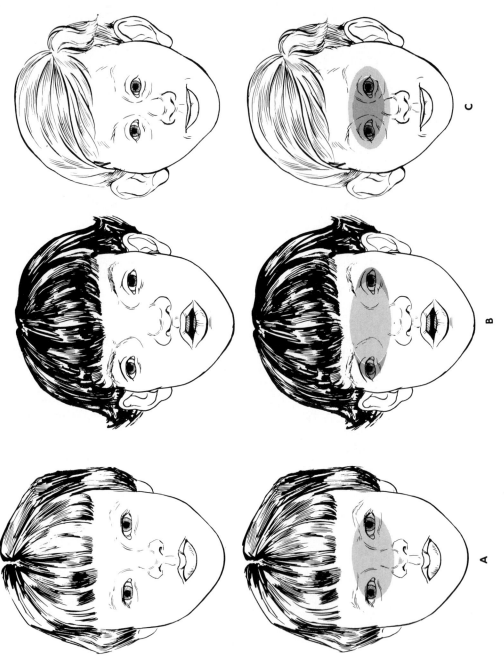

Fig. 3-8. Midface hypoplasia and hyperplasia. **A,** The normal midface. **B,** Midface hyperplasia. **C,** Midface hypoplasia. The normal midfacial area in **A** is superimposed upon the abnormal midfacial areas in **B** and **C.** Note the increase in the area that occurs in hyperplasia and the decrease that occurs in hypoplasia.

middle face in a random fashion, certain skin lesions are particularly likely to appear there. Four of the most important middle face skin blemishes are shown in Fig. 3-9. *Adenoma sebaceum* (Fig. 3-9, *A*), a characteristic of the disorder tuberous sclerosis, involves the entire malar area but usually spares the nasal base itself. Adenoma sebaceum is actually a misnomer. Historically, two types of adenoma sebaceum, neither of which is an adenoma or involves sebaceous gland tissues, are identified.

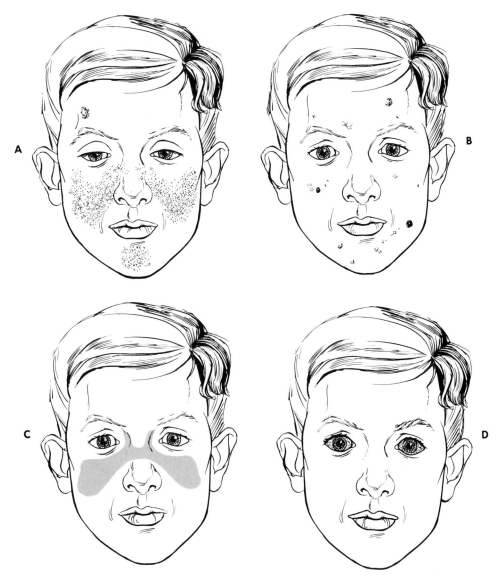

Fig. 3-9. Cutaneous lesions of the middle face. **A,** Adenoma sebaceum. **B,** Acne vulgaris, a common skin lesion of the middle face. **C,** A malar rash typical of lupus erythematosus. **D,** Telangiectasia of the conjunctiva (angeion = vessel; aktasis = dilation).

One lesion that is highly characteristic of tuberous sclerosis (see later chapters) is raised, erythematous, and fairly evenly and widely distributed in a butterfly-like pattern. This type of adenoma sebaceum is properly termed an angiofibroma because, histologically, it involves collections of fibrous and vascular elements. The second type of adenoma sebaceum is avascular and thus cannot properly be called an angiofibroma. This lesion is raised also but pale in color and not as evenly distributed. It tends to concentrate at the alae rather than to spread over the entire malar region. This second type of adenoma sebaceum is not as significantly related to tuberous sclerosis. (See Chapter 6 and Fig. 6-79 for a comparison of the two types of maculopapular lesions.)

Simple *acne vulgaris* (Fig. 3-9, *B*) is a skin lesion of the middle face that is common among teenagers. This condition can be confused with adenoma sebaceum, since both lesions are most florid in the pubescent period of life. The differentiation is usually easy because the lesions in acne vulgaris are irregular in size and distribution and acne vulgaris involves an inflammatory reaction that is not characteristic of adenoma sebaceum.

Another middle face skin lesion is the florid rash of collagen diseases (see Fig. 3-9, *C*). *Lupus erythematosus* was, after all, first distinguished as a disease by the characteristic skin lesion over the bridge of the nose. This is not a maculopapular lesion but rather a florid diffuse skin reaction resulting from inflammatory changes in the small vessels of the face. This florid butterfly rash is now known to be present in several varieties of the collagen diseases.

Another characteristic blemish of the middle face is *conjunctival telangiectasia* (Fig. 3-9, *D*). Although, technically, the conjunctiva is not skin, it is a derivative of primitive ectoderm and thus is included in this section. Telangiectasia can occur on the skin of the middle face as well. As the name implies, telangiectasia results from dilation of the small arterioles and capillaries of the involved areas (refer to the discussion in Chapter 2). Telangiectasia of the conjunctiva as well as of the skin is characteristically seen in the condition called ataxia-telangiectasia (see Chapters 6 and 8).

## NASAL BRIDGE AND TIP

The nose is an intimate part of the middle face. As mentioned in Chapter 1, the nose can be divided into proximal, middle, and distal parts. Abnormalities can occur in each part.

### Proximal nose abnormalities

The proximal part of the nose consists of the nasal base, which is the area between the bony orbits of the eyes. This area, which is entirely bony, has already been discussed. Some clinical disorders, such as the mucopolysaccharidoses, are characterized by wide nasal bases and hyperplasia in this area, while other conditions, such as the various forms of holoprosencephaly and cytogenic disturbances, involve deficient nasal bases. (See Fig. 3-8.) Disorders of an osteogenic nature tend to produce abnormalities in this part of the nose.

### Middle nose abnormalities

The middle part of the nose begins at the junction of the bony nasal base and the cartilaginous nasal bridge and extends to the part of the nose that is almost totally composed of soft tissue. Disorders of the middle nose are of several types, including abnormalities in width and in length. Abnormalities in this portion of the nose may be seen especially in cartilaginous disorders.

### Distal nose abnormalities

The distal nose comprises the skin and subcutaneous tissue that are located distal to the termination of the cartilage of the nasal bridge. There is a variety of distal nasal abnormalities, including beaked tips, bulbous and violaceous tips, and excessively broad protrusions.

• • •

A number of abnormalities of the nose do not fit into the anatomic classification we have used. These abnormalities are generally related to severe malformations that are not totally limited to the nose but that also include the rest of the face, the eyes particularly, and usually the brain as well. One such abnormality is the proboscis, which is associated with the holoprosencephalic defect. Malformed noses result from abnormalities in the frontonasal process early in gestational life (DeMyer, 1975).

Saddle nose was once thought to be pathognomonic for congenital syphilis. The nose of sarcoidosis is large and violacious. The reddened, comical nose of the alcoholic, the elephantine nose of the patient with any of a variety of neurocutaneous diseases, and the destroyed nose of the patient with lepromatous leprosy all are at least worthy of note in this section.

## ZYGOMATA AND LATERAL BONY ORBITS

As has been mentioned in Chapter 1, the slant of the palpebral fissures depends largely upon how the zygomatic processes and the lateral bony orbits develop. These structures in turn are derived from the first branchial arch on both sides. The slant of the palpebral fissures is very useful in understanding a variety of syndromes and disorders. In addition, the entire palpebral fissure is of some importance diagnostically. Normally both the medial and the lateral canthi fall on the intercanthal line, which is parallel to the other horizontal lines of the face. (See Chapter 1.)

### Mongoloid slanting

Abnormal slanting of the palpebral fissures occurs when the medial canthi and the lateral canthi are at different levels. When the medial canthi are lower than the lateral canthi, the condition is traditionally referred to as "mongoloid slant" (Fig. 3-10, *A*). Presumably this term originated because such slanting is found in Orientals. Use of the term continued after trisomy 21 was delineated as a disease entity. Since trisomy 21 patients had this tilt of the palpebral fissures and thus were called "mongols," the term "mongoloid slant" came to be associated with the facial feature. It is unfortunately too late to alter the terminology, but "V-shaped tilt" would be a more preferable designation. Exactly why mongoloid slanting occurs is uncertain. Generally speaking, there is excessive growth of the lateral middle facial structures, which are de-

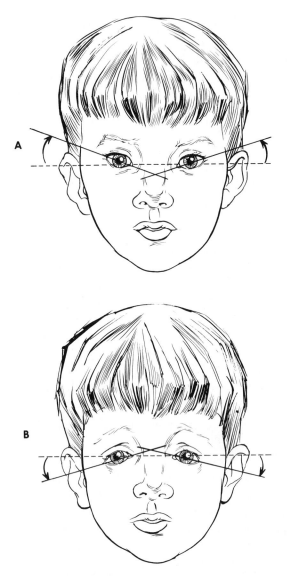

**Fig. 3-10.** Abnormal slanting of the palpebral fissures. When a line drawn through the medial and lateral canthi of each eye does not coincide with the intercanthal line, the eyes are slanted. **A,** Mongoloid slant. **B,** Antimongoloid slant.

rived from the first branchial arch, in comparison to the central middle facial structures, which are derived from the frontonasal process. When mongoloid slanting occurs, there is usually relative hypoplasia of the central face. Mild mongoloid slanting, of course, is not necessarily an abnormality. Most Western societies look upon this feature as an exotic mark of beauty, particularly in females. Females tend to have more central middle face hypoplasia than males and thus are much more likely to have mongoloid slanting. The feature is often emphasized by cosmetic companies in advertisements of facial products.

### Antimongoloid slanting

Many disorders are characterized by antimongoloid slanting of the palpebral fissures (Fig. 3-10, B). For the reasons already mentioned, a preferable term might be "tented tilt" or "A-shaped tilt." The antimongoloid slant is actually better understood than the mongoloid slant. Antimongoloid slanting is characteristically seen in disorders that involve the first branchial arch, whether they be acquired insults or cytogenic disturbances. Syndromes involving such disorders will be further delineated in subsequent chapters. The first arch syndromes all have the common denominator of hypoplasia of structures derived from the first branchial arch. The zygomatic processes and the lateral bony orbits are important first arch–derived structures. They characteristically are hypoplastic when the arch is deficient.

### Other abnormalities of the palpebral fissures

The size of palpebral fissures is important in facial diagnosis. In the fetal alcohol syndromes, particularly narrow (that is, from side to side rather than from upper lid to lower lid) palpebral fissures are common. (See Chapter 6.)

### THE EARS

The normal anatomy of the human ear has been discussed in Chapter 1. The ears are important in the diagnosis of many neurologic and dysgenic syndromes. It is important to remember, in our emphasis on the human face as viewed from the front, that the frontally viewed ear is incompletely examined. A complete examination requires direct viewing (that is, from the side of the head). Still, frontal viewing of the face can provide very useful information.

In full frontal facial viewing, the intercanthal line should fall at the point where the most anteriorly placed part of the ear joins the cranioface (that is, the aural point). Under normal circumstances the ear rises from this point to the level of the eyebrow line. When the top of the ear is at another level, there is often an abnormality in the placement of the ear. Low-set ears constitute such an abnormality. The upper ear may be malformed or traumatized. The lower aspect of the ear when viewed from the front usually falls on the nasal line.

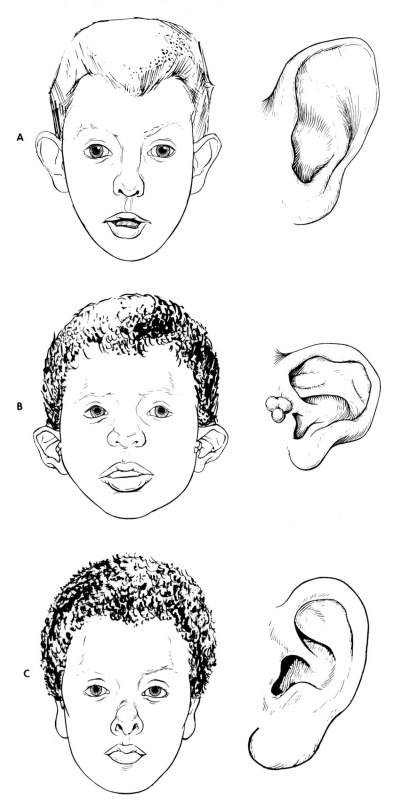

Fig. 3-11. Ear abnormalities. **A,** Protruding ears, with flattening of the tragus, antitragus, helix, and anthelix. **B,** Low-set, malformed ears with ear tags (see discussion of embryogenesis in Chapter 1). **C,** Relatively normal ear with extremely large lobules.

From a neurologic and facial diagnosis viewpoint, three major types of abnormalities need be appreciated particularly. *Protruding ears* (Fig. 3-11, *A*) are related to a variety of chronic neuromuscular diseases. The *jug ear* is associated with first- and second-branchial-arch disturbances. Anterior ear tags and lack of development of the ear, especially the rostral part, are also associated with these disturbances. (See Fig. 3-11, *B*.) The third abnormality to be carefully observed is the ear with *large lobules* (Fig. 3-11, *C*), which occur characteristically in some of the mucopolysaccharidoses.

# CHAPTER FOUR

# Lower facial segment and neck abnormalities

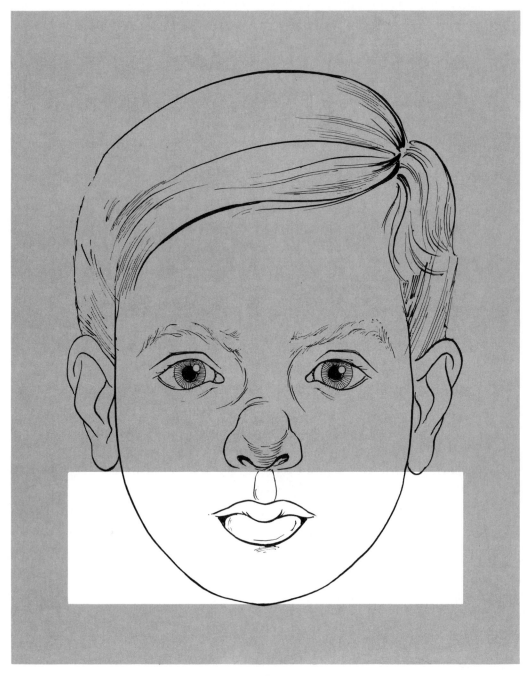

The lower facial segment has been described in Chapter 1. This segment of the cranioface includes areas readily seen by external viewing, including a central portion that consists of the mouth proper, the lips, and the cheeks and a peripheral portion that consists of the jaws and chin. The lower facial segment also includes an area not usually seen in normal facial viewing—the inner mouth, which consists of the buccal surface, the gums, the teeth, and the tongue. Since part of the neck is also seen in ordinary frontal facial viewing, abnormalities of the neck will also be discussed in this chapter. It is important to remember that many abnormalities that affect the lower face and neck are topographic and that, although such abnormalities may affect one segment primarily, they usually are not confined to it. Skin blemishes, for example, may affect more than one segment of the cranioface. Nevertheless, several topographic abnormalities will be discussed in this chapter.

## EXTERNAL LOWER FACE
### Mouth proper and cheeks (central lower face)

The central part of the lower face, discussed in Chapter 1, consists of the vermilion borders of the upper and lower lips and the immediately surrounding soft tissues.

**Cleft lip and palate.** An important abnormality of the mouth proper is cleft lip and palate. The incidence of this abnormality is estimated to be between 1 in 600 and 1 in 1250 births. Although cleft lip and cleft palate frequently occur together, it is important to remember that either cleft lip or cleft palate can occur alone. The single defect is usually not associated with coexisting deficiencies that are as severe as those found in cases involving both defects. Cleft lip may cause only a cosmetic deficit; cleft palate, especially if it is severe, may result in a cosmetic defect and the abnormal production of isolate speech sounds. Both defects, occurring alone or together, are relatively easily corrected by surgery and indeed should be corrected—the cleft lip for cosmetic reasons and the cleft palate to improve speech abilities.

Combined cleft lip and palate, however, often is associated with severe neurologic problems resulting from possible brain malformation. Functional defects caused by somatic congenital anomalies are also associated with this abnormality. The incidence of associated dysgenetic defects, neurologic as well as nonneurologic, is so great in certain variations of combined cleft lip and palate that correction of the lip and palate defect for cosmetic reasons alone is unwarranted. Many neurologically affected persons have so many additional life-threatening malformations that financial and social tragedies are possible unless a proper neurologic diagnosis is established prior to surgery.

The following rules may be helpful for the diagnostician. In general, simple cleft lip or isolated cleft palate is not usually associated with other extensive neural malformations. Next in the order of risk to the neurologic system is the so-called unilateral cleft lip and palate (see Fig.

4-1, *A*). This abnormality may be associated with neurologic defects but seldom with a regular constellation of brain malformations. The so-called bilateral lateral cleft lip and palate (Fig. 4-1, *B*) involves much more neurologic risk, since this defect may be associated with a variety of nervous system defects (see Chapter 7 and DeMyer, 1975). This type of lip and palate malformation, however, has a better prognosis from a neurologic viewpoint than a purely midline cleft lip and palate (Fig. 4-1, *C*). The midline cleft lip and palate, especially when it co-exists with abnormalities of the middle facial and upper facial segments, has a grave risk for neurologic disability.

One characteristic of human malady, however, is variability; clinical rules are not always constant. The types of cleft lip and palate shown in Figs. 4-1, *B* and *C*, do not always involve poor neurologic prognoses. However, one should be wary of implementing expensive procedures for correcting lower facial abnormalities before thorough neurologic investigations are performed (DeMyer, 1967; DeMyer, 1975; Grabb, 1965; Parkins, 1969; Sedance and others, 1970). Further discussion of cleft lip and palate may be found in Chapter 7, which presents the related syndromes of the lower face.

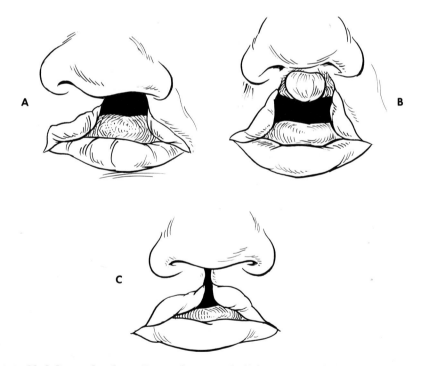

Fig. 4-1. Cleft lip and palate. Several types of clefts are possible in the embryonic development of the lower face. The types shown are presented in order of increasing severity of malformation and degree of risk. **A**, Unilateral cleft lip and palate. **B**, Bilateral lateral cleft lip and palate. **C**, Midline cleft lip and palate.

**Unilateral facial palsy and paresis.** Under normal situations the oral line is horizontal and parallel to the other important horizontal lines of the face. In unilateral facial palsy or paresis, however, there may be an abnormal tilt to this line because of a lesion involving facial nerves or muscles on one side (Fig. 4-2). The direction of the tilt may be either toward the side of the lesion or away from it, depending upon the chronicity of the asymmetrical facial lesion and whether it results from "upper-motor" neuron or "lower-motor" neuron facial weakness. A disruption can occur at any point from the neuronal body in the facial nerve nucleus in the pons to the final termination of the peripheral nerve at a muscular level.

There are two kinds of upper-motor facial nerve lesions. The "release" type lesion results from a disruption of the supranuclear cortico-pontine pathways, which arise in the primary motor area of the cerebral cortex and terminate on neurons of the facial nucleus of the pons. Such a deficit ultimately causes less severe facial muscular paresis than that caused by a lower-motor lesion, is associated with hypertonia or spasticity rather than hypotonia, and arises from dysfunction of supranuclear areas contralateral to the side of the facial paresis. The "shock" type upper-motor facial nerve lesion is believed to be caused by a disturbance to supranuclear noncorticopontine pathways. This disturbance causes acute dysfunction of the facial muscles. The functional deficit of the "shock" type lesion, also contralateral, is quite different from that of the "release" lesion. There is usually profound paresis or even palsy and fairly severe muscular hypotonia. The "shock" lesion is seldom permanent, especially in the younger child. Functional defects

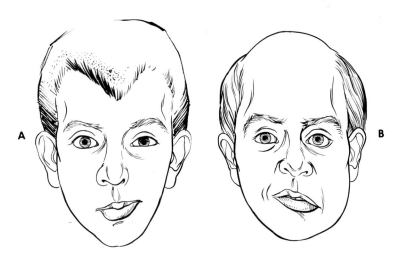

Fig. 4-2. Facial palsy. **A,** Results of a long-standing upper-motor lesion. Note that the horizontal oral line tilts upward on the side of the lesion. Note also the associated defect of the muscles of the left eye. **B,** Results of an acute lower-motor lesion. Note that the mouth tilts downward on the side of the lesion because of disruption of facial muscle function.

may last anywhere from several days to several years (Hoefnagel and Penry, 1963; Manning and Adair, 1972).

Another facial lesion, which is less easily recognized, may be produced by extrapyramidal disturbances that are usually bilateral but may be unilateral. This type of facial weakness is evident in emotional situations and seems to spare the better-defined supranuclear primary facial nerve pathways of volition.

Several other types of unilateral facial palsy or paresis are seen in clinical medicine, including common unilateral facial palsy or paresis produced by lower-motor lesions. A lower-motor (or "loss") type of facial nerve lesion affects the final neural pathway to the muscle. This "common" final pathway can be defined anatomically as the final facial neuron and the facial muscle. Functional loss consists of palsy or severe paresis and often severe hypotonia or flaccidity on the side of the lesion. Complete or peripheral facial palsy is characterized by a total loss of nervous control from the neuron to the muscle. Essentially all fibers to both the upper and the lower facial muscles on the same side as the neural lesion are affected. The functional deficit is severe; there is severe paresis, if not true palsy, and the facial muscles are very flail or floppy or severely hypotonic. On the other hand, supranuclear facial paresis—whether of the "release" type or the "shock" type—is usually contralateral and affects only the lower face. This is because the upper facial muscles are innervated bilaterally by the supranuclear fibers. Thus a supranuclear lesion on one side will cause a deficit in the contralateral lower facial muscles of expression. If acute, "shock" usually occurs, and the functional deficit consists of severe paresis and severe hypotonia. It is quite common for this type of unilateral facial paresis to be transformed over time into an upper-motor "release" facial paresis. The upper-motor "release" type of unilateral facial paresis probably is less commonly recognized than the upper-motor "shock" type of lesion. Since time seems essential for the release lesion to develop (at least a few days), when it is present it is a gauge of the degree of chronicity, in contrast to the shock lesion, which almost always is acute and occurs soon after the event that causes the disruption. Both the shock and the release types of facial paresis are partial and involve only the lower face. They are both identified as types of lower or central facial paresis. The "extrapyramidal" facial paresis or weakness, which is detected best during the expression of emotion, has been known to be unilateral, but much more commonly this rare facial paresis is bilateral.

These concepts of facial muscle physiology are very important in clinical medicine, especially during the evaluation of children who may have congenital lesions or who may develop chronic lesions. Voluntary and involuntary control of facial muscle movement and tone are important functions of the innervation of the facial muscles by facial nerves. The nerves also allow for many trophic influences that affect muscle, skin, and other tissues. In cases of long-standing neurogenic facial lesions, there often is not only atrophy of the facial muscles but also hypoplasia of the underlying osseous structures. Consequently, as an afflicted person grows, the unaffected side of the face grows normally while the affected side becomes relatively smaller.

In long-standing unilateral facial paresis, the upper lip, and therefore the horizontal oral line, is tilted upward on the affected side (in other words, the upper lip and the angle of the mouth are higher on the affected side). (See Fig. 4-2, A.) A relatively acute neurogenic lesion that produces a unilateral central or peripheral facial weakness, however, will often cause the horizontal oral line to tilt downward on the side of the lesion (Fig. 4-2, B). This is because there is a sudden disruption of function of the facial muscles on that side without a loss of trophic effect, thus resulting in a collapse of normal tone in the muscles of facial expression on the affected side. This collapse causes drooping of the upper lip, the mouth, and the entire face on that side. It is difficult to distinguish central from peripheral acute neurogenic facial lesion on the basis of the position of the mouth. However, in central facial palsy, which results from a supranuclear neural lesion, the upper face is relatively spared, whereas in peripheral facial palsy, which is caused by a lesion at the facial nerve nucleus or below, the upper face is not spared. In a central type of long-standing unilateral facial paresis (such as the "release" type of lesion with atrophy), tilting of the mouth line upward on the side of the lesion may be encountered. Such tilting indicates that an upper-motor release type of neurologic dysfunction has occurred and that there has been loss of the trophic effect.

The nasolabial fold is an important landmark of the lower face because it separates the mouth proper from the cheeks (see Fig. 4-2). Although the condition of the nasolabial fold is important as a subtle clue to the normality of the facial muscles in adults, it is less important in children and infants because their skin is less wrinkled. In facial muscle weakness having neurogenic causes, the cheek, maintained primarily by the buccinator muscles, is loose and saggy. These weaknesses are usually unilateral and thus asymmetrical, as opposed to myopathic facial weaknesses, which are usually bilateral or symmetrical. Not only is there a flattening or even a disappearance of the nasolabial fold but there is also sagging of the bulk of the cheek on the affected side. This subtle facial change should and can be easily distinguished from a true hyperplasia of the cheek, from a soft tissue mass or malformation associated with a birthmark (Fig. 4-3, A), or from edema associated either with a cellulitis or with lymphedema, as is seen in certain types of von Recklinghausen's disease (Fig. 4-3, B).

**Facial diplegia and diparesis.** Long-standing bilateral weakness and hypoplasia of the facial muscles are associated with a fairly characteristic malformation of the mouth and lips. This malformation, which has been called "tenting" of the upper lip (Fig. 4-4, A), is related to several diseases and syndromes that will be further discussed later in this book.

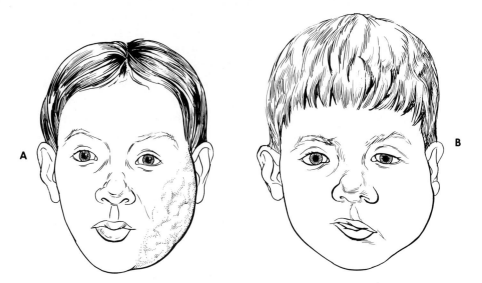

Fig. 4-3. Abnormalities of the cheeks. A flattening of the nasolabial fold can result from muscle weakness or from hyperplasia of the cheek. **A,** Cavernous hemangioma. **B,** Hyperplasia or lymphedema.

Tenting is often associated with a very short philtrum that, in some cases, allows the teeth and gums to be exposed. In this abnormality there is usually severe congenital facial diparesis or even diplegia. The tented upper lip is nonspecific in that it represents only an effect of long-standing bilateral facial muscle weakness and muscular hypoplasia or hypotrophy beginning during formative years. Facial diplegia or diparesis of this type may have either neurogenic or myopathic causes and is accounted for in large part by the loss of trophic influences (Henderson, 1939).

Another mouth abnormality seen in some of the diseases that also produce the tented upper lip has been described as a "puckered" mouth (Fig. 4-4, *B*). This abnormality has more specificity in that it is often seen in myopathic processes of a more recent onset. Not only is the appearance of the lower face affected by myopathic changes but the jaw muscles are usually weakened as well and the mouth is held open. Characteristically, these stigmata are progressive and worsen as the disease worsens. The puckered appearance of the lips results from the voluntary effort of the patient to keep saliva within the mouth. This lateral type of recently acquired facial diparesis is frequently associated with other lower facial segment abnormalities involving the muscles of mastication (that is, the masseter and pterygoid muscles), which accounts for a narrowing of the angle of the jaws when seen from the front and for an appearance of dolichofacies (Dodge and others, 1965; Harper and Dyken, 1972; Fundel and Tyler, 1965).

**Other mouth abnormalities.** There has been a wealth of literature con-

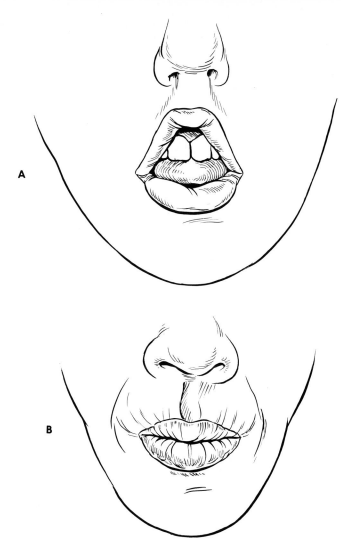

Fig. 4-4. Abnormalities of the lips. **A,** Tented upper lip common in congenital dystrophia myotonica. The tented upper lip often results from long-standing bilateral facial muscle weakness. **B,** Pursed lips, which result from a voluntary effort to keep the mouth closed and which are associated with acquired facial diparesis, as in adult-onset dystrophia myotonica.

cerning the association of certain types of mouths and lips with various neurologic and other genetic syndromes. "Fish mouths," "down-turned mouths," and thin upper lips have been written about especially often. Further study is needed, however, to determine whether these types of mouths are true abnormalities or merely variations of normal.

One should always pay attention to an extreme form of a characteristic, whether it represents a specific abnormality or merely a familial variation. This is particularly true of big and thick lips. Recognition of abnormally large lips may be extremely important in diagnosis of a wide range of neurologic syndromes, including the mucopolysaccharidoses. These syndromes will be discussed in more detail in later chapters.

### Chin and jaws (peripheral lower face)

The chin and jaw are not best viewed with the "frontal" approach that we have emphasized in this book. Protruding and receding chins (Fig. 4-5) are perhaps best appreciated in profile. Prognathism is the term most commonly used to denote an abnormally large or jutting chin and jaw, and micrognathia is used to denote an abnormally small or receding chin and jaw.

A small pointed chin may be seen even though there is no receding

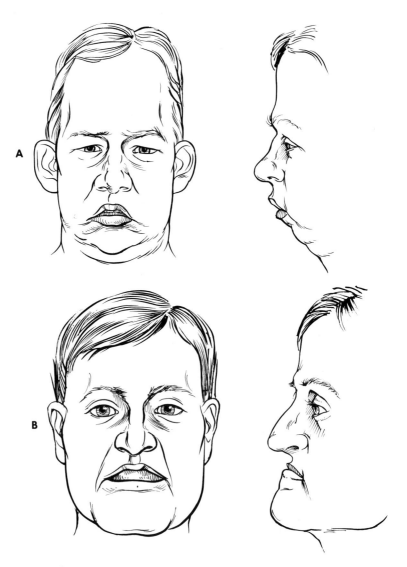

Fig. 4-5. Abnormalities of the chin. A, Micrognathia. B, Prognathism.

chin. A small, fragile, and somewhat triangularly shaped chin has less diagnostic importance than a receding chin, which is often associated with a wide variety of other defects (deGrouchey, 1969; Dennison, 1965; Fazen and others, 1967).

**First-branchial-arch abnormalities.** Knowledge of the embryogenesis of the derivatives of the first branchial arch is important for full understanding of abnormalities of the lower face. The mouth represents the first branchial cleft, the cleft that is surrounded by the first branchial arch in the embryo. Both the maxilla and the mandible are derivatives of the first branchial arch. Thus, the zygomatic arches, most of the lateral wall of the orbit, and the ear all are derived from this embryonic structure. Many noxious agents have effects upon the formation of these first branchial arch derivatives in early embryogenesis. Extrinsic noxious insults include those caused by toxins, viruses, and drugs. Intrinsic disturbances, such as those caused by chromosomal abnormalities, also can occur. A first branchial arch disturbance in the lower face may be manifested by a wide variety of deficits, one of which is micrognathia.

Not all first-arch derivatives, of course, are associated exclusively with the lower face. Many, such as the zygomatic arches, the orbits, and the ears, are associated with the middle face as we have defined it. Branchial arch deficits involving these structures have been discussed in the chapter dealing with the middle facial segment. The number of first branchial arch defects possible is virtually unlimited and includes many well-recognized combinations of symptoms and signs that will be discussed in later chapters.

**Topographic abnormalities.** Many birthmarks involve the lower face and neck, but none is characteristically limited to this segment.

Absence of lower facial hair in a postpubescent male might suggest a feminizing endocrinopathy. Similarly, excessive facial hair in an adult female may suggest masculinization. Excessive facial hair is always abnormal in a prepubescent child, regardless of sex.

**Other chin and jaw abnormalities.** Angled jaws are encountered frequently in patients who are normal as well as in those with neurologic handicaps. Although an angled jaw is not always significant, such a jaw becomes meaningful if signs of deficits involving the branchial arch are present. Persons with angled jaws that are narrow and symmetrical may have extreme dolichofacies. There is a correlation between narrow angled jaws, micrognathia, and pointed chins. An angled jaw that is narrow therefore may be characteristic of many myopathic, neurogenic, dysplastic, and metabolic disorders that will be described further in subsequent chapters. An angled jaw that is excessively wide, however, may be a normal variation rather than a true abnormality. Nevertheless, this condition, which can be detected only through frontal facial viewing, frequently is associated with at least a degree of prognathism (see Fig. 4-5, *B*) and with square chins. Certain other chin conditions are characterized by excessive overgrowth of the mandibular bone.

## INTERNAL LOWER FACE
### Buccal surface and gums

The inside of the mouth is not readily assessed in ordinary facial viewing. Under normal circumstances, even in early infancy, the mouth usually is not held open unless a person is engaged in an activity requiring facial movement such as crying, talking, laughing, eating, or teething. In abnormal situations, however, the mouth may be held open, allowing glimpses of the buccal surface and gums in addition to the other structures that have been discussed previously. In neurologic practice certain anticonvulsant medications, such as phenytoin, can produce hyperplasia of the gums. This condition occurs frequently enough that it should be considered along with the wide variety of gingival abnormalities that are related to syndrome diagnosis. Among these abnormalities are certain birthmarks that are related to neurocutaneous diseases such as tuberous sclerosis, Sturge-Weber disease, and neurofibromatosis. For example, small well-demarcated plaques of the gingivae (Fig. 4-6, A) may be of great diagnostic importance in the diagnosis of tuberous sclerosis. Other abnormalities include the many discolorations of the gums that result from exposure to various toxic substances, such as lead and arsenic. Various parainflammatory diseases, such as systemic lupus erythematosus, produce visual as well as histologic abnormalities of the

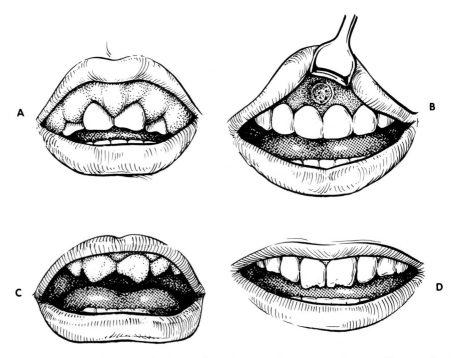

Fig. 4-6. Abnormalities of the buccal surface and gums. **A,** Gingival hyperplasia. **B,** Herpes lesion on gingival surface. **C,** Enamel dysplasia. **D,** Notched incisors.

gums. These abnormalities have similarities to what one sees in chronic phenytoin reaction. The vesicular lesions of the gums resulting from herpes simplex may occur externally as well as on the buccal surface. Stomatitis of the buccal surface is seen in several diseases, including some that are primarily infectious and some that are parainflammatory such as histiocytosis X and Behçet's syndrome (Fienman and Yakover, 1970; Lagos and Gomez, 1967).

## The teeth

A vast literature has developed concerning abnormalities of the teeth as they relate to diagnosis of systemic diseases. There are many common tooth problems related specifically to neurologic syndromes that will be discussed in this book. The facial viewer should be particularly concerned with the following dental abnormalities, which may be obvious even on frontal facial examination: (1) excessively small or unusually shaped teeth, which might be a clue to enamel dysplasia (Fig. 4-6, B); (2) excessively large incisors, occurring either with or without excessive enlargement of all teeth; (3) notched teeth, which suggest previous in utero infections (Fig. 4-6, D); and (4) abnormally chipped or absent teeth, which suggest trauma. Chipped or absent teeth are of great importance in pediatric practice, particularly as a gauge of facial trauma inflicted by self or by others (Goltz, 1962; Rossman, 1968).

## The tongue

Unlike the masticator muscles and the other muscles of the face, the tongue is embryogenically derived from cranial somitic muscle. The tongue can be said to have two parts, each of which is composed of a different type of muscle: (1) intrinsic muscles make up the bulk of the tongue as we see it when a person opens his mouth and the tongue is lying quietly in the floor of the mouth, and (2) extrinsic muscles are important in protruding the tongue.

**Macroglossia.** There is variation in the size of the tongue among individuals, and no "normal" measurements have been established. Most pediatricians, however, have established their own "norms" for children. Detection of a large tongue, or macroglossia (Fig. 4-7, A), is important, especially in the neonatal and infantile periods, to allow early diagnosis of certain conditions, such as cretinism, that must be treated before irreparable damage to the child occurs. In true macroglossia there is usually enlargement in all directions—anteriorly, posteriorly, superiorly, inferiorly, and laterally. Certain conditions, however, may give the impression of macroglossia:

1. An illusion of a large tongue might be seen in a disorder (such as trisomy 21 or mongolism) that is characterized by a small oral cavity but a relatively normal-sized tongue (Fig. 4-7, B).
2. The tongue is a site of congenital vascular malformations, which produce an appearance of a large tongue.

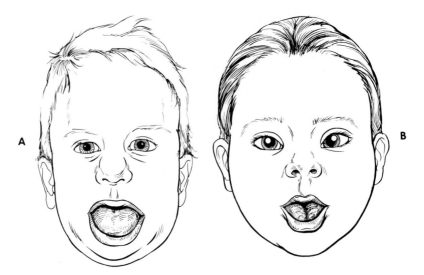

**Fig. 4-7.** Abnormalities of the tongue. **A,** True macroglossia, as might be seen in Beckwith's syndrome. **B,** Small oral cavity. A small oral cavity and mouth with a normal-sized tongue may result in an appearance of a large tongue, a condition known as pseudomacroglossia.

3. Especially in persons with epilepsy, who may injure the mouth in a seizure, apparent macroglossia may be the result of trauma to the tongue or surrounding intraoral tissues and of bleeding into those tissues. Hematoma plus edema of the tongue may be considered true macroglossia even though the intrinsic tongue tissues themselves are not large. In oral trauma, however, the tongue may be totally unaffected and appear to be large because it is caused to protrude anteriorly by edema or hemorrhage in surrounding tissues.

4. In some allergic reactions, such as angioneurotic edema, the tongue may become quite massive and even threaten to close the oral airway.

These latter "acquired" forms of macroglossia need to be differentiated from the congenital forms not only for understanding of the pathogenesis of the disorder causing the macroglossia but also for reasons of treatment and prognosis. The acquired macroglossias tend to be more asymmetrical and acute than the congenital macroglossias and thus may be greater threats to the airway and to life. Many syndromes associated with metabolic disturbances are characterized by congenital or insidious enlargement of the tongue.

In considering the tongue in facial diagnosis, a physician should remember that largeness is not necessarily the same as protrusion and that all large tongues are not necessarily long tongues.

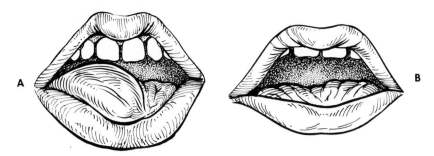

Fig. 4-8. Atrophy and hypoplasia of the tongue. A, Unilateral atrophy. B, Bilateral atrophy.

**Atrophy and hypoplasia.** The opposite of macroglossia is possible. From a medical viewpoint diminished bulk of the tongue is usually associated with an atrophic process. The term atrophy means "without nourishment" and connotes a loss of muscle bulk after the muscle has reached a volume that is normal for its age. In other words, atrophy is a wasting or deteriorating process. Tongue atrophy is an extremely important clinical sign and usually indicates a lower motor neuron lesion or a direct disturbance in the intrinsic tongue musculature.

It is very important to distinguish between bilateral atrophy, or atrophy of the tongue as a whole (Fig. 4-8, *B*), and unilateral atrophy (Fig. 4-8, *A*). The tongue is innervated by neurons that arise in the hypoglossal nucleus of the medulla. Since this nucleus receives bilateral supranuclear innervation, it is rare for there to be functional deficits of the whole tongue when the supranuclear pathways are disturbed, unless there are bilateral supranuclear lesions (such as bilateral cerebrovascular lesions, which produce a condition called "pseudobulbar palsy"). The hypoglossal nuclei are situated very close together in the floor of the fourth ventricle close to the midline. Disorders causing destruction of the hypoglossal nuclei, such as strokes, neoplasms, or degenerative diseases, rarely affect only one nucleus without simultaneously involving the other. Thus the entire intrinsic tongue musculature becomes atrophic and the tongue appears shriveled and wrinkled rather than normally contoured (see Fig. 4-8, *B*). Since denervation occurs, there is often an associated quivering or fasciculation of the intrinsic muscles of the tongue when atrophy takes place. Fasciculations, representing intrinsic irritability of denervated muscle, are characteristic of lower-motor lesions. Although atrophy and fasciculations of the tongue in general are characteristic of hypoglossal nuclear lesions, generalized atrophy, and rarely fasciculations, also can occur in primary tongue muscular disorders (a rare example may be infantile acid maltase deficiency, or Pompe's disease).

Unilateral atrophic involvement of the tongue with or without fasciculations usually is not seen in nuclear disturbances. Unilateral involvement is seen much more often in disturbances of one of the hypoglossal nerves after it has exited from the medulla and usually is not seen in intrinsic medullar or muscular disorders. A unilateral lesion may be produced by neoplasms such as meningiomas or leukemic infiltrations in the foramen magnum or at the cranial exit of the hypoglossal nerve. Disturbance of one hypoglossal nerve is rarely seen but may sometimes occur in skull fractures, other cranial traumas, and basilar meningitides. Such a disturbance also may occur as an isolated cranial nerve palsy in postimmunization periods or as a cranial nerve mononeuropathy associated with systemic metabolic diseases (such as diabetes mellitus or "osseous" mucopolysaccharidosis [Morquio's syndrome]).

Although largeness of the tongue is easily detected, smallness of the tongue is difficult to detect unless a person opens his mouth. Symmetrical hypoplasia of the tongue is rarely recognized unless it is severe. The term aglossia refers to the absence of the tongue, although it is probable that some rudiments of the tongue are present in all individuals, even those with apparent absence of all normal tongue structures. Aglossia, probably preferably called severe hypoglossia, has been described as a feature of some syndromes that will be discussed in later chapters.

**Abnormalities involving posture and protrusion.** One should be aware of abnormal postures of the tongue or an inability to protrude. Certain syndromes are characterized by protrusion of the tongue even when such protrusion has no apparent function. In severely unresponsive and generally weakened persons, the tongue may fall outside when the mouth is opened. This sign is often seen by medical house officers on geriatric wards and has been unceremoniously called the "Q" sign. This sign has no specific scientific meaning, although it is seen particularly in older debilitated persons who have had strokes and are semicomatose. The side on which the tongue protrudes does not necessarily direct one's attention to the side of a central facial palsy and hemiparesis (as has been sometimes maintained). The position of the tongue is purely the result of gravity.

A curious abnormality, which will be mentioned in the chapter on syndromes of the lower face, is associated with a rare childhood condition called the "happy puppet" syndrome. The tongue is usually long and narrow and often is protruded during paroxysms of unexplained laughter.

A banded tongue has some diagnostic importance. Such a tongue often has an extensively developed frenulum, which results in a relative inability to move the tongue forward. This condition may have an influence on speech patterns but is not associated with a specific neurologic syndrome.

**Topographic tongue abnormalities.** The furrowed tongue should be distinguished from the atrophic tongue. Deep furrows are seen in the tongues of persons with any of several syndromes as well as in some otherwise normal individuals. Geographic tongue patterns are characteristic of some diseases, as are a great number of other topographic abnormalities. Few, however, have specific meaning, and many exist as isolated abnormalities in otherwise normal persons and will not be further mentioned (Bower and Jeavons, 1967; Cohen and Cohen, 1971).

**Other tongue abnormalities.** Lobulated tongues, scarred tongues, and asymmetrical fibrous bands of the tongue are related to some of the syndromes that will be discussed later. These abnormal tongue conditions should be closely watched for.

# THE NECK

The objective of this section is not to discuss the neck as a whole but rather to dwell upon a few selected abnormalities that can be seen easily when the face is viewed from the front.

## Torticollis, retrocollis, antecollis, and head tilt

The position of the head in relation to the external environment is of great importance; maintaining the proper position is one of the major functions of the neck muscles. The primary neck muscles consist of the sternocleidomastoid muscles, the trapezius muscles, and the cervical paraspinal muscles. These muscles, acting synergistically, allow a person to react to his environment in an efficient fashion. Although head movement is a complex function, for the sake of simplicity one can think it as follows: The cervical paraspinal muscles act to stabilize the neck and are the primary extenders of the head. The sternocleidomastoid muscles are situated in such a fashion that, when working asymmetrically, they turn the head. When the sternocleidomastoid muscles act together, they are the primary flexors of the head. The trapezius muscles also are torters or turners of the head on the fixed body and tend to tilt the head to one side or the other. The trapezius muscles also shrug the shoulders. These important muscles are usually well developed, relatively strong, and symmetrical. Variations, of course, occur between individuals.

When these muscles are disturbed for any reason, abnormalities in the position of the head can be detected. Such abnormalities may be apparent in ordinary frontal facial viewing even though the basic site of the disturbance is within the neck rather than the face or the head.

Abnormal head position is involved in many neck abnormalities, the most common of which is torticollis. Although torticollis literally means "turned neck," the term has come to mean an abnormal contraction of neck musculature. The turn or torsion can be to the left or to the right. Torticollis may result from excessive involuntary contraction of one of the sternocleidomastoid muscles in relation to the other neck muscles. In torticollis resulting from dystonia, a type of organic involuntary movement, abnormal contraction is not limited to one sternocleidomastoid. All the neck muscles are abnormally contracted, with one torter or group of torters predominating. Torticollis may also be associated with functional or nonorganic mechanisms such as those seen in hysteria and in malingerers or persons with other psychiatric disturbances. Occasionally, local neck malformations cause the head to be abnormally torted.

One such malformation is the congenital absence of one of the neck torters. The resulting asymmetrical hypofunction allows the unimpeded action of the remaining torter and leads to a turned-head posture. In true torticollis, however, there is usually an excessive, sustained contraction of one of the neck torter muscles for either organic or functional reasons. There is often hypertrophy of the affected sternocleidomastoid muscle and occasionally hypertrophy of all neck muscles. Seldom is the contraction on one side only. Physiologic studies of patients with torticollis seem to indicate that both torters show sustained muscular contraction. Usually one predominates to produce the final functional deficit (Fig. 4-9, *E*).

In addition to torticollis, which is most commonly encountered, almost any head posture can be observed in dystonia or hysteria. Two such postures are retrocollis (head thrust backward) and antecollis (head thrust forward). (See Fig. 4-9, *B*.)

Tilting of the head also may be seen in dystonic movement disorders when one of the trapezius muscles overcomes the action of the other neck muscles. More commonly, however, a tilted head suggests a somewhat different cause. Simple head tilts are seen commonly in young children with ocular torter heterotropias. In such a situation, there is a malalignment of the eyes, which causes the child to tilt the head to minimize diplopia. A head tilt from an ocular problem can be diagnosed easily enough by standard ophthalmologic procedures. A more serious childhood problem that results in head tilt is a disturbance of proprioceptive and vestibular pathways within the cranium. A grave cause of head tilt is an expanding neoplasm of the cerebellum and fourth ventricle—usually a medulloblastoma.

### Other neck abnormalities

Structural abnormalities of the neck not related to tone and contraction of neck muscles and not resulting in abnormal head position are also seen and may be associated with a host of neurologic syndromes and defects. These abnormalities subtly alter the facial appearance and are important for the facial diagnostician. The three most commonly encountered neck abnormalities of this sort are shown in Fig. 4-9, *A, C,* and *D*. An extremely long neck may be a specific dysplastic feature but has not been studied to any great extent.

One of us (PRD) encountered five adult, mentally retarded, asthenic appearing individuals at a state institution. These patients were found to have extremely long and thin necks that were out of proportion with the rest of their bodies. X-ray study showed that one person had an extra cervical vertebra but no other bony abnormality. All five persons had very long and unusually appearing cervical vertebral bodies. One person had other dysplastic features that, phenotypically, suggested trisomy 21, even though long necks are not usually a feature of that disorder. Chromosome analysis was normal, however, in this patient, as it was in two

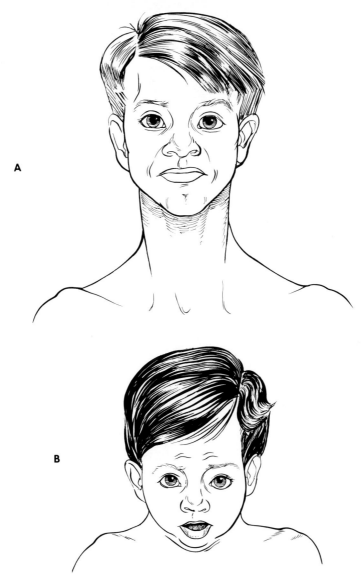

**Fig. 4-9.** Abnormalities of the neck. **A**, Dolicocollis (long neck). **B**, Antecollis (neck flexed in an anterior direction).

*Continued.*

patients without the phenotypic features of mongolism. None of the five had a muscular disorder. A survey of over 3,000 mentally retarded, institutionalized patients, which included all age groups and all varieties of retardation, uncovered no patients with conditions similar to that of the five. Further details of this syndrome, which we have tentatively called giraffism, are found in Chapter 7.

A neck that is long and thin when witnessed from both the front and

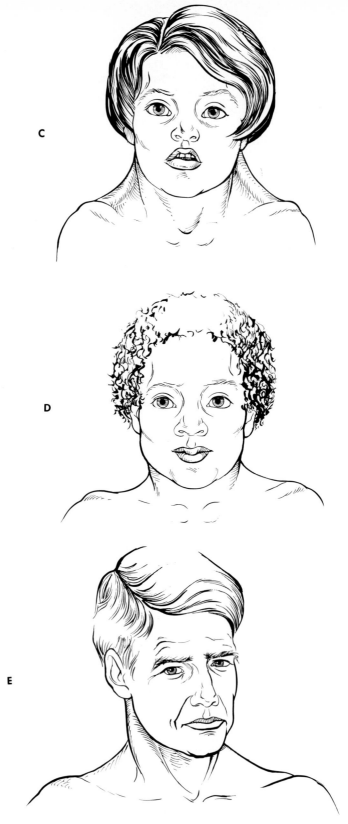

**Fig. 4-9, cont'd. C,** Pterygium colli (webbed neck). **D,** Brachycollis (wide and short neck). **E,** Torticollis (turned neck).

the side is a feature of some of the muscular dystrophies that selectively affect the anterior neck muscles. Some of the chromosomal disturbances are also characterized by abnormally long and thin necks (Fig. 4-9, *A*).

Excessively short and broad necks also should be recognized as abnormalities. Broad necks, however, may result from certain types of exercise and are seen as a normal variation in mesomorphic individuals. Excessively short necks suggest bony malformations of the cervical vertebrae. Absent vertebrae, fused vertebrae, or malformed vertebrae are possibilities. (See Fig. 4-9, *D*.)

Another neck abnormality, called pterygium colli or webbed neck (literally, the term means "winged neck"), is a disorder of the subcutaneous tissue and skin and not necessarily of the bone (see Fig. 4-9, *C*). This unusual dysplastic condition characteristic of several syndromes that will be discussed in later chapters. The short neck and the webbed neck may occur together.

# CHAPTER FIVE

# Syndromes of the upper facial and cranial segment

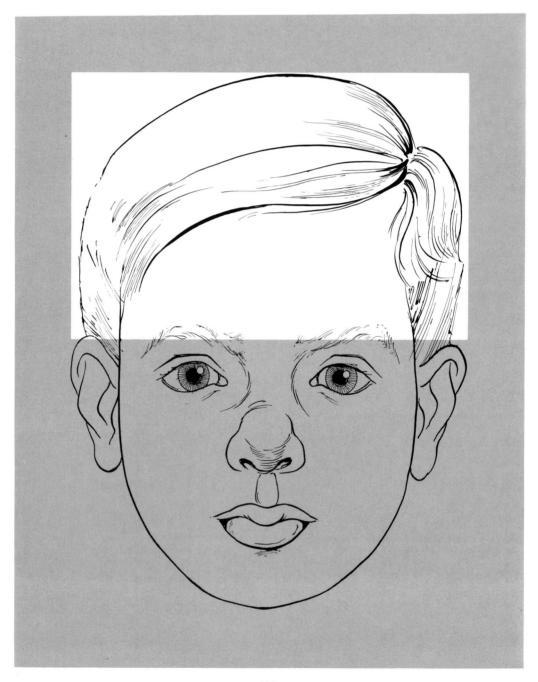

A syndrome is a grouping of two or more signs and/or symptoms into a characteristic constellation that allows the medical and psychological course of a disorder to be predicted. For syndrome diagnosis to be of any value, the signs and symptoms must be fairly consistent, characteristic, and reproducible from one patient to another. A disease, on the other hand, is a morbid condition with a proved or suspected cause and a well-defined pathogenesis. While certain disorders are both syndromes and diseases, not all syndromes represent diseases. Most diseases, however, represent syndromes. Therefore, in this restricted sense a syndrome is considered of lower diagnostic order than a disease.

Most of the features illustrated in previous chapters are definite deviations from normal or from the range of normal. An abnormality may be either a sign or a symptom but by itself is not a syndrome or a disease. For example, fever—defined as an excessively elevated temperature—is both a sign and a symptom; it definitely is an abnormality. An elevation in temperature, on the other hand, is not necessarily an abnormality. Before being able to conclude that an elevation is abnormal, one must consider the method by which the temperature was taken, the age of the patient, and any other relevant information (during ovulation, for example, an elevation in temperature is normal). When fever is associated with another sign or symptom, such as sore throat, a syndrome can be said to exist. The syndrome of fever and sore throat may be related to many diseases. If other characteristic features or abnormalities, such as enlarged and reddened tonsils, are also present, the syndrome becomes more specific and may be identified as tonsillitis. If a characteristic bacterial exudate is identified on and within the tonsils, a physician may be quite accurate in making the diagnosis of a specific disease—streptococcal tonsillitis. It is not until group A, beta-hemolytic streptococcus has been cultured from the tonsils, however, that the existence of the specific disease can be confirmed. Then the disease streptococcal tonsillitis can be treated with antibiotics and cured. At each point in this simple train of events, there is an increase in the degree of accuracy. This diagnostic process is the basis of medical practice.

Several important syndromes of the upper facial and cranial segment will be presented in this chapter. However, it is unusual for any syndrome involving facial abnormalities to be limited to the face, or, if it is so limited, to be confined to only one segment. Syndromes tend to cross the borders of facial segments and to be related to signs and symptoms not limited to the cranioface. Most syndromes have related somatic and neurologic symptoms or signs. The reader should remember that the segment involved in this chapter is the part of the cranioface situated above the eyebrow line and that most of the syndromes discussed have their basis in the concepts of abnormality described in Chapter 2. It is also pertinent to remember that abnormalities involving the frontonasal process of the embryo may have a tendency to produce abnormalities in this segment.

## SYNDROMES CHARACTERIZED BY PREMATURE CLOSURES OF CRANIAL SUTURES
### The dolichoscaphocephalies

Scaphocephaly, or boat-like skull, is a pathologic condition related to premature closure of the sagittal suture. Of the craniosynostoses, this form is probably the most common. However, physicians who see many patients with neurologic disabilities encounter this form of craniosynostosis less often than other cranial abnormalities because it is associated with fewer facial and somatic defects.

Dolichoscaphocephaly (as this condition is also known) is less of a threat to life and residual brain damage than the other craniosynostoses if the other cranial sutures remain open to allow continued expansion of the growing brain. With the closing of the sagittal suture, the growth of the cranium is predominantly in the anterior/posterior direction, resulting in an elongation of the skull. To a lesser extent, the growth is upward. (See Chapter 2 and Fig. 2-1.) Mental retardation is not a consistent finding in scaphocephaly, except in those cases in which there has been significant cerebral compression. Occasionally, full sagittal suture closure does not occur, resulting in some asymmetrical lateral cranial growth. Persons with premature closure of the sagittal suture often go through infancy and early childhood with no clinical manifestations. If such persons are recognized as abnormal, they are thought of as having merely a harmless deformity. Only during times of stress, which can produce elevations in intracranial pressure, do major symptoms develop.

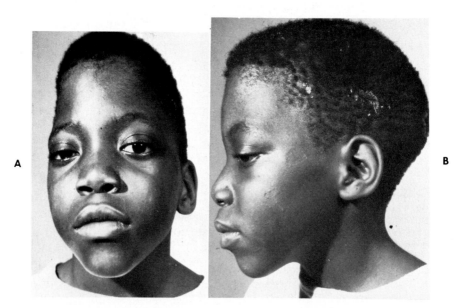

Fig. 5-1. Fourteen-year-old with dolichoscaphocephaly. A, Observe narrowed and slightly high cranial vault. Facial view is not exactly frontal; chin is tipped upward, giving illusion of low-set ears. B, Lateral view showing dolichocephaly and normally positioned ears. This child was mildly mentally retarded. During periods of stress (one occurred just before this photograph was taken), he would develop signs of increased intracranial pressure from which there would be full recovery.

These stress periods usually occur in the juvenile or adult periods of life rather than in infancy when the cranium is more pliable. The patient in Fig. 5-1 represents such a situation. He was born with the cranial defect but had no difficulties except during periods of high fever, such as during a febrile illness that occurred not long before the photograph was taken. At that time he became comatose and showed other signs of cerebral decompensation from brain herniation. After recovery he was normal again except for mild mental retardation.

Although craniofacial and somatic abnormalities have been associated with simple scaphocephaly, they are not consistent enough to constitute a separate syndrome. One possible exception is what is called the *midline hemangioma-scaphocephaly syndrome*, one of the signs of which is the persistent midline forehead capillary hemangioma, or rose wine nevus flammeus. A persistent birthmark in a mother and her three children was identified as an autosomal dominant trait. In addition to the rose wine midline nevus flammeus, twin brothers in this family had early "detected" scaphocephaly and symptoms of increasing intracranial pressure in the first few months of life (Fig. 5-2). X-ray film of their skulls

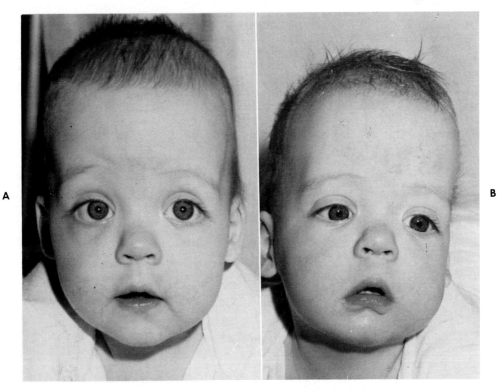

A

B

Fig. 5-2. Twins with midline hemangioma-scaphocephaly syndrome. **A,** More mildly affected twin with extensive V-shaped, midline forehead, pink-red nevus flammeus. Observe the slightly narrowed and high cranium. Photograph was taken after a craniectomy had been performed. **B,** More severely affected twin with same syndrome. The nevus is faint but slightly more extensive than in the other twin.

showed that each twin had premature closure of the sagittal suture (Fig. 5-3, *A*). Both twins underwent surgery to correct the premature suture closure, and good cosmetic results were obtained. Postoperative skull x-ray films are shown in Fig. 5-2, *B*. Later computed tomography (CT) scan study showed that one twin also had dilated ventricles (Fig. 5-4). At the time of the last examination, both patients, then over 2 years old, were considered normal neurologically and showed only mild cranial abnormality (Fig. 5-5).

If the other sutures are patent, persons with scaphocephaly usually have no other facial stigmata. Proptosis is rare, as are the other facial characteristics so common in acrobrachycephaly and turricephaly.

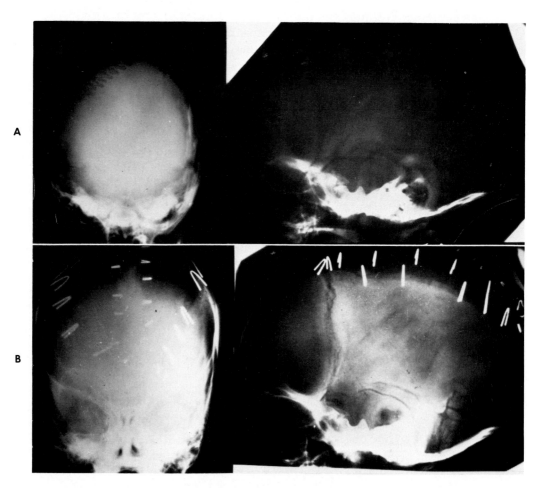

Fig. 5-3. **A,** Anterior/posterior and lateral skull roentgenograms of patient in Fig. 5-2, *A,* who had the midline hemangioma-scaphocephaly syndrome, prior to parasagittal craniectomy and insertion of Teflon. Observe the hyperostosis and complete closure of the sagittal suture. **B,** Anterior/posterior and lateral skull roentgenograms of same patient after craniectomy. Similar findings were seen in a twin seen in Fig. 5-2, *B.*

## The acrobrachycephalies

Acrobrachycephaly is a condition of extreme broadness of the head or cephalus. Apert in 1906 defined a syndrome of acrobrachycephaly that was associated with a variety of abnormalities of the hands and toes. The major abnormality consisted of webbing of the fingers or toes, which is called syndactyly (Apert, 1906; 1923). Several varieties of acrobrachycephaly and syndactyly subsequently have been described, and a classification of such syndromes has been suggested (Goodman and Gorlin, 1977; Holmes and others, 1972). It should be emphasized that not all patients with acrobrachycephaly have associated syndactyly and that not all patients with craniosynostoses with syndactyly necessarily have acrobrachycephaly (at least in the more restricted sense that we are using). It is accepted that most patients with craniosynostosis tend more toward a degree of acrobrachycephaly than a degree of dolichoscaphocephaly. Those with other types of craniosynostoses will be discussed later. A con-

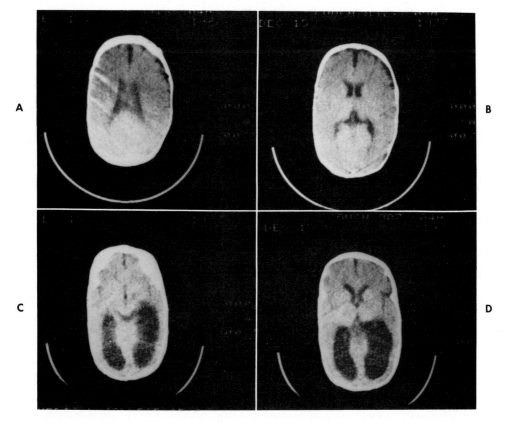

Fig. 5-4. CT scan of twins with midline hemangioma and dolichoscaphocephaly. A and B, Different cranial levels of less severely affected twin, showing only mildly dilated ventricles. C and D, Different cranial levels of more severely affected twin, showing marked enlargement of the posterior horns of the lateral ventricles.

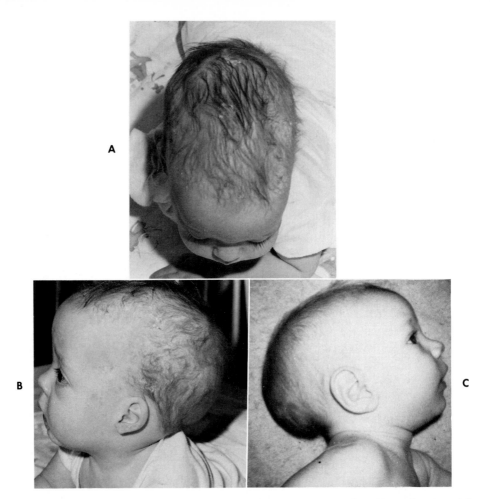

Fig. 5-5. A and B, Postoperative photographs of more severely affected twin with the midline hemangioma-scaphocephaly syndrome. A, View from top of the head, showing relatively narrow and long cranium. B, View from side, showing dolichocephaly. C, Side view of cranium of another patient for comparison, showing a bulging posterior occiput but no dolichocephaly. This cranial configuration, which is called bathrocephaly, should be distinguished from dolichoscaphocephaly. Bathrocephaly has cosmetic but no other clinical significance. (C, Courtesy of Dr. Patricia Hartlage, Medical College of Georgia.)

fusing term that appears in the literature is "acrocephaly," or "extreme cephalus," which is used to describe extremely high, long, wide, or towered heads. Many authors have used this term to refer to what we would prefer to call turricephaly or oxycephaly.

We do not agree with the "acrocephalosyndactyly" classification, which is accepted by some authors, because it includes a few conditions that do not seem to be related to acrobrachycephaly per se. According to Holmes and associates (1972), the "acrocephalosyndactylies" consist of six types. Type I, which has been called *Apert's syndrome* (Fig. 5-6), is characterized by acrobrachycephaly and syndactyly of all five digits of both hands and feet to form "mitten" hands and "sock" feet (Fig. 5-7).

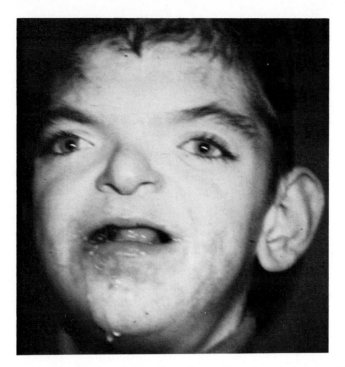

Fig. 5-6. Patient with acrobrachysyndactyly or Apert's syndrome. Observe the broadened facies as well as brachycephaly. This patient is severely retarded. The nose is small, and the forehead (although short because of a low anterior hairline) is flat and broad. The ears appear large. (Courtesy of Dr. Patricia Hartlage, Medical College of Georgia.)

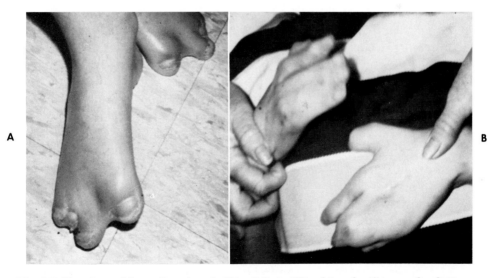

Fig. 5-7. Hands and feet of patient in Fig. 5-6. A, "Stocking feet" type of soft tissue and partial bony syndactyly of all five digits of the feet. B, Partial "mitten" type defect of the hands, with syndactyly of all fingers of both hands. The tip of the thumb had been lost in an accident. (Courtesy of Dr. Patricia Hartlage, Medical College of Georgia.)

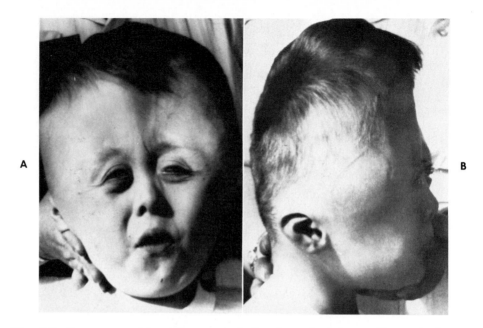

Fig. 5-8. Seven-year-old with acrocephalopolysyndactyly or Carpenter's syndrome. A, Full facial view showing broad, rounded face, broad and towered cranium, bulging of the temporal fossae, antimongoloid slant, small nose, metopic hyperostosis, and flattened to depressed nasal base. B, Side view showing extreme shortening and towering of the cranium. Observe the posterior tilt of the ears caused by the temporal bulging. The face is very flat, and the nasal base is hypoplastic and sunken.

Type II, also referred to by Holmes and associates as Apert's syndrome, consists of much the same craniofacial appearance but involves complete syndactyly only of digits 2, 3, and 4 and partial syndactyly of either or both digits 1 and 5. The validity of such an arbitrary division of Apert's syndrome is uncertain. Indeed, some authors (Goodman and Gorlin, 1977) prefer to identify type II acrocephalosyndactyly as Carpenter's syndrome (Carpenter, 1901). This syndrome, which has also been called acrocephalopolysyndactyly, is inherited as an autosomal recessive trait (Tenitancy, 1966). Persons with this disease usually have severe acrobrachycephaly due to premature closure of primarily the coronal and lambdoid sutures. Those affected have a characteristic facial appearance that is similar to but somewhat different from that seen in classic Apert's syndrome (compare Figs. 5-6 and 5-8). These persons have a more flattened facial profile, with a flat nasal base, a wide forehead, laterally displaced canthi, and mild antimongoloid slant (see Fig. 5-7.) There is often a mid-forehead ridge caused by hyperostosis of the metopic suture. In addition, in Carpenter's syndrome (Fig. 5-8) there is a tendency toward somatic abnormalities, such as genu valgum and obesity, (See Fig. 5-9 and note the skull roentgenogram in Fig. 5-10.) The biggest

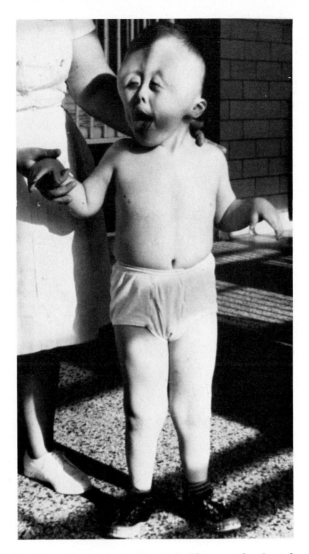

Fig. 5-9. Full-body view of patient in Fig. 5-8. Observe the facial and cranial features in relationship to the body. Patient shows obesity and genu valgum. In addition, moderate mental retardation and mild hypogonadism were suspected.

difference, however, is the presence of polydactyly, especially of the feet; syndactyly also is particularly evident between the third and fourth digits of the hands. (See Fig. 5-11.) Type III, or *Chotzen's* or *Saethre-Chotzen syndrome,* shows only mild acrobrachycephaly, as well as mild syndactyly (usually involving soft tissue alone and only isolated digits such as the fourth and fifth digits of the foot). This syndrome is also characterized by flat high eyebrows, hypertelorism, ptosis, and prognathism (see Chapter 7). Type IV acrocephalosyndactyly, or *Mohr's syndrome,* is the name now usually applied to the orofaciodigital syndromes (or OFD II).

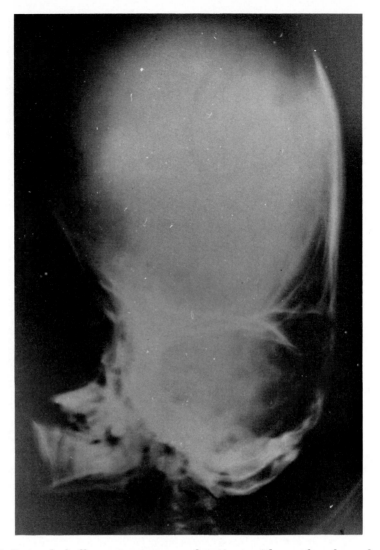

Fig. 5-10. Lateral skull roentgenogram of patient with acrobrachycephaly. Observe towered and shortened skull and obliteration of coronal sutures. Also, the temporal fossa is bulging downward and outward.

A person with this syndrome has a broad bifid tip of the nose, a midline cleft lip, normal hair, bilateral polysyndactyly of the great toe, loss of hearing, and autosomal recessive inheritance (see Chapter 7). Those with the Mohr's syndrome have few facial characteristics common to the acrobrachycephalies, although "acrocephaly" has been used as a description of their crania in several instances. Type V acrocephalo-syndactyly was reportedly described by Waardenburg (Holmes and others, 1972). This condition is characterized by plagiocephaly, buphthal-mos, bifid terminal phalanges of digits 2 and 3, elbow and knee contractures, and cardiac malformations. Persons with this syndrome do not

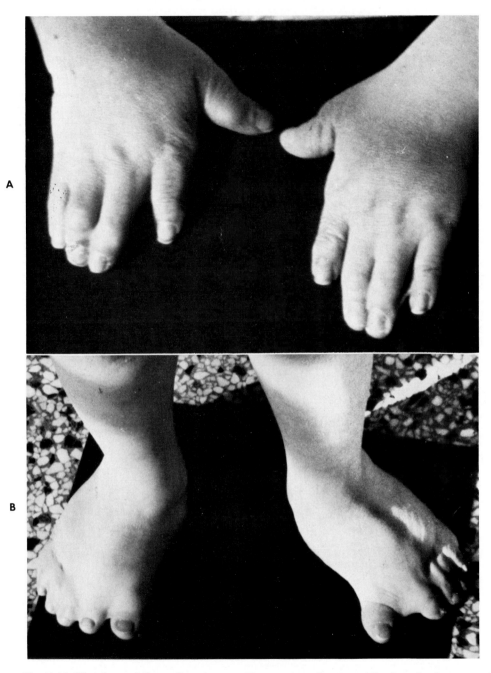

Fig. 5-11. Hands and feet of patient in Figs. 5-8 and 5-9. **A,** The hands show syndactyly between the third and fourth digits and the fourth and fifth digits. This child was born with an extra digit on the ulnar side of each hand. These extra digits were amputated. **B,** The feet show a partial stocking-type of syndactyly that involves all five digits.

have acrobrachycephaly. Type VI is also called *Pfeiffer's syndrome*. A person with this syndrome has a craniosynostosis that usually takes the form of a mild acrobrachycephaly. Syndactyly can occur in this syndrome, but more often one finds broad thumbs and big toes. Some of these digits could represent an extreme form of syndactyly involving almost total fusion of an extra digit with the thumb or big toe only. Pfeiffer's syndrome is not usually associated with mental retardation and is an autosomal dominantly inherited disorder. It is of interest not only because of its relationship to acrobrachycephaly but also because of its possible relationship to the Rubinstein-Taybi syndrome (see Chapter 6). As is evident in this review, only acrocephaloscyndactyly types I, II, and VI, and possibly III, can be considered acrobrachycephalies. Even some of these are questionable because they result from frank craniosynostotic abnormalities affecting primarily the coronal suture.

Variations of acrobrachycephaly without pronounced digital deformity also have been described. A patient with such a condition is shown in Figs. 5-12 and 5-13. This patient has severe acrobrachycephaly but only mild syndactyly in the second digital space of each foot (Fig. 5-11). The patient in this series of photographs could very well have had Pfeiffer's syndrome of acrobrachycephaly, although not all of the features were

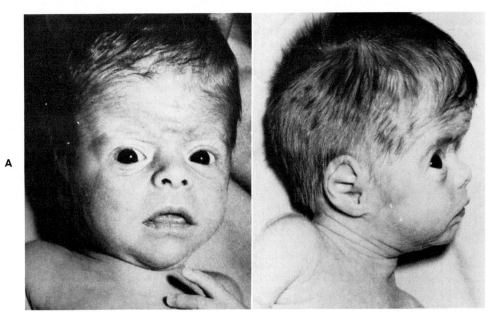

Fig. 5-12. Six-month-old infant with acrobrachycephaly. A, Full facial view showing broad and slightly towered cranium, small nose, and frightened expression. Syndactyly was not observed in digits of the left hand. B, Side view showing normal ears, brachycephaly, low forehead with hirsutism, and frightened facial expression. Nose is not beaked, and proptosis is not present. (Courtesy of Dr. Charles Linder, Medical College of Georgia.)

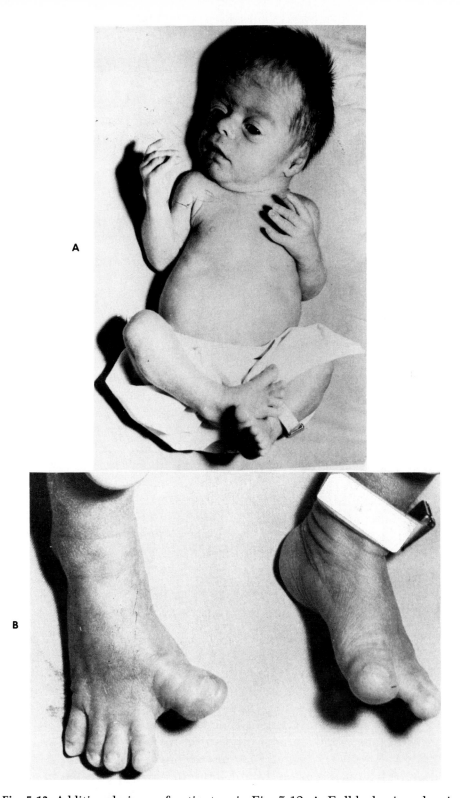

**Fig. 5-13.** Additional views of patient as in Fig. 5-12. **A,** Full-body view showing absence of syndactyly of the hands but a mild "common" type of soft-tissue syndactyly of the second, third, and fourth toes. Observe the broad halluces. **B,** Close-up view of feet, showing extremely broad big toes, syndactyly of the second and third digits, and abnormal big toe deviation. (Courtesy of Dr. Charles Linder, Medical College of Georgia.)

classic. He did have enlarged big toes. One can consider a spectrum of associated extremity deformity ranging from slight deformity (or even none) to the most severe.

One can see differences between the facial appearance of the patient having Apert's syndrome with typical facial features (Fig. 5-6) and that of the patient with Carpenter's syndrome (Fig. 5-8). In the latter patient one can see a broader forehead, metopic ridging, a "flat" face and nasal base rather than a "scooped out" face, and more of a tendency to anti-mongoloid slanting of the palpebral fissures. In addition, as shown in Fig. 5-9, there is prominent genu valgum, pes planus, and obesity. This patient was also mentally retarded. It is obvious from these two series of photographs that the two craniosynostoses have much in common yet have definite differences. Fig. 5-11 shows the hands and feet of the patient with Carpenter's syndrome. No polydactyly is evident because cosmetic surgery had been performed in infancy. But one can still see the results of scarring on the lateral aspects of both feet where the extra digits had been removed.

The syndromes of acrocephalosyndactyly should be considered whenever acrobrachycephaly occurs. An affected person is born with what is easily recognized as a deformity, if not immediately classified as acrobrachycephaly. The appearance of the face in later life depends largely upon the extent of premature closure of the coronal suture. On occasion, other sutures close prematurely as well, but they are usually the lambdoidal suture and the other sutures that are partially involved in anterior/posterior head growth.

Other facial abnormalities — also dependent upon the growth status of the brain and whether complications such as increased intracranial pressure occur — might develop. Some of these abnormalities are not limited to the upper facial and cranial segment. For example, if the metopic and squamousal sutures are patent, they act as a safety valve for the expanding brain, and considerable lateral (or transverse) and inferior cranial growth is possible. The forehead is usually quite broad. This variation usually occurs in Apert's syndrome or type I acrobrachycephaly. A very wide cranium develops, along with some middle facial deformity. If the metopic and squamous sutures are only marginally patent, if the growth character of the brain exceeds the capacity of these sutures to act as a safety valve, or if for other reasons rapidly increasing intracranial pressure develops, more grotesque facial deformities may occur. The patient in Fig. 5-8 has a considerable deformity of the middle face as well as acrobrachycephaly. In this patient cranial growth did not keep up with intracranial growth, and the orbits, the temporal fossae, the zygomatic processes, and the ears are secondarily deformed. It is not uncommon to find effects of chronic intracranial hypertension in patients with such severe suture synostosis, although frank proptosis is rare. However, acute increased intracranial pressure is seldom a feature of this syndrome. Strangely, many patients with the severe craniofacial deformity of acrobrachycephalosyndactyly are not taken to physicians early in life. The cosmetic aspects of the syndrome could be handled more appropriately early in life before severe, irreparable deformity has been established. It is believed that cosmetic handling of the craniofacial and digital deformity of these syndromes should be attempted early in life because some of the persons affected have essentially normal neurologic systems, at least until secondary brain effects become established.

The patients in Fig. 5-14, A, have mild degrees of acrobrachycephaly without extensive facial deformity. There is no syndactyly, and only mild neurologic deficits are present. The patient in Fig. 5-14, A, who probably has a mild coronal suture synostosis, is contrasted to the infant in Fig. 5-14, B, who has a greater degree of acrobrachycephaly. This latter cranial deformity was related not to a dysostosis of the coronal suture but to severe repeated head trauma, bilateral subdural hemmorrhage, and resultant microcephaly.

Although the basic malformations are very consistent from one patient to the next in the various syndromes of true acrobrachycephalosyndactyly, the degree of each malformation is extremely variable. It has been suggested that the syndromes represent various degrees of a systemic ossification defect that is not limited to the cranium. Patients with these syndromes frequently have other osseous deformities such as pes planus, genu valgum, scoliosis, kyphosis, lordosis, and deformities of the wrists and elbows. The syndromes are also associated with malformations of tissues other than bone and of organs other than the brain. Congenital heart disease, congenital cardiopulmonary abnormalities, and hypogenitalism have been reported.

Surprisingly, of all the organs, the brain (and the central nervous system) is relatively spared of malformation, although secondary neurologic deficits are common. In any suture disorder, mental abilities frequently depend upon the extent of secondary damage to the central nervous system from the cranial dysostosis and, presumably, from the effects of chronic increased intracranial pressure. The mental abilities of persons with these syndromes, however, are relatively spared. Mental retardation is not necessarily present. In fact, it is not unheard of for patients to be quite intelligent, particularly if they have milder forms of the syndromes. The social implications of their facial deformities and their other deformities are extensive, however.

## The turricephalies

The term "turricephaly" means towered or high cephalus, and, along with "oxycephaly," is preferable to the term "acrocephaly" because it avoids confusion with "acrobrachycephaly." Most of the acrobrachycephalies involve some towering or increase in height of the cranium, but extreme towering occurs when other sutures in addition to the coronal and lambdoid are prematurely closed.

In 1912, Crouzon reported that a mother and her son each had a

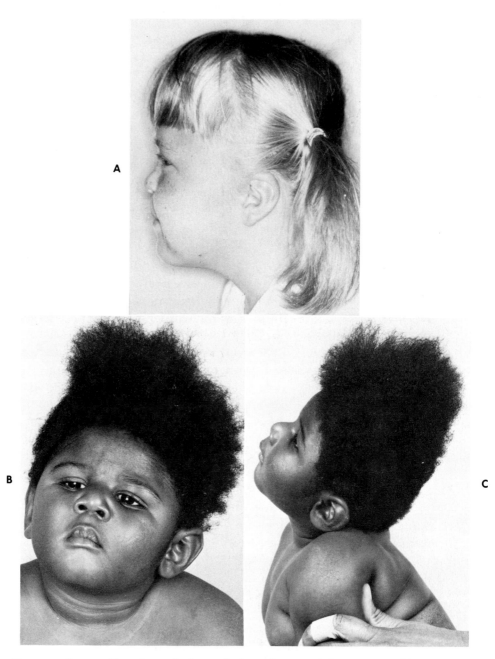

Fig. 5-14. Cases of brachycephaly not believed to result from a specific craniosyn-ostosis. **A,** Mildly retarded patient with central facial lentiginosis who also had rather severe brachycephaly of unknown cause. **B,** Facial view of severely re-tarded 12-month-old infant who had suffered from repeated head trauma during early infancy and who had had chronic bilateral subdural effusions. Observe the small cranium with short forehead. **C,** Lateral view of same patient showing pronounced brachycephaly as well as microcephaly. Craniotomies had been per-formed in the past.

slightly widened but also towered skull. In addition, each patient had a protrusion in the region of the anterior fontanel, proptosis, a beak nose, and hypoplasia of the maxilla (Crouzon, 1912). Many similar patients have been reported since this original description (Dodge et al., 1959; Jones and Cohen, 1973).

The condition called *craniofacial dysostosis* or *Crouzon's syndrome* is believed to result from premature closure of all the major cranial sutures and is the prime example of oxyturricephaly.

Many variations of the shape of the head and of the face have been written about, although the consistent feature of abnormality has been towering, or increase in the height of the cranium. One of the more common variations consists of a flat, wide forehead with slightly more increase in transverse skull diameter than in anterior/posterior diameter. This variation occurs more often in patients with predominantly coronal and lambdoid synostosis than in patients with predominantly sagittal and metopic suture dysostosis. The premature suture closure is often irregular and spares especially the parts of the sagittal and coronal sutures that border the anterior fontanel. This results in a somewhat pointed contour of the cranium around the remnants of this fontanel in later life. Because of the early closure of cranial sutures, patients with Crouzon's syndrome frequently develop both acute and chronic signs of increased intracranial pressure early in life. Proptosis is an early and consistent abnormality, because of the effect of the bulging intracranial contents on the still-pliable bony orbits. A variety of ocular abnormalities associated with the proptosis has been related to this syndrome, including heterotropias, inability to converge or fixate the eyes, optic atrophy, and acute and chronic papilledema. The palpebral fissures may be slanted in an antimongoloid fashion, but this sign is necessarily a feature of the syndrome. Facial abnormalities that are occasionally associated with this syndrome, such as maxillary and zygomatic process hypoplasia or beaked nose and flattened nasal base, are more difficult to explain purely on the basis of chronic increased intracranial pressure in early life. Hearing loss has been reported in the syndrome. The palate is often described as abnormally high and narrow, and malocclusion of the teeth is common. The tongue may be large. Refer to Fig. 5-15. The patient in these illustrations has had advanced chronic increased intracranial pressure and is severely mentally retarded. Proptosis is less evident than in the other examples of this syndrome shown in Figs. 5-16 to 5-18.

Somatic findings seem to be inconsistent in Crouzon's syndrome, although bilateral anterior subluxation of the head of the radius is occasionally present (Flippen, 1950). Patients with this syndrome often have mental retardation, the degree of which seems to be directly related to the extent and treatment of the associated increased intracranial pressure. Almost any neurologic abnormality or deficit is possible in this syndrome because of the extent of premature suture closures. X-ray films show prominent convolutional markings in the areas of the prematurely fixed sutures. The orbits and the maxilla are relatively small.

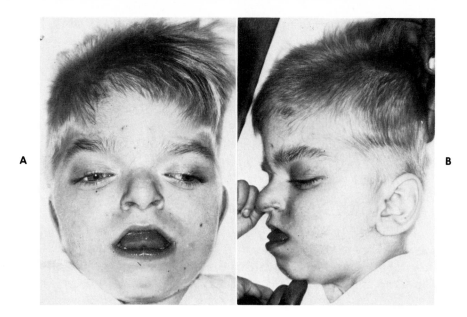

**Fig. 5-15.** Five-year-old child with Crouzon's syndrome. He had chronic increased intracranial pressure, which in the past had been relieved by craniotomy and shunting procedures. **A,** Facial view showing prominent eyes (but not frank proptosis), narrow, somewhat beaked nose, large mouth and tongue, low forehead with hirsutism, and mild hypertelorism. The cranium is high and somewhat broad. **B,** Lateral view showing turricephaly, mild brachycephaly, low-set ears, prominent forward-thrusting but narrow nose, midface hypoplasia, and large eyes. The tongue is protuberant, and there is mild prognathism.

It is important to recognize Couzon's syndrome early. The synostosis can be corrected by means of a craniectomy. Failure to correct the condition has been repeatedly shown to affect intelligence and to result in other neurologic *residuals* (such as reduced visual acuity) that are secondary to chronic or acute increased intracranial pressure.

This disorder appears to be inherited as an autosomal dominant trait with a wide range of penetrance (Shiller, 1959).

Examples of milder forms of Crouzon's syndrome can be viewed in the relatively alert-appearing infants and children in Figs. 5-16 to 5-18, all of whom, however, are mentally retarded and have mild to severe residual neurologic effects. The youngest child in the series of photographs (Fig. 5-16) had prominent proptosis, a wide forehead, and a tendency toward acrobrachycephaly, although the predominant cranial abnormality was the towered cranium. This patient, who had impending increased intracranial pressure, had craniectomies and did quite well. The second and slightly older child (Fig. 5-17) also has bilateral proptosis and a towered cranium. The third patient, a child of 8 years of age (Fig. 5-18), was only mildly mentally retarded. The chronic increased intracranial pressure was compensated.

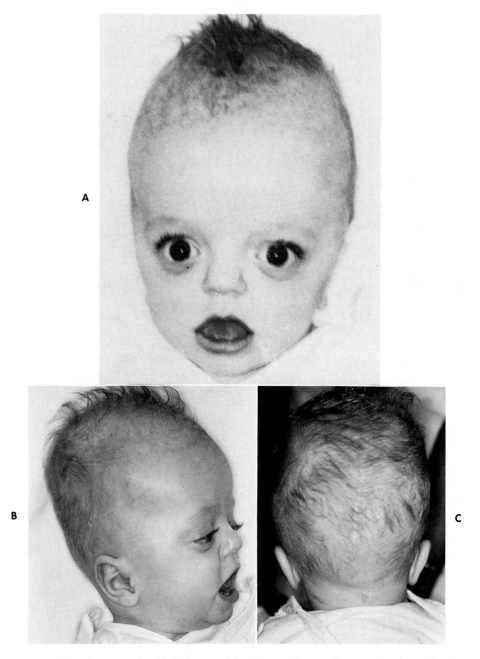

Fig. 5-16. Twelve-month-old infant with Crouzon's syndrome. A, Frontal view showing bilateral proptosis, small nose, and large tongue. B, Lateral view showing high, steepled cranium, prominent eyes, small narrow nose, and mild midface retraction. C, Posterior view showing steepled cranium.

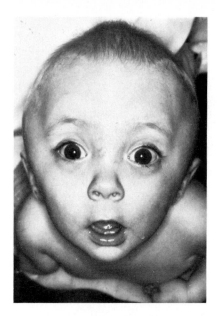

Fig. 5-17. Two-year-old with Crouzon's syndrome with oxyturricephaly. Note the high, somewhat rounded upper cranium with mild temporal bulging. The eyes are proptotic bilaterally, and the nose is narrow but short.

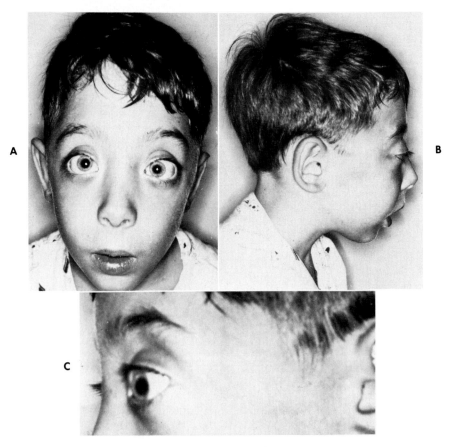

Fig. 5-18. Eight-year-old youngster with Crouzon's syndrome who has ocular as well as cranial abnormalities. A, Frontal view showing proptosis and oxyturricephaly. B, Lateral view showing steepled cranium and proptotic eyes. C, Close-up lateral view of eyes showing retraction of the eyelid over the globe. This was the usual posture of the eyelids in this patient, who at a relatively late age developed decompensated increased intracranial pressure.

# SYNDROMES CHARACTERIZED BY OTHER SUTURE DISTURBANCES

## Cleidocranial dysostosis

The cleidocranial dysostosis syndrome was originally described in a patient who had faultily developed clavicles and a large cranium (Marie and Sainton, 1897). Many cases have been described since (Smith, 1970).

The syndrome is associated with many abnormalities that are important to the physician. The essential defect in the syndrome appears to be improper ossification of membranous bone. Thus the bones of the cranial vault remain soft for an extremely long time, and the sutures may remain widely separated for the life of the individual. The anterior fontanel remains open, occasionally into adult life. The lateral aspects of the clavicles, especially, are characteristically hypo-ossified and/or poorly formed. The relationship between the osseous defect in the cartilaginous clavicle and that in the membranous cranial bones is uncertain. The pathogenesis is unexplained. Although mental retardation is sometimes present, not all patients with this syndrome have mental defects; in fact, it would appear that the majority of affected persons are intellectually normal. Macrocephaly is usually associated with the syndrome. In some instances the macrocephaly has been shown to result from hydrocephalus, but in others no cause has been found (Kalliala and Taskinen, 1962). Fig. 5-19 shows a young patient with the cleidocranial dysostosis syndrome. Because of lack of ossification of the lateral aspects of both clavicles, the youngster can practically put her shoulders together so that they touch in front of her. In addition to this defect, observe the characteristic broad forehead and enlarged cranium, which result not from unusually early closure of the coronal suture but rather from lack of closure and the macrocephaly that therefore occur. Fig. 5-20 shows a mildly mentally retarded man of 48 years who had the syndrome. He was institutionalized.

## Cloverleaf dysostosis

The cloverleaf dysostosis is quite rare. It was first described in clear terms by Holtermüller and Wiedermann and was called the Kleeblättschadel syndrome (Holtermüller and Wiedermann, 1960). The essential feature of this defect is persistent opening of the squamous suture with premature closure of other sutures, which seems to occur in utero. Some patients also have poor ossification of the entire temporal bone. The result is trilobular enlargement of the head because of the continued expansion of the cranial contents laterally from the middle cranial compartment. The outward movement of the temporal fossae results in downward tilting of the ears. In this situation the *direction* of growth of the brain changes without affecting the ultimate brain volume. Thus, persons with this deformity may have few neurologic defects. The grotesquely deformed young patient in Fig. 5-21 was reasonably normal neurologically.

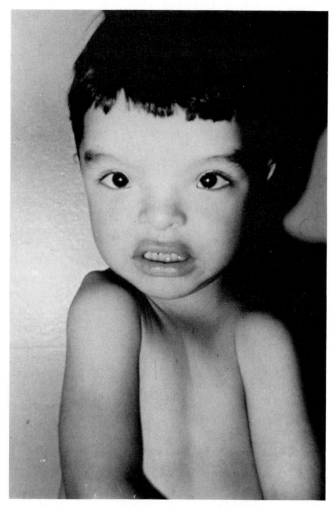

Fig. 5-19. Five-year-old youngster with cleidocranial dysostosis. Observe the abnormal position of the shoulders caused by the failure of the medial halves of the clavicles to ossify. In addition, the forehead and the cranium are very broad, and hypertelorism is present. These cranial abnormalities result from faulty ossification of the sutures and of cranial bone in general. (Courtesy of Dr. Charles Linder, Medical College of Georgia.)

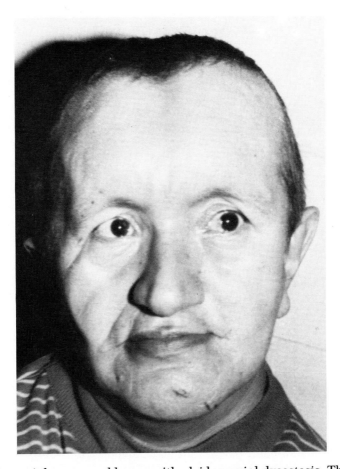

**Fig. 5-20.** Forty-eight–year–old man with cleidocranial dysostosis. There is lack of ossification of the medial halves of the clavicles, as well as macrocephaly associated with late closure of all cranial sutures and the anterior fontanel. Observe the V-shaped depression in the midline of the forehead, which corresponds to the persistently open metopic suture and the anterior fontanel. The ears are very large. This patient is mildly mentally retarded.

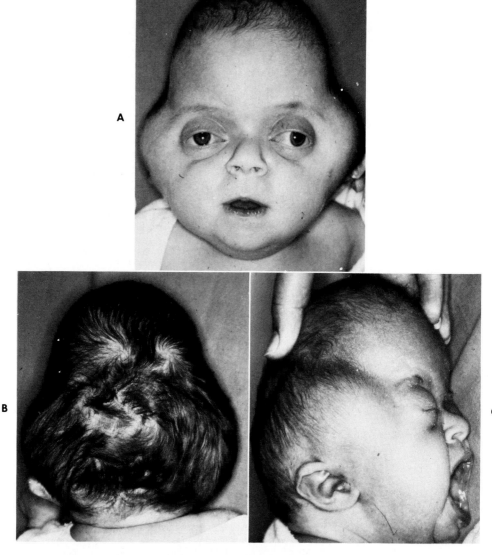

Fig. 5-21. Two-month-old infant with cloverleaf deformity. A, Frontal view show-ing protruding temporal area, steepled vertex, prominent eyes, and left exotropia. B, Posterior view showing characteristic cloverleaf configuration. Ears protrude downward. C, Lateral view showing brachycephaly, posteriorly tilted ears, and nasal hypoplasia.

## Frontal bossing syndromes

There are a variety of syndromes that involve the anterior cranium. *Encephaloceles* (Fig. 5-22) are frequently encountered protruding for-ward in the anterior cranium because of faulty midline closure in early embryogenesis. Another frequent site of encephalocele is the occiput.

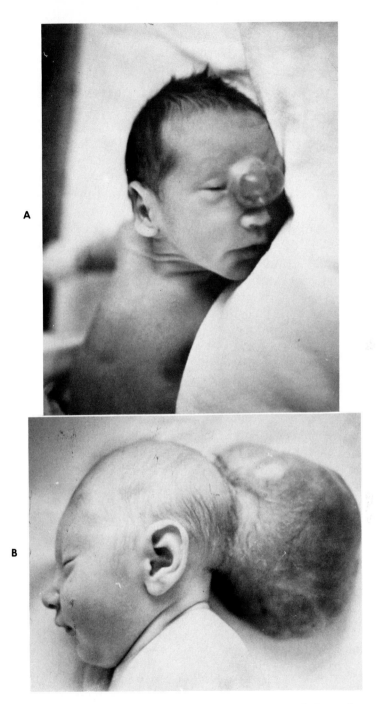

**Fig. 5-22.** Two patients with encephalocele. **A,** Newborn with frontal, nasal, interocular encephalocele. Note relative normality of other cranial structures, including nose, ear, and mouth. **B,** Occipital encephalocele in newborn. The volume of this large encephalocele is equal to, if not greater than, the remaining intracranial volume. Note sloping forehead and relative microcephaly. Ears appear large because of relative smallness of cranium. Note also the mild mongoloid slant. (Courtesy of Dr. Charles Linder, Medical College of Georgia.)

*The median cleft face syndrome* with hypertelorism (Fig. 5-23) results in a grotesque appearance but, surprisingly, is not consistently associated with subnormal intelligence. Many persons with the syndrome have normal intelligence, although the incidence of mental retardation among them is greater than in the general population. There are a number of variations of the median cleft face syndrome with hypertelorism, some of which involve frontal bossing. DeMyer believes this syndrome to be an excellent example of a disorder that results from an early defect in the frontonasal process in the embryo (DeMyer, 1972). Some, in fact, have suggested that this condition be called "frontonasal dysplasia" (Sedano and others, 1970). DeMyer rightfully contends, however, that this term is not specific enough, since there are several frontonasal dysplasia syndromes, including the holoprosencephalies. To name this disorder "frontonasal dysplasia" would represent a regression similar to calling the Rubinstein-Taybi syndrome "the first-arch syndrome." The condition may be inherited as an autosomal dominant trait. Other facial features (besides hypertelorism) sometimes associated with the median cleft face syndrome are proptosis, antimongoloid slant, and abnormal development of the bone structures of the orbits, the nose, and the jaw.

Somatic features of the syndrome sometimes may resemble an achondroplastic picture (Cohen and Cohen, 1971; DeMyer, 1967; Kurlander and others, 1967).

*Craniotelencephalic dysplasia* is a syndrome described by Jabbour and Taybi (1964). This extremely rare and unusual syndrome, originally delineated by Daum and associates (1958), is an unusual form of frontal dysostosis that is associated with exostosis in the upper forehead, premature closure of many of the major cranial sutures, and a high degree of mental retardation. Hydrocephalus may be associated with this syndrome as well. Jabbour and Taybi's case involved a mid-forehead nevus flammeus as well. Fig. 5-24 shows a mildly retarded young patient who had been treated with an ventriculoatrial shunt for hydrocephalus. Even before treatment, a "protrusion" of the upper forehead and frontal region was observed and was falsely believed to result from frontal ventricular enlargement. This type of frontal abnormality can be seen in the median cleft face syndrome as well.

•  •  •

Goodman and Gorlin (1977) list fourteen additional syndromes that are characterized by suture synostosis: Armendares' syndrome, Baller-Gerold syndrome, Berant's syndrome, Christian-Andrews-Conneally-Muller syndrome, Fairbanks' syndrome, Gorlin-Chaudhry-Moss syndrome, Herrmann-Opitz syndrome, Herrmann-Pallister-Opitz syndrome, Lowry's syndrome, Sakati-Nyhan-Tisdale syndrome, Summitt's syndrome, thanatophoric dwarfism, 5 p+ syndrome, and Weiss' syndrome. These syndromes are quite rare.

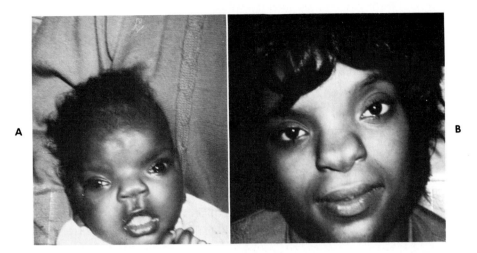

Fig. 5-23. Median cleft face syndrome. **A,** Six-month-old with pronounced hypertelorism, protruding and V-shaped forehead, cleft in approximate middle of nose, and excavation in middle of upper lip at philtrum. This baby is normal neurologically. An illusion of exotropia is produced by the corneal reflection. **B,** Mother of patient in **A.** Note similar upper and middle facial abnormalities. This woman does not have exotropia and is normal neurologically and mentally. (Courtesy of Dr. Patricia Hartlage, Medical College of Georgia.)

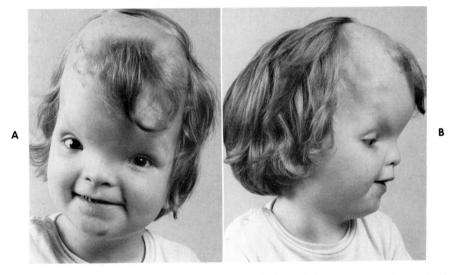

Fig. 5-24. Four-year-old patient with macrocephaly resulting from hydrocephalus and from protrusion of frontal bone and forehead. This patient was considered to have craniotelencephalic dysplasia. **A,** Frontal view. Observe frontal protrusion, hypertelorism, hypoplastic nasal base, and epicanthal folds. Patient is moderately mentally retarded. **B,** Lateral view. Note alopecia over frontal protrusion. Posterior bossing is also evident.

## SYNDROMES CHARACTERIZED BY SIMPLE MACROCEPHALY
### The hydrocephalies

The term hydrocephalus means "water head" but actually refers to the excessive accumulation of cerebrospinal fluid. There are many types of hydrocephalus, and providing detailed descriptions of each of them is not an objective of this text. Attention will be given here to the types of hydrocephalus that produce craniofacial stigmata. Essentially, these types are the ones that are progressive and that occur when the sutures are still open so that enlargement of the cranium is possible. Besides macrocephaly, craniofacial abnormalities associated with acute progressive hydrocephalus regardless of cause include proptosis, engorged cranial veins, bulging fontanels, heterotropias, spread cranial sutures, setting sun sign, and a host of other neurologic and ophthalmologic features that are not readily evident to the examiner during simple facial viewing. Although the onset of a form of hydrocephalus that produces characteristic craniofacial abnormalities usually occurs in utero, in infancy, or in early childhood (before the major sutures are completely closed) and the condition is progressive, the process may stop at any time, even without treatment, and leave residual craniofacial abnormalities that are still visible years afterward. (See Figs. 5-25 and 5-26.)

Many of the conditions that produce these stigmata are congenital. It is generally agreed that the most frequent cause of hydrocephalus is congenital malformation (Edwards and others, 1961; Gibson, 1955). The three most commonly encountered congenital malformation syndromes causing hydrocephalus are (in decreasing order of prevalence) the Arnold-Chiari syndrome or malformation, aqueductal stenosis, and the Dandy-Walker syndrome. The same craniofacial stigmata, however, can also develop in infancy and early childhood as a result of other conditions. Hydrocephalus that begins at such an age may be caused by obstruction of the foramina or the aqueduct as a result of fibrosis or by exudate and granulations secondary to infections like the bacterial, fungal, and viral meningoencephalitides. Blockage of the foramina and the aqueduct also may result from hemorrhage associated with birth or postnatal trauma, from neoplasms, or from the very rare overproduction of cerebrospinal fluid, which is speculated to be related to choroid plexus papilloma. (See Fig. 5-27.)

On rare occasions obstructive hydrocephalus in infancy and childhood is related to mechanical factors such as those occurring in achondroplasia or to changes in the meninges of the base of the brain, as occurs in some rare metabolic diseases such as acute infantile Gaucher's disease (Herrlin and Hillborg, 1962).

The *Arnold-Chiari syndrome* is perhaps the most common of the obstructive hydrocephalies. This syndrome is of several types according to some authors (Peush, 1965; Wright and others, 1975). In the usual type, there is mild to severe caudal displacement of the cerebellum and brain stem below the lip of the foramen magnum and occlusion of the foramen

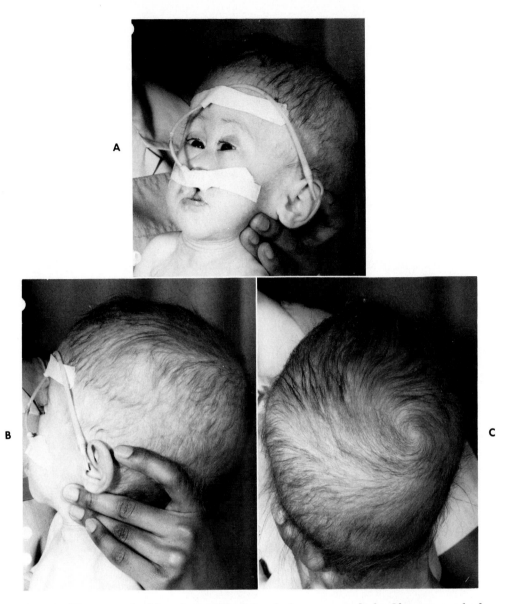

Fig. 5-25. Five-month-old patient with alobar holoprosencephaly. Observe marked hydrocephalus in addition to characteristic features of holoprosencephaly. A, Oblique view. B, Lateral view. C, Posterior view.

of the fourth ventricle. This syndrome is associated usually with a meningomyelocele or meningocele in the lumbar area or elsewhere in the midline neural axis. The hydrocephalus may be severe and rapid in its development. Fig. 5-28 shows two patients with Arnold-Chiari malformation with arrested hydrocephalus. These patients are moderately to severely debilitated.

*Congenital aqueductal stenosis* is the next most frequently encoun-

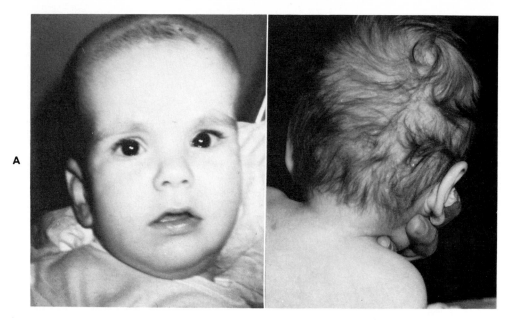

Fig. 5-26. A, Six-month-old patient, without pronounced facial stigmata, who has alobar holoprosencephaly, as shown by CT scan. Observe left esotropia and mild stigmata of hydrocephalus. B, Different patient with mildly hydrocephalic contour. (Courtesy of Dr. Patricia Hartlage, Medical College of Georgia.)

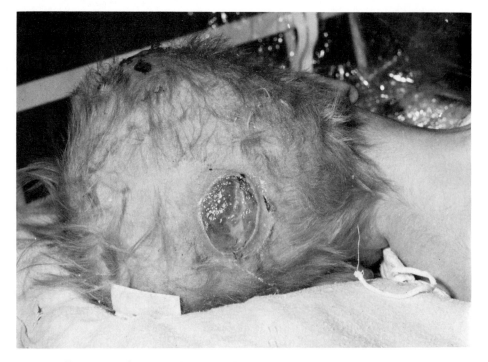

Fig. 5-27. Patient with severe hydrocephalus resulting from congenital aqueductal stenosis. Decubitus ulcer on occiput is caused by constant positioning on back. (Courtesy of Dr. Theo Thevaos, Gracewood State Hospital and Training Center.)

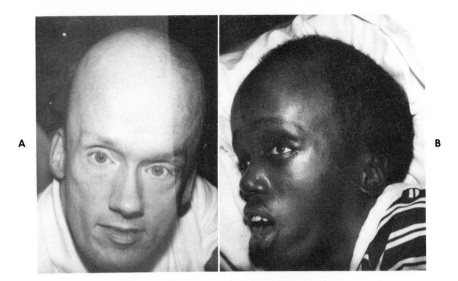

Fig. 5-28. Two patients with hydrocephalus associated with the Arnold-Chiari malformation. A, Mildly retarded 34-year-old man with cranial alopecia universalis. B, Severely retarded adult with frontal baldness and cranial stigmata of hydrocephalus.

tered malformation causing congenital hydrocephalus (Milhorat, 1978). This defect results from an aqueduct not being fully patent. Rarely will pathologic studies show a total occlusion; more commonly there is only mild stenosis of the aqueduct, which is much more compatible with late presentation of hydrocephalus as a means of compensation for poor flow of cerebrospinal fluid. *Acquired aqueductal stenosis* also can occur. In a young infant, one has great difficulty distinguishing this condition from dysgenetic malformations of the aqueduct. Common causes of such an acquired lesion are mumps and other viral illnesses.

Frequently encountered in the infantile period is another form of hydrocephalus. This form results from a congenital vascular malformation, which has been called aneurysm, in the area of the great vein of Galen. It is believed that the basic defect in this condition is a *deep arteriovenous malformation* and that the "galenic aneurysm" is merely a secondary dilation of the vessel. Regardless of the basic pathogenesis, the galenic vein enlarges massively and produces secondary hydrocephalus by exerting pressure on the underlying aqueduct. Hydrocephalus caused by a galenic aneurysm is a relatively late manifestation, occurring in late infancy. In the neonatal period the major clinical manifestation of this lesion is congestive heart failure. The infant in Fig. 5-29 has acute hydrocephalus due to a large galenic aneurysm.

The *Dandy-Walker syndrome* is believed to result from agenesis of all or part of the roof of the fourth ventricle. This syndrome is often associ-

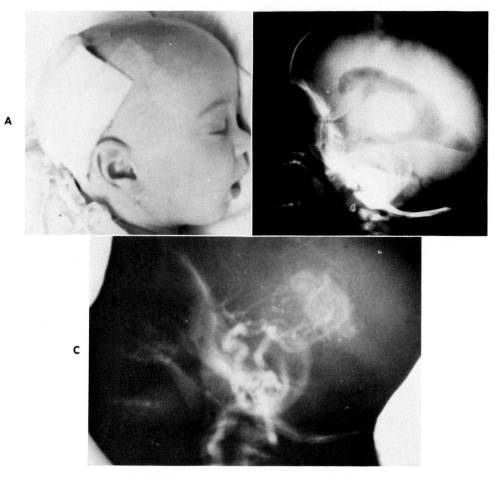

Fig. 5-29. Three-month-old patient with early hydrocephalus associated with arteriovenous malformation in region of great vein of Galen, A, Side view showing mildly hydrocephalic contour. Note presence of ventriculoatrial shunt. B, Lateral-view pneumoencephalogram showing mild ventricular enlargement compatible with cranial enlargement and depression in trigone area of lateral ventricle resulting from arteriovenous malformation. C, Lateral-view carotid angiogram showing arteriovenous malformation in region of great vein of Galen.

ated with some occlusion of the foramen at the base of the skull. The occlusion causes a large cyst to form in the posterior fossa, and hydrocephalus is common (Hart and others, 1972).

In none of the malformation syndromes are specific craniofacial stigmata necessarily seen. In the Arnold-Chiari and Dandy-Walker syndromes, one often encounters oversized posterior fossae. In the Arnold-Chiari malformation, a short and broad upper neck is common in addition to the frequently encountered meningomyelocele, usually in the lumbosacral area. Aqueductal stenosis has no pathognomonic facial or somatic stigmata, but joint and digital abnormalities, including arachnodactyly and bony anomalies at the base of the skull, have been reported in this intraventricular malformation (Mackenzie and Emery, 1972).

A neoplasm in infancy that is characterized by hydrocephalus is *choroid plexus papilloma*. It is believed that this intracranial tumor can produce hydrocephalus by two mechanisms. Probably the most common is obstruction of flow of cerebrospinal fluid at the various intraventricular foramina. Since the tumor usually arises from the choroid plexus of the lateral ventricles, the most common site of obstruction is the foramen of Munro. One frequently encounters an asymmetrical enlargement of the lateral ventricles because of obstruction at this site. (See Fig. 5-30.) Secondary obstructions at other critical ventricular sites, distant from the main obstruction, also may contribute to hydrocephalic phenomena. The possibility that choroid plexus papilloma contributes to hydrocephalus by stimulating the overproduction of cerebrospinal fluid is an intriguing theory that was originally suggested by Dandy (1921). It is improbable, however, that this mechanism is a major source of hydrocephalus in children with choroid plexus papilloma (Bohm and Strong, 1961). The head of the patient in Fig. 5-30 is mildly hydrocephalic in contour and size. This child was 14 months old when the photograph was taken but only 5 months old when infantile spasms occurred and left-sided choroid plexus papilloma was diagnosed. Spasms are unusual in infants with choroid plexus papilloma.

The terms anencephaly, hydrocephalus, holoprosencephaly, and hydranencephaly should not be confused, although they (and the conditions they represent) actually are often confused by the clinicians who use them. Anencephaly literally means "no brain," hydrocephalus means "water head," and holosprosencephaly means "whole forebrain." The term hydranencephaly was coined to refer to a condition of combined hydrocephalus and anencephaly. In hydranencephaly the cerebral hemispheres are almost, if not totally, replaced by membranous sacs (Crome and Sylvester, 1958). In this condition the meninges, cranium, and scalp are usually intact. Although at birth the affected infant may appear normal, a generalized enlargement of the head soon occurs. This macrocephaly, which usually becomes evident in the first weeks or months of life, is caused by progressive hydrocephalus, usually of an obstructive type.

Much confusion exists about the true nature of hydranencephaly. It is probable that the condition results from a severe, acquired, destructive insult to the brain in utero at a stage after most major differentiation of the brain has occurred or, in some instances at least, from an unrecognized, latent, but then rapidly progressive, congenital hydrocephalus. It is extremely doubtful that hydranencephaly has a consistent cause or pathogenesis, as is usually true of the anencephalies and the holoprosencephalic malformations. In many instances hydranencephaly results from the same mechanisms that produce some of the forms of congenital hydrocephalus previously discussed.

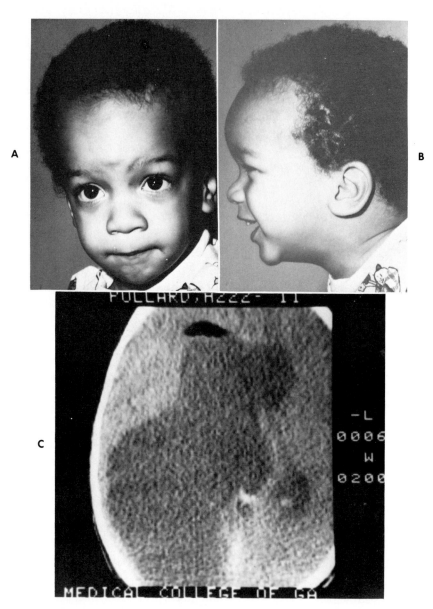

Fig. 5-30. Fourteen-month-old patient approximately 7 months after craniotomy for removal of choroid plexus papilloma that produced infantile spasms and obstructive intraventricular hydrocephalus. A, Frontal view showing mild forehead and cranial stigmata of hydrocephalus. B, Lateral view showing frontal bossing and mild posterior tilt of ears. C, CT scan shows pronounced ventricular enlargement, especially on the left. Observe the displaced left choroid plexus. (Procedure performed with contrast material.)

Hydranencephaly is not incompatible with several years of life. One patient, in fact, was reported to have an intelligence quotient of 74 at 5 years of age (Holmes and others, 1972). Nevertheless, it is doubtful that hydranencephaly was the proper designation for this child's condition, since the diagnosis was based upon only a brain biopsy and pneumoencephalographic evidence (Lorber, 1965). It was believed at one time that transillumination was a fairly specific sign for hydranencephaly. Many diagnoses of hydranencephaly were based on the presence of this sign alone without other laboratory or pathologic confirmation. Transillumination, however, is little more specific than clinical judgment. (See Fig. 5-31.) Even pneumoencephalography may not allow absolute distinction between hydranencephaly and severe forms of simple hydrocephalus. The final diagnostic distinction between hydranencephaly and hydrocephalus rests appropriately with the pathologist. That is not to say that physical stigmata, transillumination, pneumoencephalography, or computerized tomography cannot suggest one condition over another. In hydranencephaly the cerebral hemispheres are almost, if not entirely, absent. There is usually a large, thin-walled sac of fluid surrounded by a membrane of leptomeninges and a layer of glial tissue, whereas extremely thin brain tissue composes the sac in severe hydrocephalies. In severe forms of long-standing hydrocephalus, it may be extremely difficult to determine, even pathologically, whether brain tissue exists in the fluid covering. It is of interest that some subcortical optic and auditory reflexes are preserved in reportedly hydranencephalic infants,

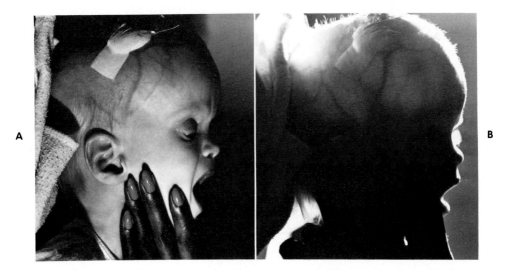

Fig. 5-31. Seven-month-old child with severe hydrocephalus caused by aqueductal stenosis. A, Lateral view showing hydrocephalic contour of cranium with frontal bossing and engorged cranial vessels (ordinary light). B, Pronounced transillumination occurred after high-intensity light was placed on other side of head. Patient had had ventricular tap.

including the optic and auditory blink reflexes. These reflexes are not dependent upon the cerebral hemispheres.

## Achondroplasia (chondrodystrophy)

Achondroplasia, the most common type of dwarfism, has been known since the early history of man and is probably neither less common nor more common now than in ancient times. Medical writings on this condition have accumulated over the years, but there still is no absolutely known cause or any specific treatment. There undoubtedly are many forms and variations of the condition.

It would appear that the fundamental defect is a disturbance in cartilaginous bone. The long bones of the body are cartilaginous and normally grow by expansion at the epiphyseal plate, where, it is presumed, the defect occurs. Longitudinal growth in the bone is not allowed because of the defect. The bones of the face are cartilaginous and thus would be expected to be (and are) involved in achondroplasia. The bones of the cranial vault, however, are not involved in achondroplasia because they are membranous.

Craniofacial abnormalities in achondroplasia include a broadened appearance of the nasal base, hypoplasia of the nasal bone, mild superciliary hyperplasia, a relatively large cranium, and somewhat grotesque facial features in general. (See Fig. 5-32.) The basic problem in achondroplasia is a tendency of bones to expand laterally at the epiphysis to compensate for an inability to expand longitudinally. For the same reasons that the wrists are thick and somewhat broad, the face is thick and somewhat broad. The inhibition of longitudinal expansion, however, does not account for the mild macrocephaly that characteristically is associated with achondroplasia. This macrocephaly may be related to hydrocephalus caused by impaction of both neural and nonneural elements at the foramen magnum as a result of the odontoid process, the neural axis, the arachnoid foramina, and the meninges all being squeezed into a relatively small space. This situation produces intermittent obstruction of cerebrospinal fluid flow and thus an obstructive extraventricular type of hydrocephalus. The macrocephaly in achondroplasia also may be related to true megalencephaly, which is of an anatomic nature. True megalencephaly may result from increases in number and size of cellular and noncellular parenchymal components rather than from metabolic or storage phenomena.

The somatic features of achondroplasia, which are well known, offer

Fig. 5-32. Ten-month-old infant with shortened limbs and deformities suggesting achondroplasia. A, Note facial stigmata, including macrocephaly and squat and thick facial features, and deformed limbs. B, Note contour of cranium. C, Roentgenographic appearance of limbs in achondroplasia.

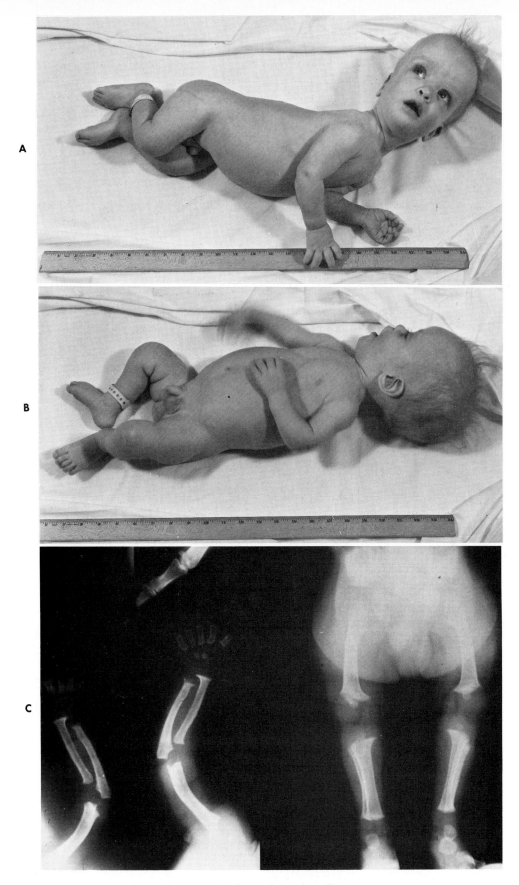

**Fig. 5-32.** For legend see opposite page.

the easiest and most consistent way to make the diagnosis in older children and adults. Because the diagnosis of achondroplasia can be exceedingly difficult in early infancy, knowledge of the characteristic facial abnormalities may be of primary importance in first suggesting the condition. (See Fig. 5-33.)

Mental retardation is not uncommon in achondroplasia. However, individuals having the conditions are markedly delayed developmentally, and thus may be erroneously termed mentally retarded (Morris and MacGillivray, 1953). Careful neuropsychologic evaluation is necessary to determine whether mental retardation actually exists.

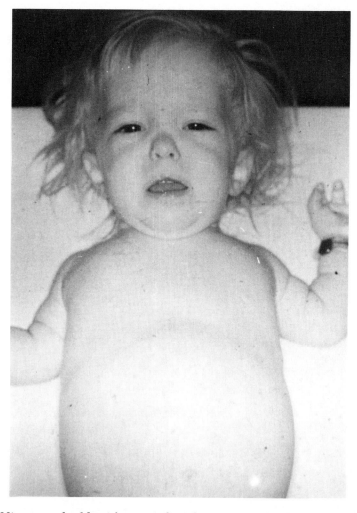

Fig. 5-33. Nine-month-old with craniofacial stigmata of achondroplasia, including macrocephaly, frontal bossing, pug nose, and mildly thickened lips. Macroglossia and large ear lobules, however, are not present. Note also the shortened upper extremity.

# The megalencephalies

Megalencephaly is a type of macrocephaly caused by enlargement of the brain parenchyma as a result of either metabolic or anatomic changes. For example, many of the inborn errors of metabolism involve megalencephaly associated with an abnormal accumulation of metabolites and other substances. In contrast, anatomic megalencephaly results from large cells or increased total numbers of cells.

It is not a purpose of this chapter to dwell in length on the specifics of diseases but rather to emphasize the craniofacial features that, if not unique to a syndrome, should distinguish it from other disorders characterized by megalencephaly. In most instances the patients who suffer from the diseases included in this section are acutely ill and in obvious discomfort. They usually show various signs of a diffuse central nervous system disturbance and may have facial stigmata and general features that suggest dementia, extreme irritability, or specific defects in various segments of their faces. Yet the most characteristic abnormal craniofacial feature is the megalencephaly, which involves the upper facial and cranial segment and is therefore included here.

There is a large group of syndromes and diseases characterized by or associated with megalencephaly. Many of them will be discussed more fully in more appropriate places in this book. Examples include the *mucopolysaccharidoses*, the prototype syndromes of which, for the most part, are associated with true and extensive megalencephaly. For example, in the *Hunter-Hurler varieties* there is a massive accumulation of glycolipids in the neurons of the central nervous system. Disorders such as the mucolipidoses and the sialase deficiencies will be discussed elsewhere even though megalencephaly would appear to be present in at least several varieties of these syndromes. All these syndromes represent possibly important links—not only clinically but also biochemically—to another vast variety of syndromes that now have been proved to have a metabolic basis. These disorders have been called the *lipidoses* or, more specifically, the *sphingolipidoses*. The sphingolipidoses, whose classification seems to change almost daily, are diseases that are strongly suspected (or, in some instances, proved) to represent deficiencies in the action of enzymes having to do with the catabolic breakdown of sphingolipids. Most of these disorders are neurologically oriented diseases, but a few are without severe neurologic manifestations.

The sphingolipidoses consist of the *gangliosidoses*, the *sphingomyelinoses*, and the *cerebrosidoses*. The gangliosidoses are traditionally divided into three main types: *the GM$_2$ gangliosidoses, the GM$_1$ gangliosidoses*, and others. *The GM$_2$ gangliosidoses* include *type I* or *classic Tay-Sachs disease* (caused by the absence of the heat-labile enzyme hexosaminidase A), *type II* or *Sandhoff's disease* (caused by the absence of both heat-labile and heat-stabile hexosaminidase A and B), and *type III* or *atypical forms* (caused by partial deficiencies in hexosaminidase A and B) of which there are several clinical types.

*Tay-Sachs disease* was originally described in 1876 by the British ophthalmologist Warren Tay (1881) and was later studied more extensively by the first American pediatric neurologist, Bernard Sachs (1887). The disease shows a very characteristic clinical picture resulting from the deterioration in neuronal function associated with an extensive accumulation of $GM_2$ ganglioside in neurons of the brain and the ganglion

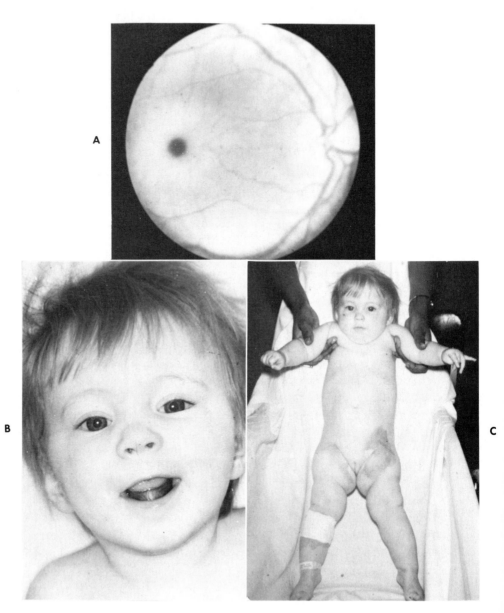

Fig. 5-34. A, Optic fundus photograph with macular region on left and papilla on right. The cherry-red spot is in the exact center of the macula and is surrounded by a halo of milky opacity representing $GM_2$ ganglioside accumulated in the ganglion centers of the surrounding macular region. B, Frontal view of six-month-old patient with classical Tay-Sachs disease. At this early stage of the disease, no craniofacial stigmata are present. C, Full-body view of same patient, showing hypotonia.

cell layer of the retina. Lipid accumulation in the retina is manifested as an almost pathognomonic abnormality that Tay called a "cherry-red spot" (Fig. 5-34). Affected patients are usually relatively normal until several months of age. Then irritability, searching eye movements, progressive hypotonia, and developmental standstill, followed by progressive loss of psychomotor milestones, hyperreactivity (such as in hyperacusis, an abnormal reaction to auditory stimuli or to almost any stimulus) occur over a period of several months. Along with these neuro-ophthalmologic symptoms, one observes a characteristic enlargement of the cranium because of megalencephaly, which is caused in turn by the progressive accumulation of ganglioside in neurons of the brain. The lipid accumulation tends to be greater in the rostral nervous system, but spinal cord neurons and peripheral ganglion cells also are affected. All symptoms are progressive. In time the infant becomes severely debilitated, and death usually occurs before 5 years of age. Although systemic signs and symptoms have been reported in this disease, including addisonian bronzing, mild liver dysfunctions, and severe eosinophilia (Dyken and Zeman, 1964) (see Chapter 8), the neurologic and ophthalmologic systems are more dramatically affected. (See Figs. 5-35 and 5-36.)

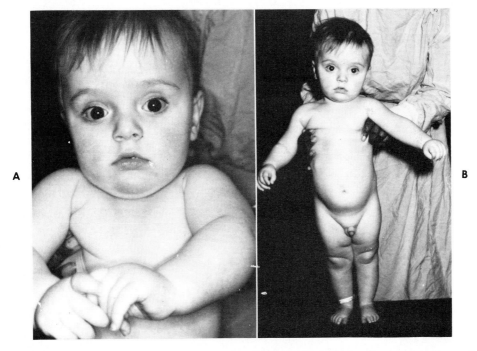

**Fig. 5-35.** Twelve-month-old patient with classical Tay-Sachs disease. **A,** Frontal view showing expressionless, blank facial appearance, mild eyelid retraction, and relatively mild macrocephaly. The degree of hypotonia of the musculature of the shoulder girdle can be estimated by the result of the pressure of the helper's fingers in the axillae. **B,** Full-body view. Observe the indirect signs of muscular hypotonia (indentation of helper's fingers, pes planus, protuberant abdomen, and so on). The craniofacial stigmata are also evident in this view.

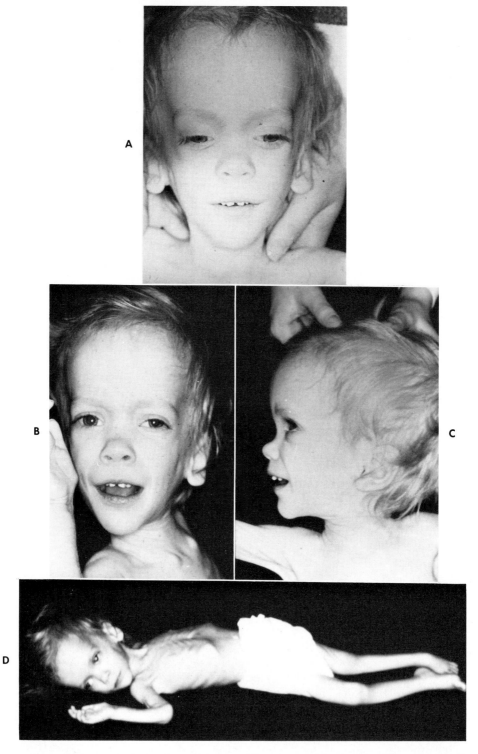

**Fig. 5-36.** Twenty-six–month–old terminal patient with classical Tay-Sachs disease. **A,** Facial view showing pronounced macrocephaly resulting from megalencephaly. The facies is dull and wasted. **B,** Note the irritability characteristic of this disease. **C,** Lateral view showing all the characteristic features of macrocephaly, including frontal bossing and engorged cranial vessels. **D,** Full-body view showing severe somatic wasting. Patient died within two weeks of this photograph.

The *GM₁ gangliosidoses*, also called the *generalized gangliosidoses*, are another form of the gangliosidoses. Affected patients have mucopolysaccharide accumulation in the systemic organs and clinical features that are similar to those of the mucopolysaccharidoses. There are two clinical types, both of which are characterized by galactosaminidase deficiency. Type I involves hepatosplenomegaly, coarse facial features, and skeletal abnormalities that are absent in type II (Goodman and Gorlin, 1977).

Closely related biochemically to the gangliosidoses but vastly different from them clinically are the *sphingomyelinoses*. These are a group of syndromes, the prototype (type A) of which is classic acute infantile Niemann-Pick disease (Schneider and Kennedy, 1967). These syndromes result from sphingomyelinase deficiency and do not always involve prominent neurologic or facial stigmata. Yet in the classic forms (which may be closely related to the mucolipidoses and the sialase deficiencies) certain common clinical features, such as cherry-red spot, dementia, and seizures, may occur. Megalencephaly, however, is seldom a prominent feature.

There are also several forms of the *cerebrosidoses*, or *Gaucher's disease*, including acute infantile and chronic juvenile cerebral types and a noncerebral adult form. The acute infantile form characteristically has neurologic symptoms even though facial stigmata are not always present, as in the patient viewed in Fig. 5-37. A rare complication of the acute form of Gaucher's disease consists of impaction of structures in the area of the foramen magnum because of the accumulation of lipid-laden macrophages in the meninges and other structures. This reaction supposedly accounts for the opisthotonic posturing characteristic of children with acute Gaucher's disease and theoretically could produce an obstructive type of hydrocephalus. The enzyme lacking in all forms of Gaucher's disease is glucocerebrosidase.

The *sulfatide lipidoses*, or *metachromatic leukodystrophy*, occur in at least three clinical forms that differ from each other in the total amount of the enzyme arylsulfatidase present. The most severe form, which begins in late infancy, is associated with many craniofacial abnormalities, of which macrocephaly caused by true megalencephaly predominates (see Fig. 5-38.) In the second form, the first major neurologic symptoms usually develop between 5 and 15 years of age. The third form, which has more slowly progressive oligosymptoms, usually has its onset in adulthood and may not involve any particular facial stigmata (Prensky, 1975).

In 1916 Krabbe described two siblings in whom rapid deterioration in neurologic functions began in early infancy and led to their deaths by the second year of life (Krabbe, 1916). Severe demyelination was observed as well as the accumulation in the brain of multinucleated globoid cells. It has subsequently been shown that *Krabbe's disease* results from deficient activity of the enzyme galactocerebroside beta-galactosidase

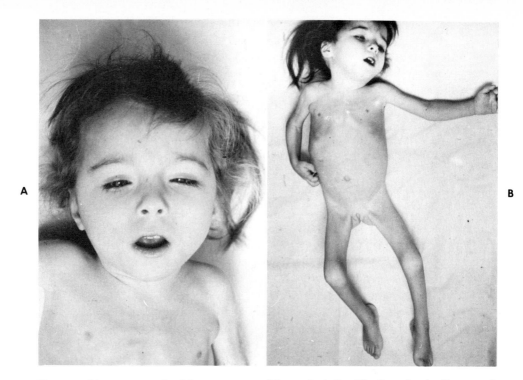

Fig. 5-37. Sixteen-month-old youngster with acute infantile Gaucher's disease. **A,** Facial view showing dull expression, mild cranial retraction, and axillary lymphadenopathy. **B,** Full-body view showing opisthotonos, general body wasting, and protuberant abdomen. Macrocephaly is not present.

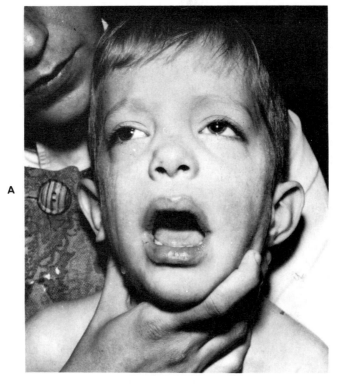

Fig. 5-38. Twenty-month-old patient with infantile metachromatic leukodystrophy. **A,** Full facial view showing macrocephaly, exotropia, and irritability early in disease.

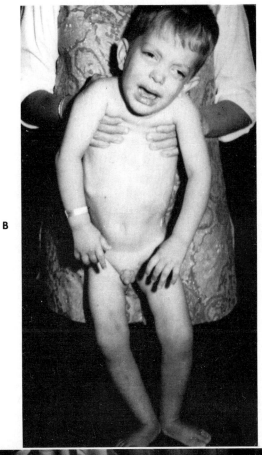

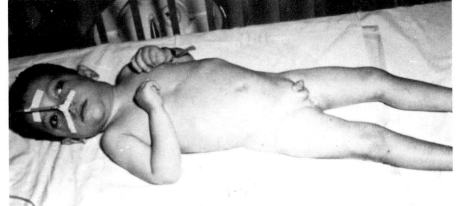

Fig. 5-38, cont'd. B, Frontal body view early in disease process showing cranio-facial stigmata and severe muscular hypotonia. C, Full body view of same patient 3 months later in a terminal stage of the disease. Observe replacement of severe hypotonia with decorticate posturing and spasticity. Relative macrocephaly from megalencephaly is still present.

(Austin and others, 1970; Suzuki and Suzuki, 1970). Although patients with this disease have severe neurologic deficiencies, there are few craniofacial stigmata. (See Chapter 6 and Fig. 6-2.) Megalencephaly is not a characteristic feature of this disease. (The patient in Fig. 6-2 showed mild proptosis, which was a transient sign of functional hyperthyroidism rather than megalencephaly or hydrocephalus with increasing intracranial pressure.)

There is additionally a wide range of diseases that are related to the sphingolipidoses. Mention has been made already of the mucolipidoses and the sialase deficiencies. *Farber's lipogranulomatosis* has few specific facial stigmata but characteristically involves progressively tender and swollen joints, a hoarse and weak cry, and neurologic deterioration (Moser and others, 1969). Persons with this disease are thought to have an inborn error of metabolism related to free ceramide and ganglioside. One patient was reported to have communicating hydrocephalus. *Wolman's xanthomatosis with adrenal involvement* is believed to be caused by acid lipase deficiency. This interesting but rare disorder is not associated with craniofacial abnormalities. Neurologic symptoms and neuropathologic abnormalities per se are not predominant (Wolman and others, 1961). *Tangier disease* is characterized by orange tonsils. The defect is believed to be due to a lipoprotein deficiency (Swaiman, 1975). *Fabry's disease* may involve cutaneous facial lesions, but they more often occur over the body as well. Persons with this disease also have mental deficiency and peripheral neuropathy. None of these rarer sphingolipidoses is actually characterized by megalencephaly.

The sphingolipidoses are grouped together for mainly biochemical rather than clinical reasons. The clinical features vary greatly, from the very typical appearance of a patient with Tay-Sachs disease, to the neurologically normal but severely systemically affected Niemann-Pick patient, to the patient with infantile metachromatic leukodystrophy, and perhaps including grotesquely deformed persons with Hurler's syndrome or absolutely normal-appearing persons with Tangier disease. These diseases involves such a wide range of possible clinical expressions that it is difficult to discuss them in the segmental approach being used in this book. The problem is further complicated by the uncertain relationships of the rarer, incompletely categorized disorders to the more typical ones. In the immediate future the rare disorders may be grouped separately for biochemical reasons.

Megalencephaly, it should be mentioned, is not a characteristic of some of the diseases that have mistakenly been considered to be related to the *amaurotic familial idiocies.* This outdated term, used originally for Tay-Sachs disease, also included the syndromes described by Batten, Mayou, Spielmeyer, Vogt, Sjögren, Bielschowsky, Jansky, Kufs, and Hallervorden, all of which are now more appropriately classified as forms of the neuronal ceroid-lipofuscinoses (Zeman and Dyken, 1969). Most of these syndromes — especially the ones having early onset — are characterized not by macrocephaly but rather by microcephaly.

*Alexander's disease* (megalencephaly associated with hyaline neuropathy) is an infantile-onset, slowly progressive type of leukodystrophy. Pathologically, one finds characteristic abnormalities in the white matter. These abnormalities are hyaline or eosinophilic bodies that appear to represent degenerative products of fibrillary astrocytes (that is, Rosenthal-like fibers) and a severe deficiency of myelin. (See Fig. 5-39.) Not only eosinophilic bodies but also ballooned axons and osmophilic bodies are seen during ultrastructural study.

The intriguing possibility that relationships exist between the mucopolysaccharidoses and the gangliosidoses type of sphingolipidoses suggests the further possibility that a relationship exists between the other leukodystrophies in general and the sphingolipidoses characterized by sulfatide disturbances. (See Fig. 5-40.)

*Canavan's disease* is another rare form of leukodystrophy that has an infantile onset but that generally has a more acute and fulminating downhill course than Alexander's disease. The brain is larger and heavier than normal, but the ventricles, although sometimes large, are never of the size associated with obstructive hydrocephalus. Spongiform changes occur usually at the junction of the lower cerebral cortex and the underlying white matter. This latter finding is the opposite of the situation in Alper's disease, which is invariably associated with microcephaly as a result of giant cystic changes throughout the central nervous system. Megalencephaly in Canavan's disease is usually not as extensive as in Alexander's disease, possibly because the more rapid course of Canavan's disease removes the opportunity for more extensive parenchymal accumulation (Banker and others, 1964).

Closely related, perhaps, to the rare Canavan's disease, which to this juncture is still of uncertain origin, may be *maple syrup urine disease.* This metabolic error of branched, chained amino acid catabolism, is characterized by rapid neurologic deterioration, hypertonia, seizures, and death. Several patients recently have been reported to have survived into childhood with relatively few neurologic residual effects after receiving, early in their lives, diets that are low in branched chained amino acids. In untreated patients, who succumb invariably, the neuropathologic findings are very similar to those in Canavan's disease. Although megalencephaly has not been a consistent clinical feature of maple syrup urine disease, it is intriguing to think of a possible link between the conditions. The patient in Fig. 5-41 is thought to have maple syrup urine disease. He has opisthotonos, cortical thumbs, and irritability but does not have macrocephaly. There are now several variant forms of maple syrup urine disease as well as several closely related abnormalities in amino acid metabolism.

## Macrocephaly resulting from subdural accumulations

The subdural space is an intracranial compartment where expansion potentially can occur. The space is relatively smaller and more limited in the adult than in the newborn, in whom it can become quite large. Var-

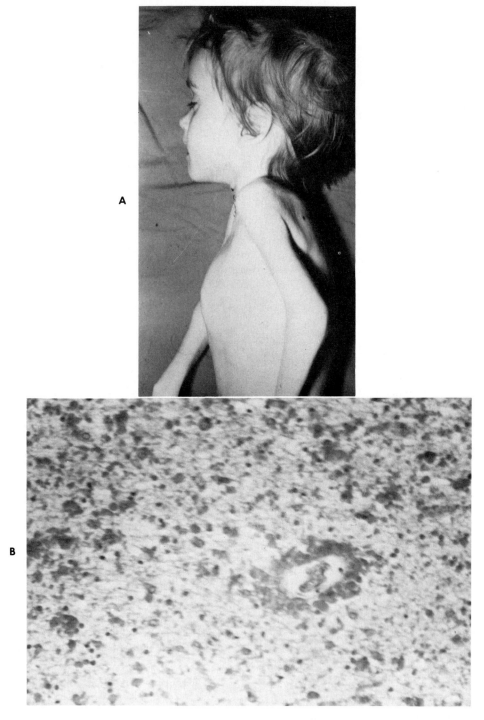

Fig. 5-39. A, Postmortem photograph of 4-year-old child who died after a disease falsely believed to be congenital hydrocephalus. Postmortem examination showed the disorder to be Alexander's type of leukodystrophy. Observe emaciation and macrocephaly. B, Low-power microphotograph of white matter of brain showing numerous Rosenthal fibers or hyaline bodies characteristic of this disease. (Courtesy of Dr. Farivar Yghamai, Medical College of Georgia.)

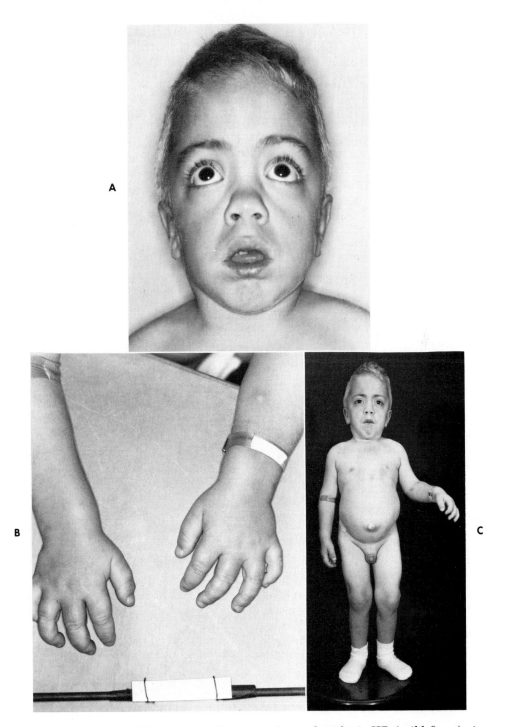

Fig. 5-40. Five-year-old patient with mucopolysaccharidosis IIB (mild form). A, Frontal view showing the mildly coarse facial features of the mucopolysaccharidoses. Observe relative macrocephaly, superciliary hyperplasia, broad nose and lips, and large ear lobule. B, Hands show spade-like features with mild ulnar deviation. C, Full-body view showing other features of mucopolysaccharidoses. (See also Fig. 8-12, C.)

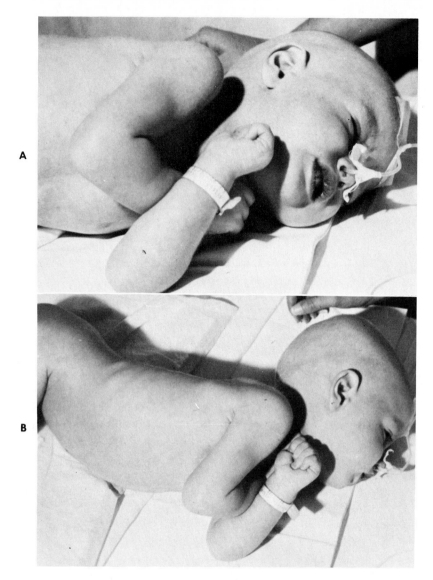

Fig. 5-41. Three-month-old patient with maple syrup urine disease, moderately advanced. A, Close-up view of face and upper torso showing retroflexion of head and irritability. There is no obvious macrocephaly, but the cranium is relatively large. Observe decorticate hand posture. B, Lateral body view showing opisthotonic posturing. This view allows better appreciation of cranial contour and decorticate posturing of upper extremities and hands.

ious types of fluid can accumulate in this space, depending on the pathologic process involved. Although neoplastic tissue can infiltrate the subdural space, as in leukemia and other metastatic neoplasms, this is rare. It has been argued that cerebrospinal fluid may accumulate there after subdural taps, but the accumulation generally consists of blood or pus or a serosanguinous material that is simply called an effusion. The most common causes of subdural fluid accumulation are trauma and infections.

The symptoms of subdural effusions result from pressure being transmitted from the closed, compartmentalized subdural space to either the underlying brain or the overlying skull. This pressure results primarily from the fact that the subdural space does not freely communicate with the other nonneural (that is, osseous) structures of the head (see the explanation of the development of the meninges from the cranial envelope). Which symptoms develop following significant accumulation of fluid in the subdural space depends upon (1) the amount of fluid that accumulates (it is generally assumed that from 1 to 2 ml of fluid may normally exist in the space), (2) the rapidity with which fluid accumulates (the slower the accumulation, the better the organism can compensate for the increasing pressure – especially the pressure on the brain), (3) the type of fluid that accumulates, (4) the age of the person affected, and (5) the type of disease process that causes the accumulation. In chronic subdural hematoma, osmotic factors also may play an important role in the production of symptoms (Rabe, 1967).

The craniofacial abnormalities caused by subdural effusions should be separated into two groups – those related to loss of stimulation or to inhibition of innervation to craniofacial structures ("neurogenic" abnormalities) and those caused by the dysplastic action of long-standing subdural effusion upon the skull ("cranioplastic" abnormalities). The neurogenic abnormalities are important primarily in the more acute, adult-onset, traumatic types of subdural effusion, whereas the cranioplastic abnormalities are important only in chronic, pre – suture-closure periods and therefore in cases involving injuries or other insults in infancy and early childhood. In the still-pliable skull, chronic conditions can produce abnormalities in the size and shape of the cranium that are important in craniofacial diagnosis.

Traumatic subdural fluid accumulations are called hematomas, which may be separated into acute and chronic types according to how much time elapses after the injury before the symptoms appear. The symptoms of *acute subdural hematoma* may occur soon after head trauma, including birth injury. They usually are immediate and take the form of neurogenic lesions. Cranial nerve dysfunctions are common, especially of the trochlear nerve and the oculomotor nerve (see Chapter 6). After the sutures are closed, no cranioplastic abnormalities are seen. In an infant, however, before the sutures are closed, acute subdural hematoma may be associated with a hydrocephalic-like picture that results not only from an effect upon the underlying brain and from cerebral edema, which in turn produces macrocephaly but also from the direct effect of the expanding subdural space on the skull. It is difficult to distinguish the macrocephaly in this situation from the macrocephaly associated with hydrocephalus. Often, in fact, hydrocephalus occurs also.

A *chronic subdural hematoma* usually is not composed of blood at all but rather of a serosanguineous fluid. Trauma is followed by a symptom-free period that varies in length from case to case. This period is shorter in infants than in older children and adults. In the older child and the adult, the symptoms are neurogenic in origin. In the younger child, the infant, and the newborn, on the other hand, a characteristic cranial molding may occur. Chronic subdural hematoma in the infantile and early childhood periods may produce certain changes in the configuration of the skull, especially when, as is often the case, the accumulation of fluid is bilateral. There is a tendency for the cranium to appear square or box-like when viewed from the front or the top (see Fig. 5-42). The transverse distance (width) of the forehead increases because of the tendency of subdural fluid to collect in the anterior cranial compartment (see Fig. 5-43).

*Child abuse* and *child neglect* are frequent causes of chronic subdural hematoma. Abused or neglected children develop other facial stigmata as well. Physically and emotionally neglected young children may exhibit a dull "vacant" stare and show signs of poor hygiene and pallor that suggests anemia. These symptoms may be combined with the square forehead and the boxed cranium to suggest a fairly specific diagnosis. Children with facial and cranial abuse may show other signs of both recent and old injury. Old and recent ecchymoses are common. Hemorrhages into the conjunctiva and the retina are seen, as is dislocation of the lens. The nose may be injured, and deviation of the sep-

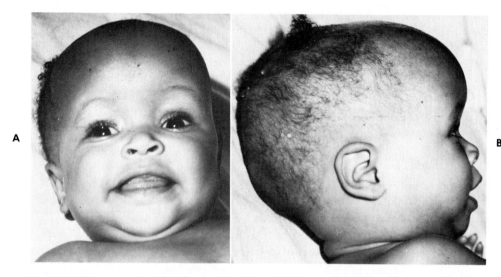

Fig. 5-42. Five-month-old infant with chronic bilateral subdural hematomas secondary to repeated head trauma (child abuse). A, Frontal view showing happy facial expression, broad and bossed forehead, mild right exotropia (observe corneal reflection). B, Lateral view showing macrocephaly. The square contour results from relative frontal protrusion.

tum is often seen. Both acute and chronic ear injuries are common. Patches of baldness, indicative of forceful pulling of the hair, are common signs of abuse in the cranial area. It has recently been pointed out that direct head trauma is not always the cause of chronic subdural hematoma or effusion in infants and children. It is highly probable that violent shaking can produce this type of injury in babies (Caffey, 1974). Since the history of a case of head trauma is difficult to obtain from a parent who, for reasons that may or may not be legitimate, is not willing to discuss the matter, a physician should be constantly on the lookout for this disorder among children with any of the stigmata mentioned.

Another significant cause of subdural effusion, particularly in infants and young children, is the bacterial meningitides, especially those caused by *Hemophilus influenzae*. The postinfectious subdural effusions that result represent a "complication" that occurs very frequently. These effusions generally have the same characteristics as acute and chronic

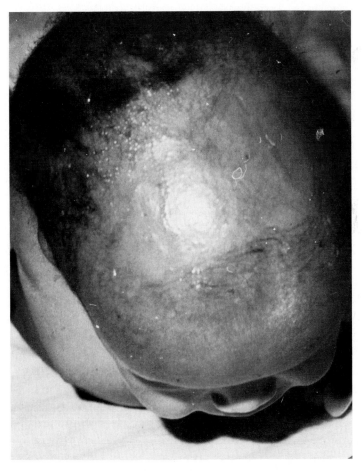

Fig. 5-43. Vertex view of cranium of child in Fig. 5-42, giving further appreciation of the square or rectangular cranial enlargement. Head has been shaven for subdural taps, which had been repeatedly performed on this infant.

subdural hematomas, with some notable exceptions. The subdural space tends to become loculate. Areas of smoldering infection thus occur and require drainage either by subdural taps or, in some instances, by craniectomy.

Rarely, *subdural empyema* may develop following a subdural effusion caused by meningitis. More commonly, however, this condition represents a complication of osteomyelitis of the skull rather than meningitis. The symptoms of subdural empyema are more constitutional than specific. Affected persons are usually very ill and have severe neurologic problems. The disease may be more smoldering than an acute subdural hematoma but still too acute and self-limited to produce cranioplastic defects. Neurogenic abnormalities, however, may be quite obvious.

## SYNDROMES CHARACTERIZED BY MICROCEPHALY
### Anencephaly

Anencephaly is the extreme form of microcephaly. This congenital anomaly is more common than is suspected in clinical medicine, since most affected infants are nonviable and, it is suspected, not reported as cases of anencephaly but simply as abortions or stillbirths. Although it is common for anencephalic infants to be preterm and nonviable, occasionally gestation is of normal length, and the infant lives for a few minutes, hours, or days. The defect is a complicated one. Seldom is there extensive functional neural tissue above the hypothalamus. Usually there are associated abnormalities of the scalp, skull, meninges, and face (see Fig. 5-44). Some of the facial abnormalities are vaguely similar to those seen in the "true" or "pure" form of primary microcephaly. Few clinical studies are available about this malformation. One of us (PRD) had the opportunity to perform detailed neurologic examinations of the anencephalic child in Fig. 5-44. This boy was a term baby and the first-born child of a young mother of low socioeconomic status who came from a large industrialized community in northern Indiana. The patient lived for 6 days after his birth. No systemic abnormalities were discovered, but he had many consistent neurologic abnormalities. All myotatic reflexes were brisk and sustained. Spinal and brainstem reflexes were present, including optic blink, auditory blink, pupillary reflexes, Doll's maneuver, caloric reflexes, and most vestibular reflexes. The somitic muscles appeared hypertrophied and were rigid to passive movement. Sustained tonic postures in decerebration were elicited. The baby showed extreme poikilothermy and hypothermia. There was an unsustained, throaty cry. There was no indication that the patient could hear or see, even though the vegetative visual and auditory responses listed above were present. Sucking and swallowing mechanisms were strong enough to maintain what was assumed to be an adequate caloric intake by mouth. The child was unexpectedly found dead in his crib. An autopsy showed no functional cerebral tissue above the diencephalon.

Study of the face of this patient shows a striking craniofacial picture.

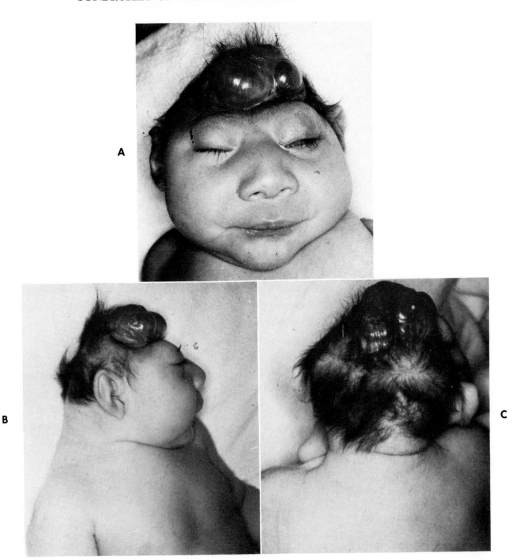

Fig. 5-44. Five-day-old full-term infant with anencephaly. A, Frontal view. Observe cystic mass of cranium, which represents rudiments of skin, subcutaneous tissue, skull meninges, and brain. The face appears abnormal, but ears, eyes, nose, and mouth are reasonably well formed. These structures appear large because of the smallness of what should have been the cranial vault. There is a mongoloid slant to the palpebral fissures. B, Lateral view. C, Posterior view.

The cystic mass over the vertex of the cranium represents the rudiments of the cerebral hemispheres. No bony elements cover the mass, although skin and cranial hair extend to the base of the lesion. One of the most striking abnormalities is the disproportion between the cranium and the face. The face appears large in the photograph but in reality is smaller than normal for infants of this age. The eyes are close-set and appear larger than normal. There is a mongoloid slant to the palpebral fissures.

The forehead is low and narrow and recedes sharply. The ears seem to be high but actually are normally placed. The nose seems broad and long, but this impression also is essentially an optical illusion resulting from the smallness of the cranium. These same features are present, although less pronounced, in the patient in Fig. 5-45, who has "pure" primary microcephaly.

### Primary microcephalies

Primary, pure, or *true microcephaly* is unexplained microcephaly that is not accompanied by other major malformations or anomalies. The condition has a genetic implication and has been reported as being both autosomal and sex-linked and both recessive and dominant (Kloepfer and others, 1964). In some instances mental retardation is not as pronounced as the degree of cranial smallness might suggest. As with anencephaly, the most striking physical characteristic is the contrast between the small size of the cranium and the normal size of the face (see Fig. 5-45). The forehead is low, narrow, and receding. In contrast, the eyebrows, the eyebrow ridges, the orbits, the nose, the mouth, and the ears are usually normal in size. The vertex thus seems pointed. The occiput is often flattened.

Usually the condition is evident at birth. After full growth, affected persons frequently are small in height and weight and in various body parts. Mental retardation is common, but there is no direct correlation between cranial size and mental functioning abilities. There may be

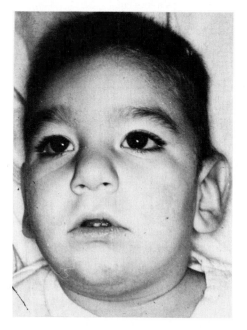

Fig. 5-45. Moderately retarded patient with primary familial microcephaly. Note shortened forehead and illusion of large face.

many neurologic symptoms and signs, especially in later life. These include a variety of cranial nerve dysfunctions, aphasia, autistic behavior reactions, spasticity, choreoathetosis, hyperreflexia, and other major dysfunctions (MacGillivray, 1967).

Another type of primary microcephaly was described by Seckel (1960) and has since come to be called *Seckel's bird-headed dwarfism.* Seckel described two children who had extreme primary microcephaly, short stature, prominent eyes, beak-like noses, narrow faces, and small chins. The term nanocephalic dwarfism has also been used to describe the syndrome. Since the original description, several other patients with similar symptoms have been reported (Harper and others, 1967). There is a wide range of associated anomalies in the reported cases. They vary from nanocephaly and dwarfism to skeletal and urogenital defects.

Some patients with Seckel's bird-headed dwarfism have severe mental retardation and limited speech abilities and are unable to care for themselves. Others have been reported to have intelligence quotients as high as 80 (Mann and Russell, 1959). Seizures have been seen in several patients. Patients with this syndrome have been reported to live as long as 75 years. The presence of similarly affected siblings in several families has suggested an autosomal recessive inheritance. Figs. 5-46 and 5-47, *A*, show two unrelated patients with the syndrome. In Fig. 5-47,

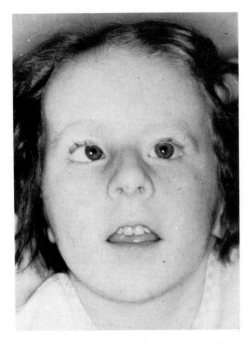

**Fig. 5-46.** Nine-year-old patient with severe dwarfism, refractive seizure disorder, severe mental retardation, heterotropia (right esotropia), microcephaly, and birdlike facial features presumed to indicate Seckel's bird-headed dwarfism.

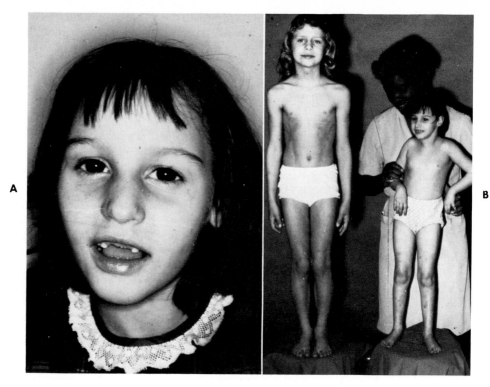

Fig. 5-47. Eight-year-old patient with Seckel's bird-headed dwarfism. A, Frontal view showing microcephaly and dainty and sharp facial features. B, Full-body view in which patient is compared to normal female child of same age. The bird-like facial features and the microcephaly are especially evident in this photograph.

*B*, the size of a severely affected patient is compared to that of a normal child of the same age. Note the narrow, bird-like face and the microcephaly. The nose tends to be long and beak-like.

The term lissencephaly, or "smooth brain," refers to a pathologic condition in which the gyri are wide and the sulci are shallow and narrow. In severe cases, both the gyri and the sulci are absent. It was pointed out by Dieker and associates (1969) that some of the patients who were discovered, during autopsies, to have this disorder seemed to have a fairly characteristic and consistent syndrome during life. The syndrome was named the *lissencephalic syndrome*. Its most characteristic feature is microcephaly. In addition, affected patients have hollowed-out temporal areas, wrinkled and hirsute facial skin, and a slanting low or high forehead with eyebrows tilted medially to give a ferret-like appearance to the face. Micrognathia is common, and the ears are usually low-set or tilted posteriorly because of deficient cartilage. Polydactyly has been reported. Infants with the syndrome are always severely affected neurologically from the earliest moments of life. At first hypotonia and weakness predominate, but later hypertonic rigidity and opisthotonos become prevalent. Psychomotor development is poor. Seizures of many types occur and are refractory to usual treatments. Electroencephalography may show a "hypsarrhythmic" pattern. All infants with the syndrome have died within the first year of life. Their lives are characterized by poor vegetative functions and severe failure to thrive. The syndrome may be inherited as an autosomal recessive trait.

Cockayne (1936) described a sibling pair, both of whom had dwarfism, microcephaly, mental retardation, abnormal retinal pigmentation, optic atrophy, exposure dermatitis, and progressive neurologic deterioration. Persons having this constellation of signs, known as *Cockayne's syndrome*, may appear normal at birth. They have gradual loss of subcutaneous fat, which first occurs in later infancy and childhood. Older patients have a senile appearance, with sunken eyes and prominence of the maxilla and nose. Eye abnormalities are common, especially in later life, and include, besides the characteristic sunken eyes, blindness, optic atrophy, pigmentary retinal degeneration, cataracts, and nystagmus. Gonadal dysfunction occurs commonly. A variety of skeletal deformities is usually present, including stooped posture, kyphosis, long arms and legs, and shortened trunk. The hands and feet seem disproportionately large. Scaly, erythematous dermatitis is especially prominent after exposure to the sun. All patients show subcutaneous atrophy and thinness.

The microcephaly may be one of the most prominent features. Psychomotor development is slow and mental deficiency is marked. Most intelligence quotients are below 50. Slow deterioration in mental and motor functioning appears (usually in the second decade), and nystagmus, ataxia, intention tremor, incoordination, reflex changes, blindness, and deafness are evident. It is believed this syndrome may represent a sudanophilic leukodystrophy. (See Chapters 6 and 8.)

## Secondary microcephalies

Secondary microcephaly is associated with an apparent cause, as opposed to primary microcephaly, which does not have an apparent cause. There are a host of environmental factors, acquired conditions, and hereditary disorders associated with secondary microcephaly.

The causes of microcephaly are many and include almost any brain insult that occurs in the major formative and growth phases of the brain, whether it be in prenatal, perinatal, or postnatal periods. An important prenatal factor is intrauterine infections such as those resulting from the so-called TORCH encephalopathies. (TORCH is an acronym for toxoplasmosis, rubella, cytomegalovirus, herpes simplex, and "other" in utero infections.) In addition, insults to the fetal brain that can produce secondary microcephaly have been associated with maternal phenylketonuria, radiation, and exposure to a variety of toxins including some medications and substances previously considered harmless, such as anticonvulsants and alcohol. (See the discussion of the fetal alcohol syndrome in Chapter 6.) Other important perinatal insults that produce microcephaly are related to the circumstances of birth, such as perinatal anoxia and birth trauma. True phenylketonuria, neonatal infection, infantile exposure to toxins, malnutrition, and many other conditions also may inhibit brain growth and thus cause microcephaly. Head trauma—especially when it is repetitive, as in *child abuse and neglect*—is an important cause of microcephaly. Various chromosome defects and abnormalities also are important causes of secondary microcephaly, with the most important example being Down's syndrome, or trisomy 21. In time, many of the hereditary microcephalies probably will be more appropriately placed in the secondary microcephaly category. The cause of the decreased brain growth and formation in these syndromes, however, is uncertain, and until such time that it is known, these syndromes generally will continue to be classified as primary microcephaly. This reasoning also holds true for most of the microcephalies that are not associated with chromosome defects. Such microcephalies are referred to as forms of "cerebral dysgenesis." (See Fig. 5-48.)

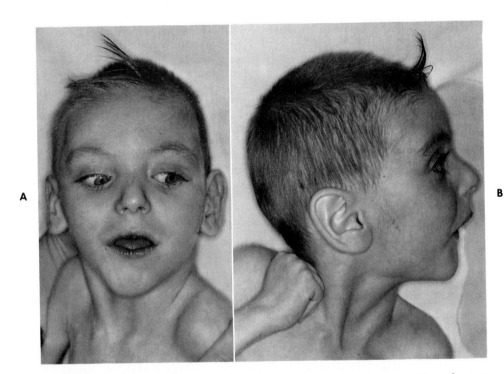

Fig. 5-48. Patient with early-onset disorder involving slow degeneration of neurologic functions, which autopsy showed to be the rare central nervous system disease called opticocochleodentatic degeneration. A, Frontal facial view. Observe features of severe "secondary" microcephaly. B, Lateral view. (Another patient with this disorder is shown in Fig. 8-34. See also Fig. 6-66.)

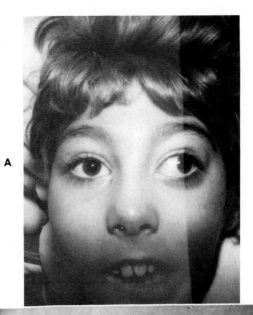

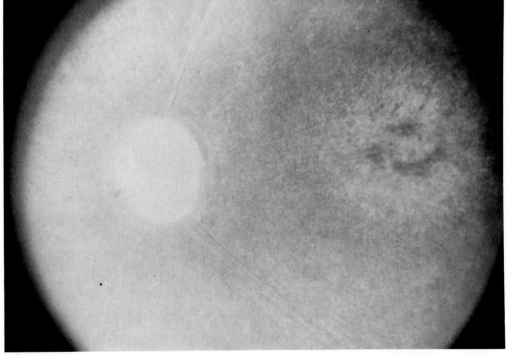

Fig. 5-49. Severely retarded and debilitated patient in her twenties who has congenital toxoplasmosis. A, Note microcephaly and pronounced left exotropia. B, Funduscopic photograph showing mild "salt and pepper" changes in the paramacular region (on the right) and optic atrophy and attentuated retinal vessels (on the left). These findings are compatible with an old chorioretinitis, as is typically seen in congenital toxoplasmosis. Skull x-ray film showed that this patient also had many periventricular calcifications.

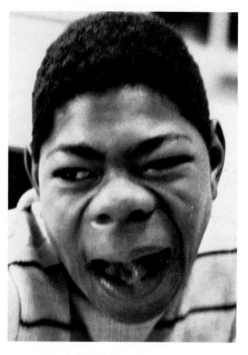

Fig. 5-50. Severely retarded and debilitated patient in his twenties who suffered from perinatal cerebral hypoxia. He has spastic quadriparesis, secondary microcephalic features, and severe exotropia on the right.

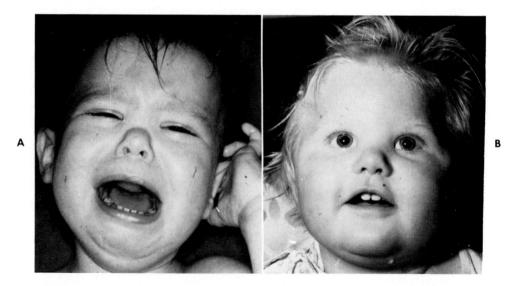

Fig. 5-51. Two infants with untreated phenylketonuria. A, Three-month-old showing extreme irritability but no other specific facial or cranial stigmata. B, Seven-month-old showing placidity and a reasonably alert facial countenance. Observe hypopigmentation, as well as eczema over one cheek.

*Congenital toxoplasmosis* was once considered to be the most common of the congenital TORCH encephalopathies. The effect on the brain results from the infestation of the fetus with *Toxoplasma gondii.* One sees a devastating meningoencephalitis with severe granulomatous and necrotic changes. These spotty but extensive patches of severe brain damage are associated with calcification, which may show up on skull x-ray films. Characteristically, the organism also affects the retina and produces a rather extensive chorioretinitis. (See Fig. 5-49, *B.*) Another preferred site of the organism is the reticuloendothelial system, especially the liver. The effect on the individual depends, of course, on the severity and the extent of the infection. Mortality in the neonatal period is high, and, if the patient survives, morbidity is also high. Persons who survive are often severely neurologically handicapped.

*Hypoxic encephalopathy* may produce severe dysfunction of the central nervous system and marked growth failure—especially of the more rostral part of the brain, which is responsible for cranial growth. Microcephaly is therefore one of the most common signs of perinatal anoxia.

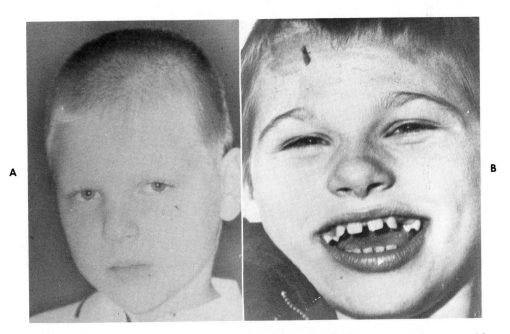

A                                                                                          B

Fig. 5-52. Two children with partially treated phenylketonuria. **A,** Five-year-old with mild facial dullness. This patient, along with an identical twin, was hyperactive and moderately mentally retarded in spite of having had a phenylalanine-restricted diet from early in infancy. Observe hypopigmentation. No microcephaly is present yet. (His identical twin is shown in Fig. 8-16, *B.*) **B,** Eight-year-old child with moderate mental retardation and severe hyperactivity requiring chronic hospitalization. He appears pleasant but was extremely aggressive and self-mutilatory. Observe abrasion on forehead and mild suggestion of microcephaly. Teeth are small and widely spaced. Patient is relatively hypopigmented in comparison to other family members, who are not affected.

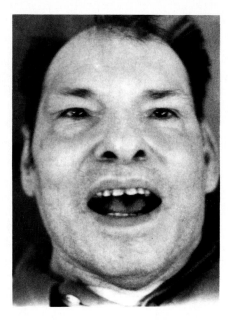

Fig. 5-53. Thirty-nine–year–old patient with trisomy 21. Observe the microcephaly, which is more obvious because of the baldness. Other facial features of Down's syndrome also are present.

Very often there is a wide variety of other neurologic symptoms such as spasticity, rigidity, cranial nerve dysfunctions, choreoathetosis, paresis, paralysis, hyperreflexia, hypotonia, mental retardation, and seizure activity. (See the example of a severely microcephalic patient in Fig. 5-50.)

Both the inborn error of metabolism called phenylketonuria, which is characterized by phenylalanine hydroxylase deficiency, and a non-enzymatic form of this disease called *maternal phenylketonuria* are associated with microcephaly. In the former condition the microcephaly usually is not evident at birth, but in the latter condition it frequently is. Both conditions in time are associated with microcephaly, but seldom of the severity found in other brain devastations mentioned previously. It has been estimated that only about 50% of untreated phenylketonuric (PKU) patients have microcephaly. (See Fig. 5-51.) Fig. 5-52 shows two PKU patients, one with microcephaly and the other without. Trisomy 21 characteristically is associated with microcephaly, as can be seen in Fig. 5-53. DeLange's syndrome (see Chapter 6) may also show a profound degree of microcephaly.

## SYNDROMES CHARACTERIZED BY ABNORMALITIES OF THE HAIR
### Baldness and alopecia

Baldness is so common that it probably would best be considered a normal variant of the aging process in males. Yet certain types of bald-

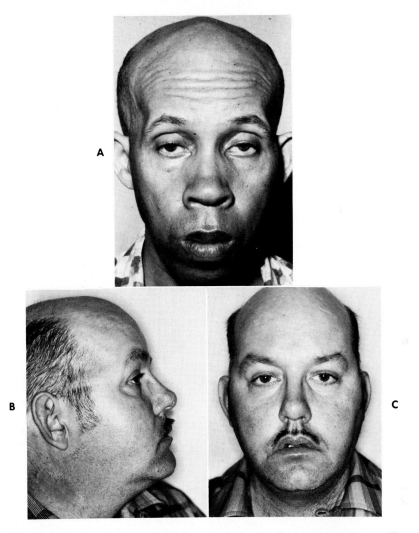

Fig. 5-54. Two male patients with classical dystrophia myotonica. A, Twenty-five–year–old. Observe the frontal baldness, temporal atrophy, bilateral ptosis, flattened lower face, pursed lips, and sagging jaw, which produce the illusion of a long facies. B, Lateral view of 32-year-old patient with dystrophia myotonica. Note the neck musculature wasting. C, Frontal view of patient in B. Note the sneering upper lip as well as other facial and nuchal abnormalities.

ness have diagnostic significance. Frontal baldness, as seen characteristically in *dystrophia myotonica*, probably is related to the multiple endocrinopathies seen so typically in this disease. Although the frontal baldness that is clearly evident in the two patients in Fig. 5-54 is seen more often in males with dystrophia myotonica, it is also seen (although rarely) in females with the disease. Besides the endocrinopathic basis for this disease, it is probable that skin and hair follicles are also abnormal. Dystrophia myotonica will be discussed in more detail in subsequent chapters of this book.

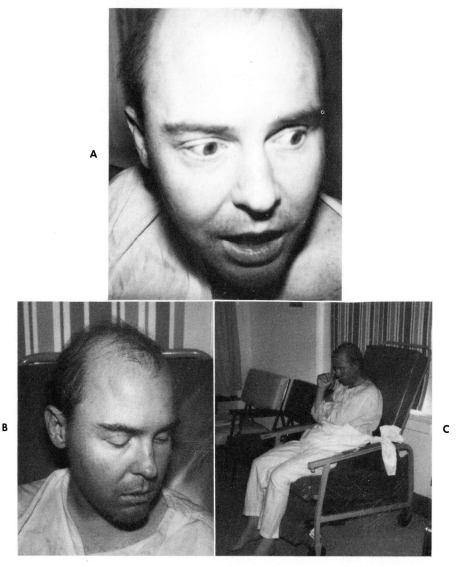

Fig. 5-55. Twenty-six–year–old patient with the clinical features of the Klüver-Bucy syndrome of docility, hypersexual behavior, polyphagia, and "psychic" blindness. All symptoms began 2 to 3 years before these photographs were taken and were progressive and coexistent with alopecia universalis. A, Close-up view showing frightened and demented facial expression. Note alopecia. B, Cranial view of distribution of alopecia. Hair was fine and had no histologic abnormalities. C, Full-body view. Patient had to be restrained because of abnormal behavior but was docile when undisturbed.

More commonly related to a variety of syndromes are the various forms of alopecia. Both *ectodermal dysplasia* and the *Hallermann-Streiff syndrome* are characterized by hypotrichosis if not frank alopecia. The *Hutchinson-Gilford type of progeria,* on the other hand, is often associated with true alopecia – that is, universal loss of cranial as well as somatic hair. The *syndrome of congenital absence of cranial skin* is usually associated with patchy alopecia, whereas *alopecia areata with mental disturbances* involves more universal cranial hair alopecia. A recently seen patient had a long history of alopecia universalis and also showed slowly progressive dementia and signs and symptoms suggesting the *Klüver-Bucy syndrome.* This patient's mental behavior was quite similar to that of persons with progressive lesions of the hypothalamus, deep temporal lobes, and limbic system. No identified toxic, vascular, or neoplastic lesion was discovered during a thorough investigation (Fig. 5-55). The hair was normal histologically.

Chronic exposure to a wide variety of toxic substances may produce loss of hair. Almost all *heavy metal poisonings* – but particularly those involving arsenic, lead, and cadmium – may have this effect. Seldom are these toxic forms of alopecia limited to the cranium, however. *Menkes' kinky hair syndrome,* now believed to result from an intrinsic disturbance in copper metabolism, is characterized by cranial hair changes of a specific type. *Monilethrix* also involves cranial alopecia. *Argininosuccinicaciduria,* an aminoacidopathy, frequently is associated with alopecia.

Patchy loss of hair related to mechanical causes seems to be related to *Albright's hereditary osteodystrophy* and *idiopathic hypoparathyroidism.* The exact reason is uncertain, but affected patients tend to purposely pull out patches of cranial hair. Loss of cranial hair is likewise not uncommon in cases of *child abuse.*

Selective loss of eyebrows characterizes lepromatous leprosy (see Fig. 5-56.)

## Facial hirsutism

Women with too much facial hair sometimes go to great expense to eliminate it. Facial hair in women is not necessarily an abnormality. Pathologic facial hirsutism, however, characterizes several syndromes. In *DeLange's syndrome,* one of the prototype facial hirsutism syndromes, hair is particularly obvious on the forehead and between the brows. Another common site of excessive hair in this syndrome is the back. (See Fig. 5-57). Excessive facial hair is also seen frequently in the classic forms of the *mucopolysaccharidoses,* namely the Hurler, Hunter, and Sanfilippo types (MPS, IH, IH/S, IS, II, and III). One of the more common examples of excessive facial hair is seen in epileptic patients who are receiving *phenytoin treatment.* A fairly rare syndrome associated with excessive facial hair is *Waterman's syndrome* (see Chapter 7). Many patients with *neuronal ceroid-lipofuscinosis* have pathologic facial and

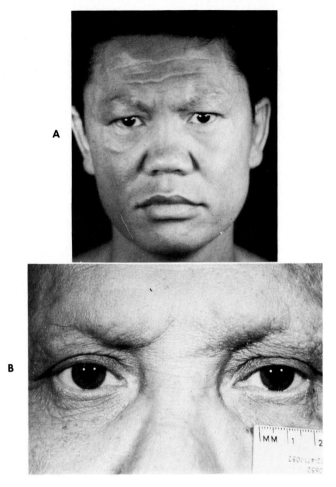

Fig. 5-56. **A,** Patient with lepromatous leprosy and diffuse infiltration of facial skin. Note alopecia of eyebrows and lashes caused by infiltration of skin appendages by cells containing *Mycobacterium leprae.* **B,** Another patient with lepromatous leprosy. Note puffiness of skin over supraorbital ridges and alopecia of brows and lashes, resulting from infiltration with *Mycobacterium leprae.* (Courtesy of United States Public Health Service Hospital, Carville, Louisiana, and Dr. Thomas Swift, Medical College of Georgia.)

somatic hirsutism. The *dementia-emaciation syndrome* (discussed in Chapter 8) is characterized by excessive facial and somatic hair (see Fig. 5-58). The *lissencephalic syndrome,* the *N syndrome, Donohue's syndrome,* and *hypertrichosis universalis congenita* are also characterized by facial and body hirsutism.

## Cranial poliosis and white forelocks

Poliosis—streaky abnormal hypopigmentation of hair—or the broader white forelock may be seen in *craniofacial leukoderma, Waardenburg's syndrome, vitiligo, tuberous sclerosis, neuronal ceroid-lipofuscinosis,*

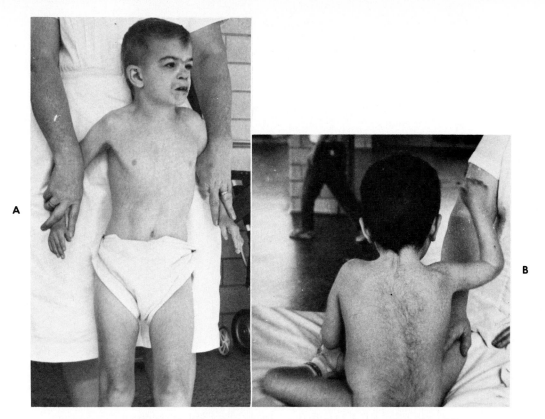

Fig. 5-57. Two patients with DeLange's syndrome. A, Eighteen-year-old severely mentally retarded and dwarfed patient. Observe the severe facial hirsutism, midline eyebrow, microcephaly, pinched and small nose, macrosomatia, and small hands with hypothenar atrophy. B, Severely dwarfed and mentally deficient 17-year-old who has the pronounced body hirsutism typical of this syndrome.

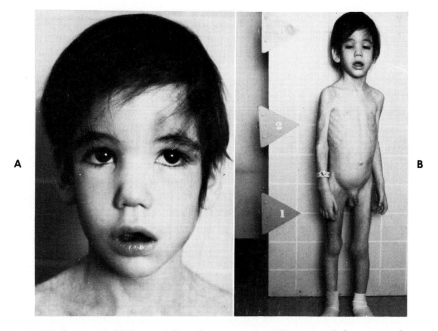

Fig. 5-58. Eight-year-old boy with a degenerative disease of the central nervous system called the dementia-emaciation syndrome. (See also Fig. 8-14.) A, Facial view showing hirsutism, subcutaneous atrophy, and dull expression. B, Full body view showing universal hirsutism and severe emaciation.

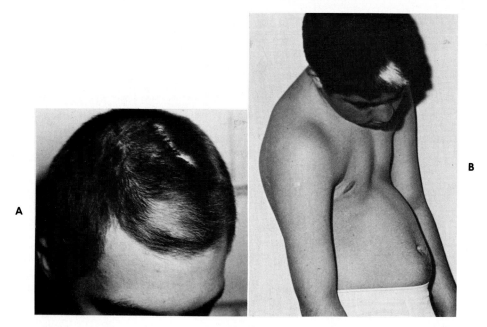

Fig. 5-59. Two patients with craniofacial leukoderma with distribution behind the hairline. A, Twenty-year-old patient with trisomy 21. White hair is growing from the congenital patch of white skin. B, Sixteen-year-old patient with many stigmata of Waardenburg's syndrome, including medial eyebrow hyperplasia, widely spaced eyeballs, and white forelock. The leukoderma is totally behind the hairline on the patient's right side. This patient also had moderate mental retardation and recurrent spasms as an infant. He was mistakenly diagnosed as having tuberous sclerosis, even though he had no adenoma sebaceum or other more diagnostic features of that disorder. (See also Fig. 6-84.)

*Turner's syndrome, phenylketonuria,* various forms of *partial albinism, Sanfilippo's type of mucopolysaccharidosis,* and many varieties of *progeria.* (See Fig. 5-59.)

## CRANIAL NEUROCUTANEOPATHIES

There is a large group of neurocutaneous diseases that affect the upper facial and cranial segment, the most frequently encountered of which is *Sturge-Weber syndrome.* The skin manifestation of this syndrome (that is, the nevus flammeus), however, seldom involves only the upper facial and cranial segment and therefore will be discussed in more detail in chapters to follow. A variation of this syndrome involves a port wine nevus flammeus in the midline of the upper face and cranium. This variation may also be associated with severe telangiectatic lesions of the conjunctiva and the midbrain. (See Fig. 5-60.) A less common cranial neurocutaneopathy is congenital absence of cranial skin as seen in

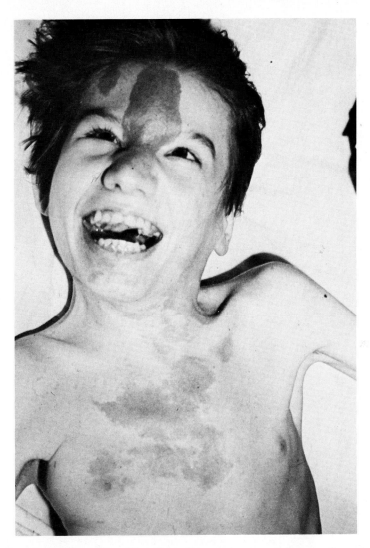

Fig. 5-60. Patient with midline-distributed port wine type of nevus flammeus. This patient was severely debilitated, mentally retarded, and quadriplegic. The nevus appears extensively on the body and spottily on the face. A telangiectatic conjunctival lesion was present in the right eye and extended into the retina and presumably into the mesencephalon. (See also Fig. 6-36.)

Fig. 5-61. Another commonly encountered neurocutaneous disease with cranial involvement is *tuberous sclerosis* (Fig. 5-62), which, however, more frequently involves the middle face. In this disease certain cutaneous lesions, though, characteristically involve the cranium and upper face. One is called a "leather patch" or a cranial shagreen patch (see Fig. 5-64, *A*). This hyperplastic skin mark usually does not involve the underlying tissue. It is often fleshy and easily movable although rough.

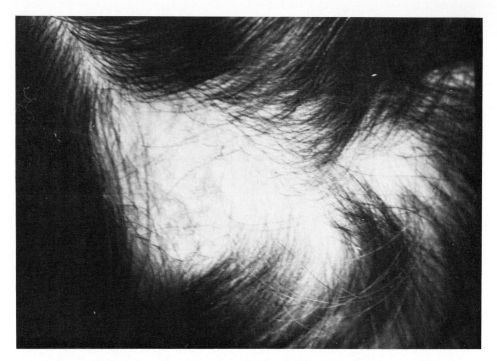

Fig. 5-61. Close-up view of patient with congenital absence of cranial skin in the left parietal region. The lesion, which is depressed and slightly hyperpigmented, is associated with mild atrophy of the underlying subcutaneous tissue and bone. This 5-year-old patient was mentally retarded and had right focal motor seizures. Electroencephalography showed a spike focus originating from an area of the brain contiguous to this skin lesion.

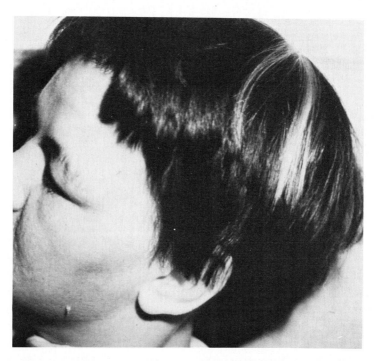

Fig. 5-62. Institutionalized woman in her fifties who has tuberous sclerosis. Note streaks of poliosis in parietal area, Balzer-type adenoma sebaceum, and scarring of upper eyelid and forehead from repeated cranial trauma secondary to seizures.

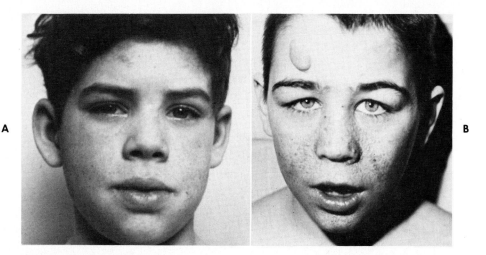

Fig. 5-63. Two patients with tuberous sclerosis. A, Eight-year-old patient, with specific learning disabilities but without mental retardation, who had seizures, adenoma sebaceum, and other cutaneous lesions of tuberous sclerosis. Observe the mild angiofibromas in the malar region and the asymmetrical sharkskin patches on the right side of the forehead. B, Twelve-year-old mentally retarded patient. Observe the even distribution of the angiofibromas over the malar region in contrast to the large, asymmetrically located fleshy lipofibroma on the right of the forehead.

Another closely related skin lesion associated occasionally with tuberous sclerosis is fibrous dysplasia. This lesion involves skin, subcutaneous tissue, and skull (see Figs. 5-63 and 5-64). Such skin lesions have also been associated with *Albright's polyostotic fibrous dysplasia* (which has more systemic involvement) and *neurofibromatosis.* Associated with leukoderma of the upper facial and cranial segment is the condition called *craniofacial leukoderma,* although the variant originally described by Sugarman and Reed (1969) involved mainly the middle face. We have encountered several forms of craniofacial leukoderma involving all three facial segments. Craniofacial leukoderma seems related to a high incidence of mental retardation and seizure disorders.

We have seen upper facial and cranial leukoderma in the *dysmigration syndrome,* which is associated with trisomy 21 (see Chapter 6), as well as in *Waardenburg's syndrome.* The latter is usually characterized by a white lock of hair, but seldom is the forehead itself involved. There are also other characteristic features of this syndrome.

Coup de sabre is believed by some to be a linear, more confined type of Parry-Romberg syndrome (Peskova and Stockar, 1961). The disorder consists, at first, of a linear skin lesion that may be congenital. Later the lesion may be progressive, with subcutaneous involvement and then involvement of underlying tissues, including the bones and muscles. Coup de sabre appears to be related in some fashion to a chronic or subacute inflammatory process and could be a manifestation of an unusual auto-

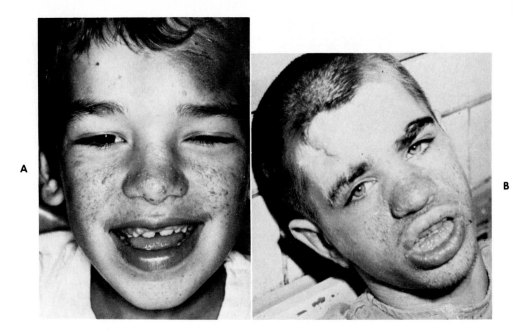

Fig. 5-64. Two patients with tuberous sclerosis. A, Eight-year-old patient. Observe extensive, evenly distributed angiofibroma of middle face and large hyperpigmented sharkskin lesion of left forehead, producing asymmetry of palpebral fissures. Leather patch is extensive and overlies a large osseous fibrous dysplasia of the frontal bone of the skull. Observe gum hyperplasia resulting from phenytoin therapy. B, Seventeen-year-old institutionalized patient. Observe large osseous fibrous dysplasia of right forehead as well as other characteristic facial stigmata of tuberous sclerosis.

immune phenomenon, as may be taking place in the collagen diseases. Other entities that are very closely related to coup de sabre, if they are not the same disease, are linear scleroderma of the face and the extremities and hemifacial atrophy. These disorders have progressions similar to that of coup de sabre. Characteristically, at least in the syndromes limited to the upper facial and cranial segment, the skin lesion begins close to the midline as a slightly pigmented and slightly depressed mark with a linear distribution. This mark looks and feels very much like a scar from a sabre slash. The cutaneous lesion progresses and next involves the underlying subcutaneous tissue. Although remissions can occur at any point in this course of development, all lesions are potentially unrelenting. There is a tendency for cranial extension to occur, at which time bone destruction usually occurs. The syndrome can be very deforming. In addition, severe neurologic manifestations may develop, such as focal motor and sensory deficits and focal seizures that are contralateral to the side of maximum involvement if the lesion extends over the cranial hemisphere. Besides coup de sabre, the patient in Fig. 5-65

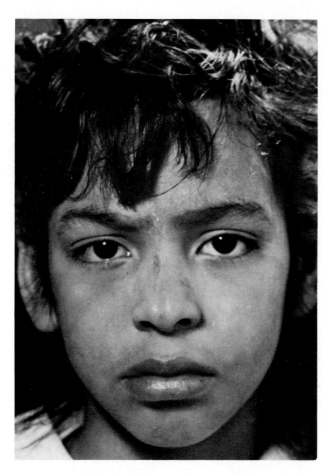

Fig. 5-65. Thirteen-year-old girl with complex syndrome consisting of recently acquired polyarthritis, leukopenia, recurrent pleural effusions, positive lupus erythematosus cell preparations, antinuclear antibodies, and left focal motor seizures. She was born with a thin midline scar extending from the tip of her nose to the forehead. As she grew, this lesion became more extensive and tended to mushroom in the right forehead and frontal region. Atrophic changes in the skin, subcutaneous tissues, and bone were evident by the time this photograph was taken. Observe the anterior limits of the slightly hyperpigmented, scarified linear lesion, which was believed to indicate coup de sabre or Parry-Romberg syndrome. (See also Fig. 6-78.)

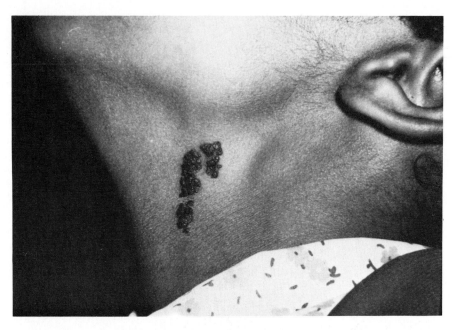

**Fig. 5-66.** Small, linear, organoid nevus located in the submandibular region on the right in a patient with mild mental retardation and idiopathic generalized tonic-clonic seizures. The patient is 8 years old and has no other cutaneous lesions. This organoid nevus is of the type called the linear sebaceus nevus of Jadassohn. When distributed in the upper facial and cranial segment, this lesion is usually associated with severe mental retardation and recurrent, refractory seizures, as described by Feuerstein and Mims.

also had symptoms of systemic lupus erythematosus, which was confirmed by appropriate laboratory examination.

Probably closely related to coup de sabre is the *linear sebaceous nevus of Jadassohn* (Holden and DeKaban, 1972). This skin lesion, limited to the face, has been described in patients with convulsions and mental retardation (see Fig. 5-66). These lesions are also called organoid nevi. Nevi are present at birth and begin usually as yellow-orange papules that become patches or linear streaks, especially when formed in the middle of the forehead. Similar in distribution to coup de sabre, the organoid nevi may extend down to the tip of the nose or up to the cranial vault. They are usually associated with alopecia. Unlike coup de sabre, these lesions involve thickening and hyperplasia of the epidermis and hyperplasia of the sebaceous glands, as shown by biopsy. In coup de sabre one sees more atrophic and mildly inflammatory changes. It has been determined that patients with the nevus of Jadassohn usually, but not always, are mentally retarded. Seizures may occur in the first months

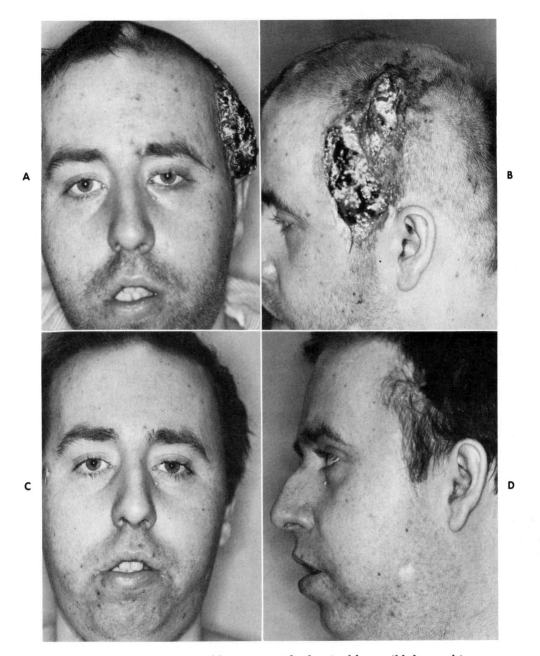

**Fig. 5-67.** Twenty-two–year–old patient with classical but mild dystrophia myotonica. **A,** Facial view of patient prior to operation to remove calcifying epithelioma from the left frontal-temporal region of the scalp. Observe mild facial stigmata of dystrophia myotonica, including facial diparesis, bilateral mild ptosis, and dull facial expression. **B,** Lateral view showing the calcifying epithelioma, which is a loculated, seeping lesion. **C,** Facial view of patient 6 months after photographs in A and B, after removal of epithelioma. Facial stigmata of dystrophia myotonica have not changed. **D,** Lateral postoperative view.

of life. One patient had severe unilateral cortical atrophy on the side of the skin lesion.

*Calcifying epitheliomas* are benign but disfiguring neoplasms of the skin that recently have been shown to be related to dystrophia myotonica (see Fig. 5-67).

# CHAPTER SIX

# Syndromes of the middle facial segment

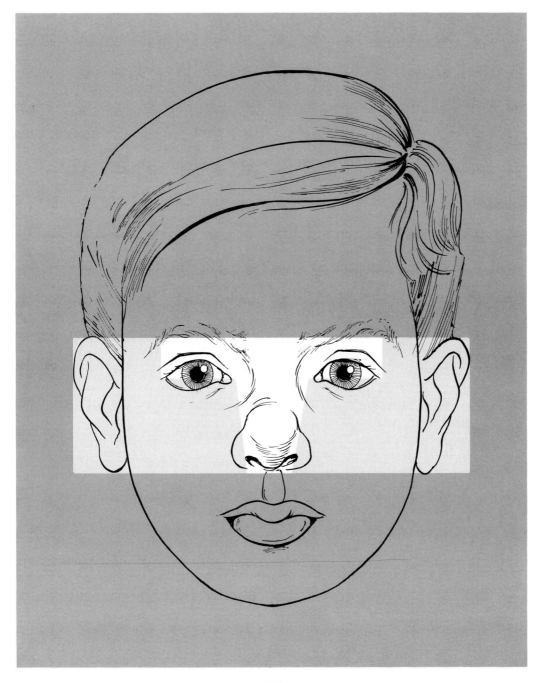

This chapter will discuss some of the more important syndromes and diseases affecting the middle face, which is delineated superiorly by the browline and inferiorly by the nasal line. The middle facial segment, which includes many important anatomic structures, usually is a focus of attention for diagnosticians as well as for the casual facial viewer. Since the syndromes involving abnormalities in this portion of the face are many, we will make no attempt to be comprehensive and will limit discussion to syndromes of greatest incidence, importance, or interest. In general, the outline followed in Chapter 3 will also be used in this chapter.

## SYNDROMES OF THE CENTRAL MIDDLE FACE
### Syndromes characterized by ocular protrusion and abnormal ocular size

Exophthalmos and proptosis are terms that many physicians have used interchangeably. We will often distinguish between the two here, however. The term exophthalmos (literally "out eyes" condition) will be used to refer to conditions that are usually fairly symmetrical and that are often associated with metabolic dysfunctions. We will use the term proptosis to mean an asymmetrical or even unilateral abnormality that is often associated with nonmetabolic disturbances.

**Exophthalmos.** Hyperthyroidism is a condition that results from excessive secretion of hormones by the thyroid gland. These hormones result in an increased rate of oxidation in tissues, disturbances in the nervous system, and other metabolic effects. Excessive secretion of thyroid hormone is frequently associated with exophthalmos and/or other ocular abnormalities. In general, hyperthyroidism seems to occur most often in females in early childhood. The condition may be exacerbated by puberty and pregnancy. In children especially, acute infections of the upper respiratory tract and tonsillitis may precede the development of the hyperthyroid state. Hyperthyroidism occurs in many instances as a normal response to the environment and to the stresses of life. The essential features of the pathologic state, known as *Graves' disease*, result not from the hyperthyroid state per se but from the continuity of hyperthyroidism over extended periods of time, even after the triggering factors that produce stress hyprethyroidism have long since been removed or controlled. The credit for the first descriptions of sustained hyperthyroidism is appropriately given to the great Irish surgeon Robert Graves (Graves, 1835). Dr. Graves was a generalist who contributed to the fields of clinical neurology, general surgery, and endocrinology. A close relationship is thought to exist between thyrotoxicosis and pituitary disturbances such as acromegaly. Exophthalmos, for example, can be produced by thyrotrophic hormone secreted by the pituitary gland and may be secondary to some purely neurologic diseases (Guyton, 1971, p. 911).

From this brief discussion it is clear that constitutional and systemic features usually herald hyperthyroidism, which can be triggered by many factors including trauma, infection, and other physical or psychic insults. Occasionally, however, the disease begins without recognizable precipitating factors. The initial symptoms usually include loss of weight and strength, fatigue, restlessness, intolerance to heat, profuse sweating, cardiac palpitation, irritability, hoarseness, difficulty in swallowing, oligomenorrhea or amenorrhea, vomiting, and diarrhea. Occasionally, behavioral changes are the early symptoms. Such changes include increasing irritability, severe emotional outbursts, uncontrollable and unexpected loss of temper, severe anxiety, and even mania or manic-depressive neurosis or psychosis. Purely neurologic symptoms also may be the presenting problems. These include progressively increasing restlessness and in the child, hyperactivity, severe tremulousness, increasing clumsiness even to the point of frank ataxia, a tendency to drop things, and choreic movements. Speech may occasionally be severely dysarthric. Weakness of skeletal muscles is present to some degree in most patients with hyperthyroidism, but occasionally fatigue and weakness may be so great as to suggest myasthenia gravis. In addition, several forms of myopathy have been shown to be associated with hyperthyroidism.

Facial stigmata suggesting hyperthyroidism are inconsistent but present in a high percentage of cases particularly in more long-standing forms. The eyes are large and shining. Staring is observed, and blinking is infrequent. The eyelids may be retracted bilaterally, causing the eyelids not to keep pace with the eyeballs when the affected person gazes downward. This lid/eye lag has been called von Graefe's sign. A person with hyperthyroidism frequently shows weakness of convergence (Moebius' sign) early. Later, when full exophthalmos develops, all eyeball movements may be impaired. In some instances an associated puffiness of the eyelids is seen, as well as hyperemia of the conjunctiva. When such ocular signs develop rapidly and are present in alarming degrees, the condition is termed malignant exophthalmos.

Hyperthyroidism is suggested by the typical clinical picture of a combination of loss of strength, loss of weight without anorexia, heat intolerance, fine tremor, and hyperkinesis. When these characteristics are accompanied by exophthalmos and goiter, little doubt about the diagnosis exists. If the symptoms are not pronounced, however, appropriate laboratory investigations are necessary to confirm the diagnosis. (See Fig. 6-1.)

It should be emphasized again that the hyperthyroid condition may exist as a reaction to many diseases — especially in neurologic disease in infants — although hyperthyroidism is not recognized as readily as it perhaps should be. Fig. 6-2 shows a child with the facial characteristics typical of hyperthyroidism. The eyes are prominent and staring because the eyelids are slightly retracted symmetrically. No other stigmata of hydrocephalus are apparent. Thyroid function tests were mildly abnormal. This facial appearance was characteristic early in the course of the disease in this child, who was ultimately determined to suffer from

Krabbe's globoid cell leukodystrophy. This disease is associated with a total absence of the enzyme galactocerebroside beta-galactocidase. The characteristic opisthotonos, signs of pyramidal tract dysfunction, and extreme irritability so characteristic of Krabbe's disease are appreciated in Fig. 6-2, C.

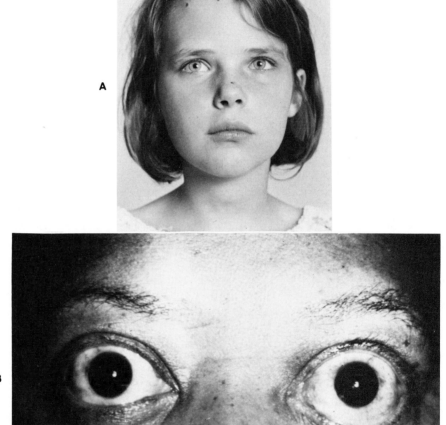

Fig. 6-1. A, Twelve-year-old girl with nonrheumatic chorea of recent onset. Note slightly retracted eyelids over mildly exophthalmic eyes. Patient was proven to have Grave's disease. B, Close-up view of greatly retracted eyelids of a patient with severe exophthalmos. (B, Courtesy of Dr. John Bigger, Augusta, Georgia.)

Other conditions that may present with exophthalmos in the infant and child particularly are the *hydrocephalies* and *craniosynostoses.* These conditions are described in more detail in Chapter 5.

**Proptosis.** The large dural sinuses may become thrombosed when there is infection in the dural spaces surrounding them. In infants this thrombosis is often related to severe dehydration or marasmus and involves especially the superior sagittal, lateral, or cavernous sinuses. *Superior sagittal sinus thrombosis* is often a complication of severe dehydration or starvation and also may be related to osteomyelitis of the skull. Afflicted persons are severely and acutely ill and have a wide range of severe neurologic abnormalities. They often have severe engorgement of the veins of the forehead and cranium and may not have severe proptosis. Persons with *lateral sinus thrombosis* are less severely ill. Affect-

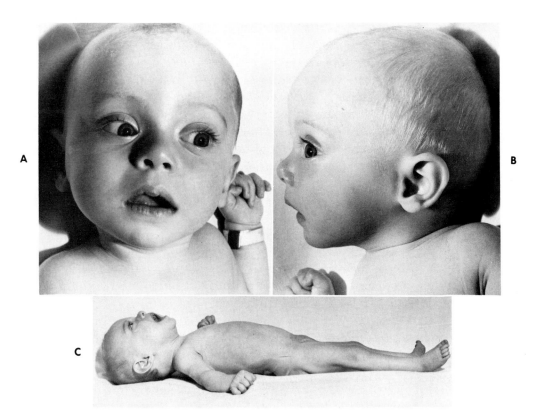

Fig. 6-2. Thirteen-month-old girl with Krabbe's leukodystrophy that was proved by fibroblast culture to be associated with an absence of galactocerebroside-β-galactosidase. The patient was also found to have mild functional hyperthyroidism. A, Frontal facial view showing dull, apathetic expression, normocephaly, and mild retraction of the eyelids over the eyeballs. Notice the "cortical" thumb of the left hand. B, Lateral view showing lid retraction. Cortical thumb of right hand can be observed. C, Lateral full-body view showing opisthotonus, decorticate posturing, and irritability, which were characteristic of this patient's usual behavior.

ed infants may have the facial stigmata of hydrocephalus, but proptosis is less prevalent than in a usual hydrocephalus. This syndrome occurs following otitis media and mastoiditis. *Cavernous sinus thrombosis,* which is frequently secondary to a suppurative process in the nasal sinuses or the upper half of the face, is usually unilateral at its onset. Patients with septic thrombosis of the cavernous sinus are acutely and severely ill. Such patients have a septic temperature and usually have severe pain in the eyes. Bilateral proptosis is often present. Usually, however, the proptosis is somewhat asymmetrical, causing diplopia. There is usually severe hyperemia of the conjunctiva and edema and redness of the eyelids. The optic discs may be swollen, and there may be hemorrhages into the retina.

An arteriovenous fistula is an abnormal communication, either single or multiple, between an artery and a vein. Arterial blood, because of its higher pressure, enters the vein directly without traversing a capillary network. Fistulas are classified as congenital (usually multiple and present from birth) or acquired (usually single and saccular and arising from trauma or, less frequently, from infection of the artery wall). *Congenital arteriovenous fistulas* occur within the central nervous system as well as systemically. Rarely do central nervous system congenital lesions connect the carotid artery and the cavernous sinus. They are more likely to occur in the subarachnoid space. If they rupture, they tend to produce massive subarachnoid hemorrhage. In children, however, they usually do not hemorrhage but rather produce symptoms either by a "stealing" mechanism that causes relative ischemia in neighboring brain areas or by a mass effect, since such lesions can become quite large. Fig. 6-3 shows a child with a large congenital arteriovenous fistula. This child had painless swelling of the right forehead and mild proptosis of the right eye for several years before she sought medical aid because of a focal motor seizure. Roentgenography, isotope brain scanning, and arteriography showed a large arteriovenous malformation of the forehead, retro-orbital space, and right frontal and temporal lobes.

*Acquired arteriovenous fistulas* of the carotid-cavernous system are quite rare in childhood. Adults may develop such lesions after bullet or stab woulds, but these causes of acquired fistulas are less likely in a child. Rarely, acquired arteriovenous fistulas may result from diseases characterized by cerebral arteritis, such as sphenoid sinusitis, osteomyelitis, syphilis, collagen disease, and mycotic arteritis.

The symptoms and signs of an *acquired cavernous-carotid arteriovenous fistula* are similar to those of cavernous sinus thrombosis. Usually, the symptoms of the former condition are also related to an inflammatory process that involves the following sequence of events: The intracavernous portion of the carotid artery becomes inflamed, the wall weakens, hemorrhage (or at least arterial leaking) occurs, and finally a cavernous-carotid fistula develops, with blood flowing from the artery (where the pressure is higher) to the venous sinus that surrounds it.

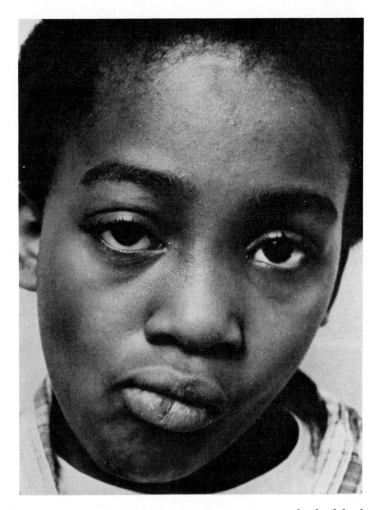

Fig. 6-3. Fourteen-year-old girl with recurrent seizures who had had an asymmetrical facies for most of her life. Shortly before this photograph was taken, she began to complain of bruits and headache and had a focal motor seizure. Note the proptotic right eyeball and tortuous arteriovenous malformation of the right forehead and upper eyelid. There is possibly megalocornea or buphthalmos of the right eyeball. The vascular malformation extended into the cranium and extensively involved the right temporal tip and frontal lobe of the brain.

Cavernous-carotid fistula and cavernous sinus thrombosis can usually be distinguished clinically by the fact that in the former (1) the proptosis tends to be pulsating, (2) there is a bruit over the eye on the side of the fistula that usually disappears with digital occlusion of the carotid artery on the same side, (3) there is more asymmetry, (4) patients complain less of pain and have fewer signs of sepsis, and (5) there is a more chronic course. (See Fig. 6-4.)

*Neurofibromatosis or von Recklinghausen's disease* is a multisystem disorder that has many facial, neurologic, and systemic features.

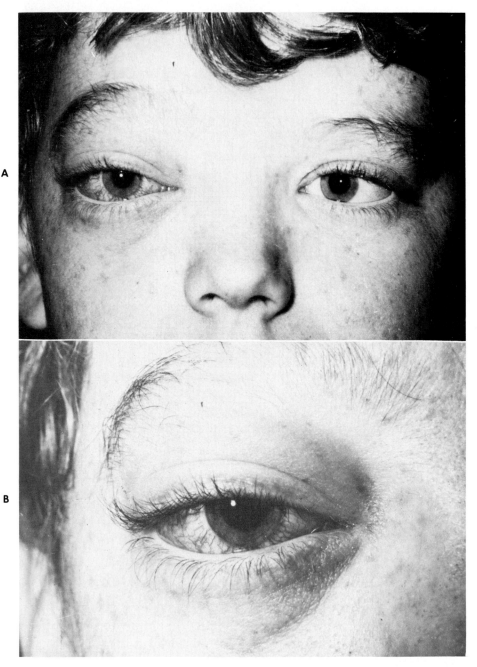

Fig. 6-4. Eleven-year-old boy who had had headaches and reddened conjunctivitis for several months. He began to have more severe headaches and to complain of bruit. He developed a unilateral proptosis of the right eye that was associated with intermittent diplopia. A, Close-up view of eyes showing proptosis and injected scleral vessels of the right eye. B, Close-up view of right eye allowing better appreciation of scleral injection. (See also Fig. 6-35.)

These features will be discussed in several chapters and sections of this book (see Chapter 7, particularly, regarding hemihypertrophy of the face). There have been arguments about who should be credited with the first descriptions of this disease. This is not surprising, since the disorder takes many forms and has been common in our society, both in the distant past and in the present. It has been claimed that Robert the Bruce did not have leprosy, as was once assumed, but rather was crippled from a form of localized neurofibromatosis (Gardner, 1952). The core abnormalities in multiple neurofibromatosis are numerous hyperpigmented cutaneous lesions, which have been called "café-au-lait spots" because of their color (a light tannish tint), and multiple neurofibromata, which may occur peripherally as well as centrally. The neurofibromata can arise from peripheral nerves at any point along a nerve's course. These stigmata, or at least the tendency to have them, are inherited as an autosomal dominant trait (Crowe and others, 1956). Various dysplasias as well as neoplasias are associated with von Recklinghausen's disease. Yet certain groups of features occur regularly enough to be considered syn-

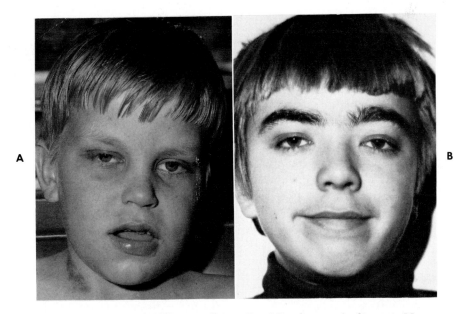

Fig. 6-5. A, Twelve-year-old boy with von Recklinghausen's disease. Note asymmetry of the eyeballs with mild proptosis of the right eyeball. Observe thickened upper eyelid on right and mildly raised right eyebrow, particularly in its lateral extension. A café-au-lait spot is visible on right neck. Patient was found to have a midbrain-diencephalic glioma, which spared the optic nerve and chiasma. B, Fourteen-year-old patient with von Recklinghausen's disease who was evaluated for mild mental retardation. The eyes are mildly asymmetrical, and the left eyeball is slightly proptotic. The space between the lateral part of the eyebrow and the lateral canthus is slightly larger on the left. Observe also the relative hyperplasia of the left eyebrow. Full investigation showed that this patient had neither brain nor otic tumor.

dromes within the entire dysplastic complex. One such syndrome of neurofibromatosis involves unilateral proptosis and usually includes a dysplasia of the sphenoid bone and other tissue in the retro-orbital space. The proptosis is usually congenital and may be either mild or severe (see Fig. 6-5). This syndrome, known as "orbital" von Reckling-hausen's disease, may be associated with malignancy of the optic nerve and the diencephalic-mesencephalic area of the brain. The resulting tumors are usually astrocytomas of an infiltrating type. Although not highly invasive, they may slowly infiltrate critical areas of the central nervous system over a period of time (see Figs. 6-5, A, and 6-6). The tumors, which may be observed to filtrate extensively the posterior hypothalamic region, account for a variety of endocrinologic symptoms and signs.

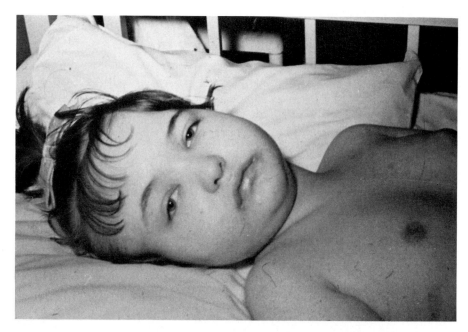

Fig. 6-6. Eight-year-old girl with a long and complicated history. She was born with multiple café-au-lait spots. At about 18 months of age, abnormal eyeball movements developed, which were soon followed by visual failure, first of the right eye and then of the left eye. The presence of an optic glioma arising on the right and extending into to the left optic nerve by way of the optic chiasm was demonstrated. A biopsy was performed, but the lesion was only observed and not removed. Soon afterward seizures developed. They were controlled by anticonvulsants. When this patient was about 6 years of age, the first signs of puberty developed with menarche but little thelarche. Just before this photograph was taken, bulging of the craniotomy site for the biopsy was observed, as well as gradual decreases in levels of activity and mental alertness and an increase in the number of seizures. Note the asymmetrical eyeballs, with the right eye showing proptosis. Observe the bulging right temporal area, which was the site of the craniotomy, and the café-au-lait spots on the body.

**Buphthalmos.** The term buphthalmos refers to the enlargement of the eyeball or globe itself and not to protrusion of the globe from pressure or mass. The distinction between it and the preceding conditions is an important one.

*Sturge-Weber disease* has been mentioned in prior chapters and will be mentioned in subsequent ones, since this disorder, like many of the neurocutaneous diseases, is characterized by extensive facial involvement. The disease typically affects the middle face, especially the eyes. The disorder was first described by Sturge in 1879 and was further delineated by Horrocks in 1883, Kalischer in 1897, Dimetri in 1923, and the great Frances Parke Weber in 1922. Weber's contribution to the understanding of this disorder admittedly was not as great as his many other contributions to the field of rare disorders. Weber described only one of the first skull x-ray films taken of this condition. The first clinical delineation, however, was undeniably Sturge's. The first pathoanatomic study was probably Kalischer's. Since the official designation "encephalotrigeminal hemangiomatosis" is nonspecific and cumbersome, we will use the name most commonly given to the condition—Sturge-Weber disease—regardless of its inaccuracy (Alexander and Norman, 1960).

The disease results from an insult early in embryogenesis at a time important in the development of the craniofacial and cerebral blood supply. The disorder is not inherited. Several necessary clinical features must be present before a diagnosis of Sturge-Weber disease can be made, but if they are present, they are quite predictive of postmortem brain pathology, on which, one would suppose, any disease diagnosis must ultimately rest. The clinical syndrome is characterized by a trigeminally distributed capillary hemangioma of the nevus flammeus type. This lesion, a port wine stain, is more extensive and deeper in color than the more common nevus flammeus seen in infancy. The port wine stain is fairly sharply demarcated from the surrounding normal skin; it is slightly raised and fairly homogeneous (see Fig. 6-7). The skin over the lesion is slightly thickened, a feature that allows further differentiation between it and other types of capillary hemangiomas. (See the discussion of the hemangioma-scaphocephaly syndrome in Chapter 5.) The distribution of the port wine hemangioma is variable but almost always corresponds to the distribution of the first division of the trigeminal nerve, which includes most of the forehead and upper face. When only partial, this hemangioma involves an area around the eye. The lesion often is characterized by some bilateral facial involvement, but even when bilateral, the stain is usually more pronounced on one side. Midline facial distribution is uncommon, if it occurs at all (see Fig. 6-36 for a possible exception to this rule). Extensive somatic port wine hemangiomas may be seen as well.

Noting the most extensive distribution of the port wine stain is important in predicting the ultimate neurologic and ophthalmologic

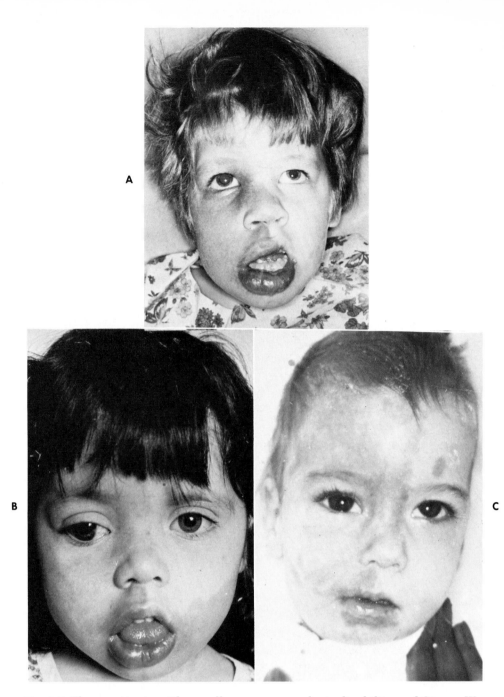

Fig. 6-7. Three patients with equally severe neurologic disability and Sturge-Weber disease. **A,** Six-year-old. Note the port wine nevus flammeus involving the upper, middle, and lower face on the right, as well as buphthalmos of the right eye. The nevus extends to midline and involves patchy areas on the left. Note also the extensive labial hyperplasia related to hemangioma and phenytoin treatment. **B,** Four-year-old. Observe the port wine nevus flammeus in a distribution similar to that in A. There is extensive buphthalmos on the right resulting from congenital glaucoma. Enlargement of globe produces illusion of exotropia on right. **C,** Six-month-old patient with Sturge-Weber disease. Observe more patchy, unilateral hemangioma on right and mild involvement on left as well. There is buphthalmos, as well as secondary malalignment, of the right eye with the enlarged eyeball tending to protrude outwardly, laterally, and especially inferiorly.

involvement. Port wine staining that extends over the face to the midline, filling most of the compartment of the first division of the trigeminal nerve on one side, indicates the presence of an extensive symptomatic lesion of the pia-arachnoid on the same side. When such a meningeal hemangioma is present, there is usually extensive neurologic symptomatology. Involvement of the pia-arachnoid in an older child or an adult can be confirmed by a skull roentgenogram that shows a typical pattern of calcification (see Fig. 6-8). The presence of Sturge-Weber disease, therefore, is established not only by the typically trigeminally distributed port wine stain but also by the pia-arachnoid hemangioma and calcification on the same side. Characteristically, x-ray films show a "double railroad track" type of configuration that is due not to the pia-arachnoid hemangioma itself but rather to calcifications in the neighboring convolutions of the brain as a result of chronic ischemia and anoxia. A diagnosis of Sturge-Weber disease cannot be made with certainty without arteriographic or postmortem confirmation of the existence of the pia-arachnoid hemangioma. Nevertheless, the presence of the facial lesion allows such a diagnosis to be made with a high percentage of accuracy.

Associated with Sturge-Weber disease is a fairly characteristic clinical syndrome that involves unilateral motor seizures, hemiplegia, hemihypoplasia, mental retardation, and glaucoma. In infants with an extensive port wine stain in the distribution area of the first division of the trigeminal nerve (which involves most of the eyelid), there may be an associated unilateral glaucoma. The increased intraocular pressure causes the infant's eye to enlarge, resulting in buphthalmos. (See Fig. 6-7, *A* and *B*.) The unilateral ocular enlargement is quite evident in even the youngest patient in Fig. 6-7, which is a series of photographs of patients of different ages with Sturge-Weber disease. The glaucoma may be treatable with surgery.

The calcification within brain tissue that occurs in Sturge-Weber disease usually affects the outermost layers of the cerebral cortex. The resulting parenchymal changes account for the sometimes severe neurologic dysfunctions. It is expected, therefore, that typically affected patients will have long-standing, contralateral hemiparesis or hemiplegia, relative hemihypoplasia of the contralateral lower face and extremities, and severe, sometimes resistant, unilateral motor seizures. Patients are frequently but not always mentally retarded. In our experience it has held true that the earlier the onset of seizures and the more refractory they are to control with anticonvulsants, the more serious the effect on subsequent motor and intellectual capacity. Early recognition and control of seizures by both medical and, if necessary, surgical means is important for the care of persons afflicted with Sturge-Weber disease.

Several other syndromes may be associated with buphthalmos. For example, another neurocutaneous disease, called *von Hippel's syndrome*, may be associated with a mild degree of buphthalmos. Von Hippel's syn-

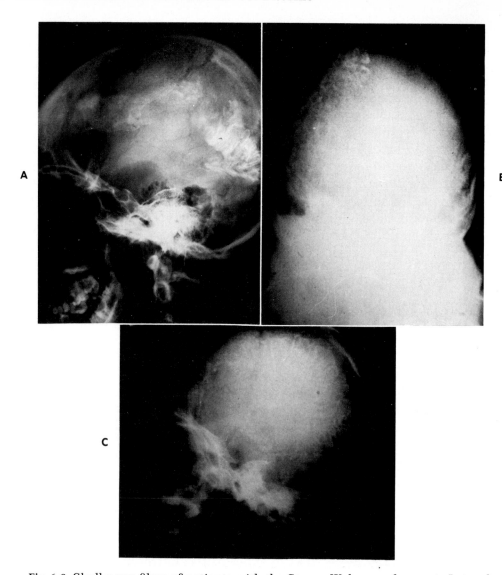

Fig. 6-8. Skull x-ray films of patients with the Sturge-Weber syndrome. A, Lateral view showing typical "railroad track" calcifications in the posterior hemisphere on one side. Less extensive calcification is seen anteriorly. This calcification represents the chronic effects of ischemia of the superficial layers of the brain and does not indicate the presence of a pia-arachnoid hemangioma, which is usually placed more anteriorly and does not typically calcify. B, Anterior/posterior (Towne) view of skull of patient in Fig. 6-7, B, showing typical convolutional calcification on one side of the cranium. The lesion is on the right, corresponding to an extensive port wine nevus flammeus on the patient's right face. C, Lateral view of skull of same patient.

drome, which tends to be inherited as an autosomal dominant trait, is also associated with cerebellar hemangiomas and other neoplastic conditions. (See Fig. 6-9.) It is said that persons with von Recklinghausen's disease can have true buphthalmos. In addition, many other forms of *congenital glaucoma* per se may involve enlargement of one or both eyes.

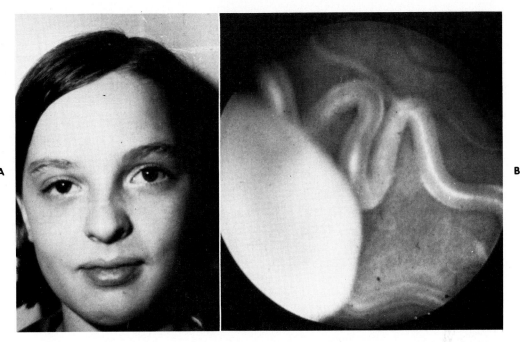

Fig. 6-9. A, Facial view of patient with visual problems in the right eye resulting from von Hippel's syndrome. For several years, patient had gradual proptosis of the right eyeball coexistent with diminished vision. Observe enlargement of right eyelid and mild relative external deviation of right eye by noting corneal reflections. B, Fundus photograph of right eye of same patient. Observe retinal angioma with extremely dilated feeding and exiting vessels. The angioma lies above and to the right of the area of the detached retina on the left. This patient's condition was extensively investigated, and at the time these photographs were taken, she did not have a lesion of the posterior fossa or the cerebellum.

**Microphthalmia.** Microphthalmia is a condition in which the eye is markedly smaller than normal. Anophthalmia, of course, would be the most severe degree of microphthalmia. According to Walsh (1957), there are three types of anophthalmia. The primary type is due to failure of the optic pit to deepen and form an outgrowth of the forebrain. Secondary anophthalmia results from absence or abnormal development of the whole forebrain. A third type of anophthalmia occurs when the optic vesicle forms but subsequently degenerates. Each type may be unilateral or bilateral. Technically, the *holoprosencephalies* are not typically associated with microphthalmia per se, yet it may be one of the features of these disorders. The most severe type of the holoprosencephalies is known as the *cyclopic monster* (DeMyer, 1972). In this condition the two eyes are partially fused to give an appearance of a single eye. True microphthalmia is also present but is secondary to the ocular fusion problem. In the other types of holoprosencephaly and in the *trisomy 13 syndrome,* anophthalmia or severe microphthalmia is said to exist. In these conditions, fusion of the eyes (synophthalmia) does not occur, although

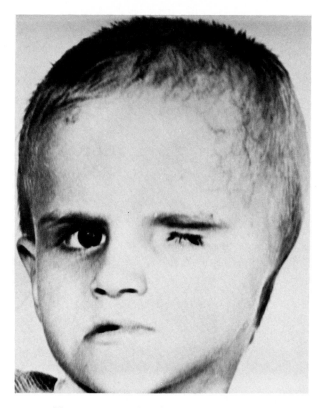

Fig. 6-10. Nine-year-old institutionalized patient with otoculomandibular hypoplasia. This syndrome also has been known by other names, such as otomandibular dysostosis and the lateral facial hypoplasia syndrome. The patient was severely hyperactive and aggressive, may have had seizures, and was profoundly mentally retarded. Note the hypoplasia of the lateral eyebrow, anophthalmia, hypoplasia of eyelid, absence of the ear, hypoplasia of the zygomatic process and mandible, and microstomia, all on the left side. The right side of the face is normal.

there are usually severe degrees of hypotelorism (Patan, 1960; Smith, 1964).

*Otoculomandibular hypoplasia (otomandibular dysostosis)* is a syndrome characterized by unilateral hypoplasia or aplasia of the eye, ear, mouth, or mandible. Rarely, the entire side of the face may be involved in the process. (See Figs. 6-10 and 6-11). The deformities are obviously secondary to an insult late in gestational life, since the affected patient is born with them and there is no progression. Although the severe forms of this syndrome are very rare, it would appear that neurologic dysfunction usually exists. The patient in Fig. 6-10 was severely retarded at 9 years of age. He was dwarfed and has paroxysmal attacks of violence and hyperactivity that vaguely resembled atypical seizures. These attacks, occurring several times per day, were resistant to standard anticonvulsants.

A somewhat similar situation occurred in the patient in Fig. 6-11.

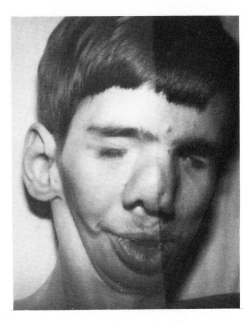

Fig. 6-11. Institutionalized 18-year-old patient with severe mental retardation, body growth failure, and severe neurologic and ocular defects. Note the abnormalities in both the central and the lateral middle face. There is a broad nasal tip with a cleft that extends down to the central lower face. A cleft lip had been corrected in the past. In addition, there is bilateral microphthalmia, as well as extensive hypoplasia of the zygomatic process, lateral bony orbit, mandible, and ear on the right. Ear tags are also present. This condition results from a combination of partial defects occurring early in the formation of the face and involving the frontonasal process (from which the midline structures are derived) and the right first and second branchial arches.

However, this patient also showed evidence of *both* lateral middle facial and central middle facial hypoplasia.

These dysplasias involving the eye are quite different from acquired lesions such as those occasionally observed in severely mentally retarded, aggressive patients who engage in self-mutilation. Such a patient is shown in Fig. 6-12.

Closely related to the syndrome we have called otoculomandibular hypoplasia is the *cryptophthalmos syndrome*, which was originally described in the nineteenth century by Zehender (1872) but detailed more recently by others including Goodman and Gorlin (1977). This condition is characterized by a "hidden eye" and is distinguished from otoculomandibular hypoplasia and simple anophthalmia by the fact that the hypoplastic eyeball is covered with skin. Persons with this syndrome, which is inherited as a recessive trait, have other dysplastic defects, including cleft lip, ankyloglossia, gonadal abnormalities, anal atresia, meningomyelocele, and syndactyly.

The *microphthalmia syndrome of Lenz* is an uncommon disorder consisting of asymmetrical or unilateral congenital hypoplasia of the

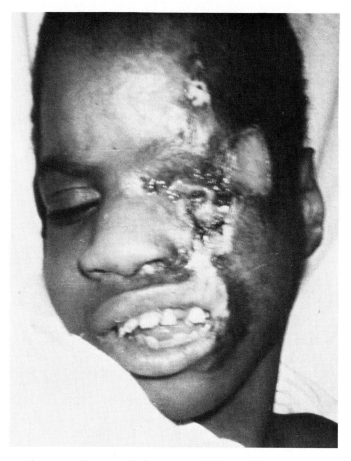

Fig. 6-12. Severely mentally retarded patient of fifteen years of age who has mutilated his face. Total enucleation of the eye and the lateral middle face has occurred. (Courtesy of Dr. Patricia Hartlage, Medical College of Georgia.)

eyeball. This disorder was first documented by Lenz (1955). The syndrome is distinguished from other syndromes of microphthalmia by the
fact that, typically, in addition to deformed auricles there is also an asthenic habitus resulting from sloping shoulders, low scapulae, and a cyl-
indrical-appearing thorax. We believe that these features sufficiently
identify the syndrome, but, in addition, patients may have other bone
and joint abnormalities, especially talipes calcaneovalgus and disorders
of the digits. Cardiovascular and genitourinary anomalies are also features of the syndrome. The disorder is inherited as a sex-linked trait. The
patient in Fig. 6-13 showed the hallmark abnormalities – microphthalmia and asthenic body build – as well as many of the associated anomalies. In addition, this patient, who was profoundly mentally retarded,
had several false-positive tests for urinary homocystinuria and secondary corneal clouding.

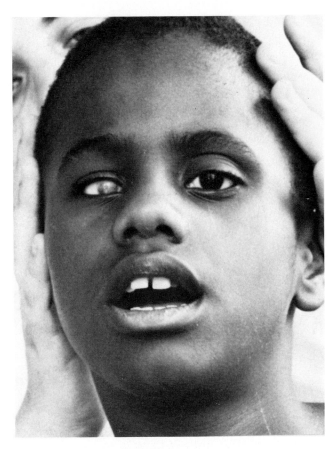

Fig. 6-13. Fourteen-year-old child with severe mental retardation, aggressive and hyperexcitable behavior, and marfanian or asthenic habitus. This patient, who also has microphthalmia of the right eye, congenital lenticular cataract, and corneal clouding, is believed to have Lenz' syndrome.

The *Hallermann-Streiff syndrome* is usually grouped with the first-branchial-arch syndromes. One of the distinctive features that separates this disorder from the many other first-arch syndromes is the consistent presence of congenital abnormalities of the eye. (See Figs. 6-14 and 6-15.) It is said that the syndrome was first reported by Aubry (1893). Hallermann (1948) and Streiff (1950) clarified the disorder and recognized the distinctive features. This syndrome consists of mandibular hypoplasia, micrognathia, long and thin beak-like nose, hypoplasia of nasal cartilages, zygomatic hypoplasia, antimongoloid slant, deafness (occasionally), high-arched and narrow palate, small mouth, and multiple dental anomalies. To us, the distinctive features, besides those suggesting the first-arch syndrome, are (1) cranial and somatic hypotrichosis or alopecia; (2) congenital ocular abnormalities such as microphthalmia, congenital cataracts, blue sclerae, nystagmus, and hetero-

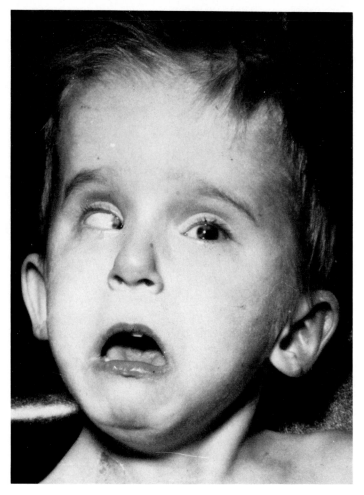

Fig. 6-14. Patient with Hallermann-Streiff syndrome. This three-year-old child has severe mental retardation, macrocephaly, relative cranial hypotrichosis, triangularly shaped facies, low-set ears with mild zygomatic micrognathia and mandibular hypoplasia, and narrow and small nose. Note also the mild microphthalmia, as well as the severe esotropia on the right.

tropia; and (3) cranial contour or size abnormalities, such as brachycephaly, frontal or parietal bossing, microcephaly, macrocephaly, and dehiscence of longitudinal and lambdoid sutures with open fontanels. Mental retardation is common, although intelligence may be normal.

Cockayne's syndrome is associated with a general senile facial appearance and other facial characteristics (Cockayne, 1936). Because these abnormalities involve the entire face, the disorder will be discussed more fully in Chapter 8. The eyeballs, are, however, characteristically small, and they appear to be sunken in the sockets. The Marinesco-Sjögren syndrome, a type of spinocerebellar degeneration, is typically associated with lenticular cararacts (Alter and Kennedy, 1968). This dis-

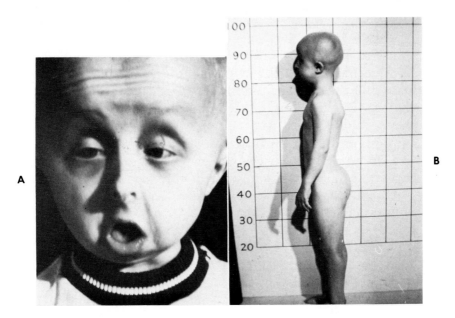

Fig. 6-15. A, Nine-year-old child with mild mental retardation, dyscephaly with bird-like face and narrow nose, triangularly shaped facies, and severe hypotrichosis. Microphthalmia is obvious. Patient had bilateral lenticular cataract. B, Lateral body view of same patient. (Courtesy of Dr. John Bigger, Augusta, Georgia.)

order will more fully be discussed later (see p. 218). The atrophic or acquired mechanism that produces microphthalmia in the Marinesco-Sjögren syndrome also occurs in *Lowe's oculocerebrorenal syndrome* (Lowe, and others, 1952). Although *Parry-Romberg syndrome* or *hemifacial atrophy* is not limited to the eye, this disorder may present as an ocular atrophic defect, since progressive atrophy often occurs of all tissues of the face (Parry, 1825; Romberg, 1846). Rarely, *septo-optic dysplasia* or *DeMorsier's syndrome*, consisting of absence of the septum pellucidum, congenital hypoplasia of the optic nerve, and hypothalmic dysfunction, can be associated with congenital microphthalmia. *Cross' syndrome*, which has been observed in three siblings, involves gingival fibromatosis, hypopigmentation, oligophrenia, and athetosis (Cross and others, 1967). This syndrome also is characterized by bilateral microphthalmia with sunken eyes. *Oculodento-osseus dysplasia* or *the ODO syndrome* also may involve microphthalmia, in addition to other dysplastic cranial and somatic features (Gorlin and others, 1963).

Microphthalmia may also be observed in persons who suffer from colobomas of the iris. This defect may be associated with a mild to moderate degree of hypoplasia of the eyeball. Syndromes characterized by iridal coloboma are *Goltz's syndrome* (also called focal dermal hypoplasia) and *the trisomy 22* or *cat's eye syndrome*. Both syndromes have many characteristic features in addition to ocular abnormalities (Goodman and Gorlin, 1977).

## Syndromes characterized by abnormalities of the iris and pupil

**Horner's syndrome.** In 1869, Horner described a syndrome in humans that was produced by the interruption of sympathetic pathways to the eye and head. Earlier, however, the great French physiologist Claude Bernard had described a similar picture in experimental studies in lower animals. The features of this syndrome include (1) miosis resulting from paresis of the pupillary dilator muscles, (2) ptosis resulting from paresis of the sympathetically innervated Müller's muscles of the upper eyelid (which help maintain the integrity of the palpebral fissure), (3) anhidrosis or hypohydrosis caused by disturbance of sympathetic fibers to the sweat glands, and (4) enophthalmos. Whether the enophthalmos is illusory or real (in which case it would be caused by paresis of Müller's retrobulbar muscle) is still in question (Walsh, 1957).

The sympathetic disturbance in Horner's syndrome may result from disruption of neurons or pathways at several anatomic levels and may occur in various degreees, depending upon the extent of the lesion. Common sites of disruption are the brainstem (particularly in the lateral medulla in the reticular formation), the upper spinal cord (cervical or high thoracic levels), the anterior spinal roots (low cervical or high thoracic levels), the cervical sympathetic trunk, and the carotid sympathetic plexus. Somewhat similar sympathetic disturbances also may occur in lesions of the suprasegmental centers in the hypothalamus.

The syndrome may be either acquired or congenital (Farmer, 1968). Both types are seen in both children and adults, although the acquired type may be more prevalent in adults because of greater incidence of vascular and neoplastic disease. The congenital form is usually caused by a lesion that occurs early in embryonic development. In both types the major pupillary symptoms result from the unopposed action of the parasympathetic system. Miosis occurs in an affected pupil because of the pupillary constriction brought about by the pupillary constrictor muscle, which is innervated by parasympathetic nerves.

*Acquired Horner's syndrome* is seen in cases of brainstem lesions, in which incomplete syndromes may occur. Hypohidrosis may extend far below the face area. Brainstem lesions are usually caused by vascular insufficiency in the distribution area of the posterior inferior cerebellar artery. This artery supplies the lateral medullary "wedge." Rarely, pontine tumors, demyelinating diseases, and encephalitis may be responsible for acquired Horner's syndrome. Syringomyelia, spinal tumor, and other high spinal cord lesions rarely may be associated with cases of partial Horner's syndrome. Lesions of the anterior spinal roots of the low cervical and high thoracic levels (from C8 to T2-3) may produce abnormalities of the pupil because of interruption of the preganglionic sympathetic fibers as they exit the spinal cord to enter the paravertebral sympathetic trunk. Other neurologic deficits also may be seen in this syndrome. The cervical sympathetic chain itself it also vulnerable to lesions caused by many of the same disorders that affect the anterior roots. These disorders may be infectious (for example, meningitis, radiculitis, or neuritis), neoplastic (for example, metastatic tumors of the mediastinum and thoracic inlet), or traumatic (for example, penetrating wounds, surgical procedures, or injury to the lower brachial plexus). These disorders also may result from pressure caused by a vascular malformation such as an aortic aneurysm. The cervical sympathetic chain is particularly susceptible to damage from an enlarged thyroid and from surgery. A rare form of disruption of sympathetic fibers to the head occurs when sympathetic postganglionic fibers are damaged after they leave the various sympathetic ganglia. Such acquired lesions at these sites may occur with internal carotid aneurysms or neoplasms. In these distal sympathetic disturbances, the anhidrosis may be partial — limited to the forehead alone, for example. Other sympathetic and neurologic functional deficits may also occur in distal disturbances.

Since acquired Horner's syndrome is almost always unilateral, a common presentation is anisocoria. Thus acquired Horner's syndrome must be differentiated from other disorders that cause anisocoria, such as direct oculomotor lesions that produce an oculomotor palsy. Such lesions are commonly associated with increased intracranial pressure, causing herniation of rostral brain contents at the supratentorial notch. In such an instance the parasympathetic fibers to the pupillary constrictor muscles are relatively depressed, and the sympathetic fibers to the pupillary dilator muscles are allowed to act unopposed. In both oculomotor palsy and Horner's syndrome, an affected pupil may still partially function and constrict when stimulated by light or during accommodation, especially early in the disease process. Although patients with Horner's syndrome have small pupils and those with oculomotor lesions have large pupils, other symptoms of both syndromes must be taken into account to differentiate them from each other, especially in unilateral conditions. In oculomotor palsy, extraocular muscle disturbances are expected as well as true ptosis on the side of the larger pupil because of the accompanying paralysis of the nerve branch travelling to the levator palpebri muscle. Other, less ominous causes of anisocoria may occur iatrogenically. Therapeutic agents such as pilocarpine may cause pupillary constriction, as in the patient in Fig. 6-16. Pupillary dilating agents that aid in examination of the retina are commonly, if not routinely, used in medicine. Particularly when long-acting pupillary dilators, such as atropine sulfate, are used, dilation and anisocoria may last for weeks. Thus, a physician who is evaluating a person with anisocoria should consider the possibility that pupillary medications may be causing the condition. Another common cause of anisocoria, especially in rural areas, is accidental instillation of gypsum weed, a commonly occurring plant that contains atropine. A physician who is unaware of this possible cause of anisocoria, especially in children, may become unduly alarmed until it is clear that no serious neurologic process is involved. In addition, one occasionally encounters persons who have mild congenital anisocoria.

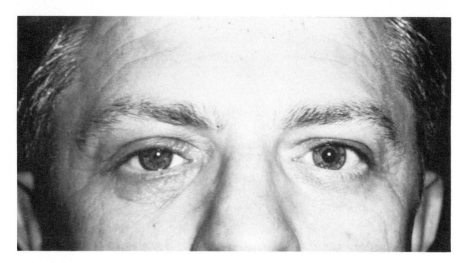

**Fig. 6-16.** Anisocoria in a patient with adult-onset glaucoma of the right eye. This condition was treated with miotic agents, which produced an inequality in pupil size. (Courtesy of Dr. John Bigger, Augusta, Georgia.)

Although many relatively innocuous conditions can cause or be associated with anisocoria, it still is a very serious ocular sign.

Differentiation between the miosis seen in Horner's syndrome and the conditions of the pupil described by Argyll Robertson, which are associated with *central nervous system syphilis*, is pertinent (Walsh, 1957). In cases of Argyll Robertson's pupil, the disorder is often bilateral even though pupillary size is frequently unequal. Patients with Argyll Robertson's pupil therefore may have anisocoria. Argyll Robertson's pupil is smaller than normal and irregular (see Fig. 3-2). Whereas the miotic pupil of Horner's syndrome reacts both to light and to accommodation, the pupil of Argyll Robertson reacts only to accommodation.

*Adie's syndrome*, which is characterized by anisocoria, involves diffuse hyporeflexia and large pupils that have been described as myotonic (see Fig. 6-17). The disorder is usually bilateral, but the pupils tend to be unequal. Mydriasis is usually present. The myotonic pupil reacts sluggishly, if at all, to light or accommodation (Walsh, 1957).

*Congenital Horner's syndrome* has basically the same features as acquired Horner's syndrome, but there are differentiating features that are important. Although the same sites of dysfunction of sympathetic neurons and pathways are probable in both syndromes, there is substantial evidence that the dysfunction in the congenital syndrome occurs because of abnormal migration of cells of the neural crest during embryogenesis—a phenomenon that has been called dysmigration. Congenital Horner's syndrome is often associated with other defects of embryogenesis and with frank malformations. What is known about the development of the sympathetic system suggests that a misdirection (or dysmi-

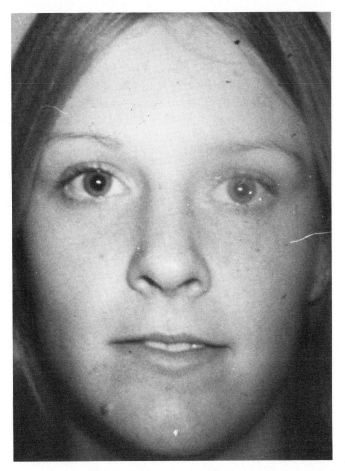

Fig. 6-17. Sixteen-year-old patient with headaches believed to be inflammatory in nature. Note the mild anisocoria. This patient's eyes tend to be mydriatic, even in bright light, and are poorly reactive to direct light stimulation. In addition, the patient has hyporeflexia, especially at the patellar areas, and is believed to have Adie's syndrome. (Courtesy of Dr. Patricia Hartlage, Medical College of Georgia.)

gration) of migrating cells arising in the fetal nervous tissue occurs. Congenital Horner's syndrome, it seems, usually results from disturbances in the differentiation of certain cells of the neural crest at a 4 to 7 somite stage of development. At this time cells of the sympathetic system begin their migration to more peripheral sites. This migration occurs in company with melanocytes, which also arise in the neural crest. In persons with congenital Horner's syndrome, it appears that a misdirection of the migration of these cells has occurred. Thus, one usually observes associated defects in pigmentation, as well as sympathetic deficits. It would appear that a variety of noxious insults to the organism at this critical time could produce a disturbance in the ultimate location of both types of cells. It is quite common in congenital Horner's syndrome to have associated pigmentation defects of the cranioface. Heterochromia (differently colored irises) is often associated with sympathetic dysfunctions. The patient in Fig. 6-18 has all the features of Horner's syndrome listed on p. 202. The history of his case indicates that the noxious insult took place in an early stage of enbryogenesis and precludes the possibility of a recently acquired sympathetic nervous system lesion.

The sympathetic fibers that innervate the cranioface also innervate the walls of the arteries that serve these structures. Sympathetic action on the arteries enables dilation and therefore flushing of the skin to occur in order to regulate temperature. Patients with Horner's syndrome, the result of a "loss" type of lesion, do not flush or sweat in the normal manner. At the same time, however, the relatively pale skin of a person with poor sympathetic supply to the skin may be quite warm to the touch. These findings are seen more often in congenital forms of Horner's syndrome than in the acquired form (see Fig. 6-18).

**Other heterochromia syndromes.** Certain conditions may be confused with Horner's syndrome. Many of the partial hypopigmentation syndromes such as *Waardenburg's syndrome, Vogt-Koyanagi syndrome, Harada's syndrome, Sugarman-Reed syndrome (craniofacial leukoderma)*, and *vitiligo* must be differentiated from each other. In addition to heterochromia, Waardenberg's syndrome is characterized by seemingly wide-set eyes (dystopia canthorum), medial eyebrow whorling and hyperplasia, deafness, and white forelock (Waardenburg, 1951). Faulty migration of neural crest cells in all the congenital syndromes characterized by heterochromia probably occurs, but this is especially true of

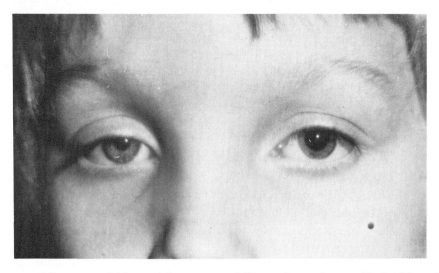

**Fig. 6-18.** Nine-year-old boy with congenital Horner's syndrome. He had hypohidrosis on the right but flushed dramatically on that side of his face during exercise, which was performed immediately before this photograph was taken. Observe anisocoria caused by miosis and pseudoptosis on the right as well as hemifacial erythema extending to midline. The irises are both light but are colored differently (heterochromia), the left being brown and the right blue.

Waardenburg's syndrome. Heterochromia and cranial leukoderma with a white lock of forehead hair have been seen in proven cases of *Down's syndrome* or *trisomy 21*. (See Fig. 6-19, *C*). Evidence of dysmigration, in fact, is not uncommon in Down's syndrome. It is common to see differently colored portions of one iris (Fig. 6-20).

One of us (PRD) has seen three patients with a rare type of reflex seizure that he has called "half-and-half seizures" (Dyken, 1969). This

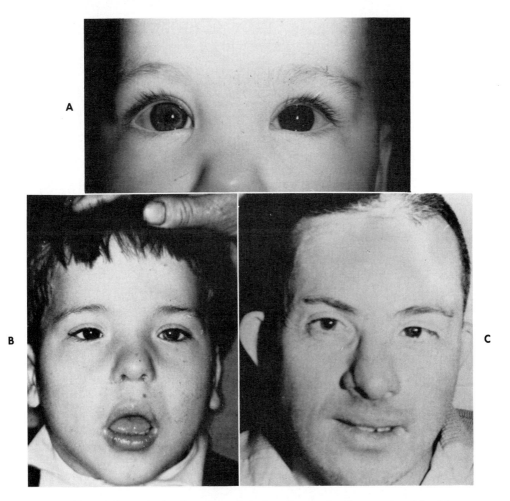

Fig. 6-19. Heterochromia in three unrelated patients. A, Three-year-old with congenital heterochromia without other abnormal features. B, Four-year-old child with severe mental retardation, deafness, midline cranial poliosis not extensive enough to be termed a white forelock, dystopia canthorum, and mild medial eyebrow hyperplasia. He was believed to suffer from Waardenburg's syndrome. Note the heterochromia, which is also a feature of this syndrome. C, Thirty-two-year-old patient with proven trisomy 21 who, besides the features typical of this syndrome, also has heterochromia and cranial leukoderma with a white lock of hair. Disorders involving heterochromia and other signs of partial depigmentation have been called dysmigration syndromes because they result from the improper migration of neural crest cells (that is, melanocytes). (A, Courtesy of Dr. John Bigger, Augusta, Georgia.)

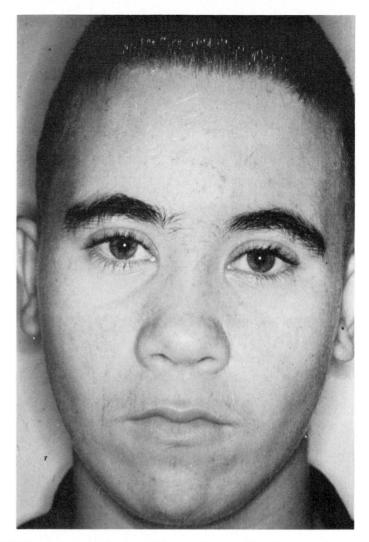

**Fig. 6-20.** Mildly retarded 15-year-old boy with some facial features reminiscent of Down's syndrome, including mongoloid slanting and epicanthal folds. Note the prominent Brushfield spots of the irises. There is no heterochromia, although areas of blue and brown appear in one iris.

syndrome involves several transient signs that suggest an intermittent sympathetic disturbance of the face. In the *half-and-half syndrome,* the patients had recurrent generalized tonic seizures, beginning in early life, which were consistently induced by some sort of sudden, alarming, or painful stimulus. Each patient was neurologically intact between seizures and showed no permanent sign of sympathetic dysfunction. After the ictus, one patient was observed to have vivid blushing over half of the face and neck (Fig. 6-21, *A*). The other patients had a broad band of blushing extending over part of the middle face (Fig. 6-22). We now believe that these patients had congenital central nervous system lesions

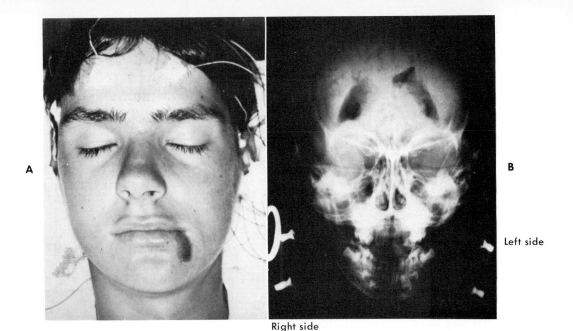

Right side                                    Left side

Fig. 6-21. Half-and-half syndrome. **A,** Fifteen-year-old patient with regular, recurrent tonic seizures, present from early infancy, that are precipitated by sudden, unexpected tactile stimuli of the face. Following the tonic seizure, the left half of the face showed vivid flushing. This half-and-half reaction extended to the thyroid cartilage. **B,** Anterior/posterior pneumoencephalogram of skull of patient in A. Note the dilation of the medial aspects of the temporal horn of the right lateral ventricle.

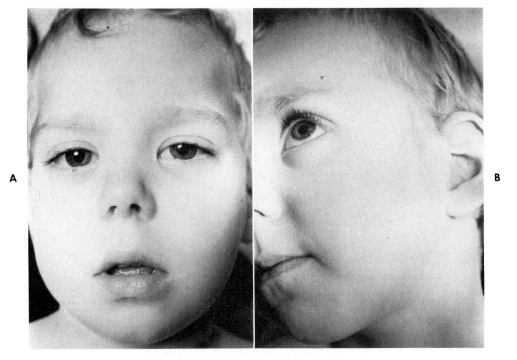

Fig. 6-22. Seven-year-old patient with a history very similar to that of the patient in Fig. 6-21. **A,** Facial appearance during recovery from a tonic seizure. Left side face is erythematous. **B,** Oblique facial view showing the broad, mildly erythematous band in the area of distribution of the second, and a portion of the third, division of the trigeminal nerve on the left.

of atrophic nature. Pneumoencephalography showed that two of the patients had asymmetrical temporal horns and dilation of the side opposite the blushing. (See Fig. 6-21, *B*.) We reason that the sites of dysfunction were in the deep temporal and/or hypothalamic areas, since these areas are known to subserve suprasegmental sympathetic functions. We speculate that these sites were the originating points of localized epileptogenic discharges that account for not only the seizures but also the transient sympathetic dysfunction that follows.

A number of other abnormalities of the pupil and iris are important in syndrome diagnosis. Colobomas of the iris, when complete, characteristically resemble a keyhole. (See Fig. 6-23.) Colobomas of the iris are found in various cytogenic syndromes, including trisomy 18.

### Syndromes characterized by abnormalities of the cornea and lens

**Wilson's hepatolenticular degeneration.** In 1912, Kinnier Wilson first documented in depth the disease that is now known by his name (Wilson, 1912). Most now consider the disease to be an inborn error of copper metabolism, usually with an autosomal recessive inheritance, that is manifested primarily by cirrhosis of the liver and neurologic signs caused by progressive damage to the lenticular nucleus, or to the putamen and globus pallidus. This dysfunction results in rigidity, tremor, and

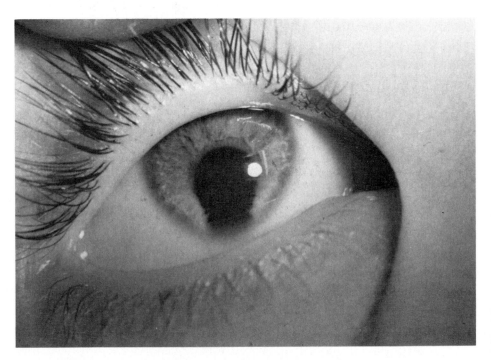

**Fig. 6-23.** Close-up view of eye of a patient with partial trisomy 18, which has resulted in iridal coloboma. Note the keyhole appearance characteristic of this abnormality. (Courtesy of Dr. John Bigger, Augusta, Georgia.)

involuntary movements. Several forms of the disease are known to exist. The classic type, which Wilson (and earlier, Wilson's mentor, Gowers), described, usually appears in childhood or early adolescence. This form of the disease is usually identified as the progressive lenticular degeneration type. It is relatively rapidly progressive and shows severe rigidity, pseudobulbar symptoms, and tremor. Another, less progressive, form has a later onset (sometimes as late as the third or fourth decade) and a longer course. This form of Wilson's disease has been called the pseudosclerotic type. Many intermediate forms also occur, as well as various formes frustes with oligosymptoms or only some of the classic symptoms. The formes frustes are of great importance and possibly account for many cases of idiopathic hepatic cirrhosis, unexplained recurrent ascites, hematemesis, jaundice, unexplained coma, mental deterioration, recurring psychotic episodes, idiopathic seizure disorders, essential tremors, and other unexplained neurologic symptoms in patients who do not have other signs of Wilson's disease. (See Fig. 6-24.)

In many instances the liver abnormalities not only occur earlier but

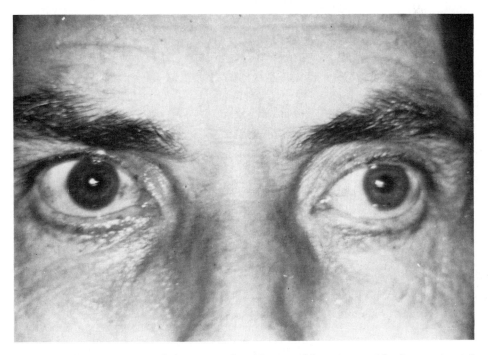

Fig. 6-24. Close-up view of the eyes of a 40-year-old patient with the untreated pseudosclerotic form of Wilson's hepatolenticular degeneration. Note the relatively broad, homogeneous, and golden-brown band that extends from the outer half of the iris to the limbus. This band, the Kayser-Fleischer ring, which is equally visible in both eyes, actually results from free copper deposits in Descemet's membrane rather than in the iris itself. This patient also has mild exotropia of the right eye. (Courtesy of Dr. Les Drew, Indiana University School of Medicine.)

also are more severe than the neurologic abnormalities (Walshe and Cumings, 1961). It is not uncommon for a patient to succumb to the effects of cirrhosis without developing neurologic symptoms other than terminal coma. A person with an almost purely nonneurologic form of the disease is shown in Fig. 6-25. Still, tremor, dystonia, dysarthria, and fixed smiling may appear even before liver symptoms. In the progressive lenticular form of Wilson's disease one usually sees relatively rapidly developing dystonic postures, choreic movements, an open-mouthed fixed smile, and difficulty in mental concentration as initial manifestations. Tremor occurs late in this form, which usually begins before the affected person is 18 years of age. An onset of neurologic symptoms after this age is characterized by tremor and dysarthria. An onset after the age of 30 or so is characterized by tremor, dysarthria, slow mental deterioration, and a more parkinsonian picture.

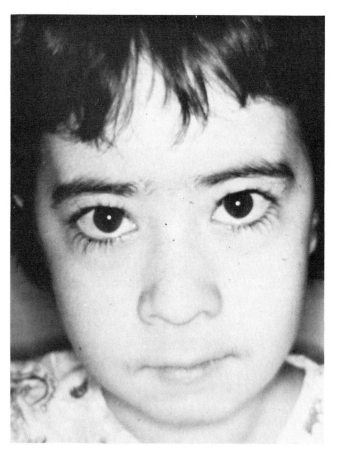

Fig. 6-25. Eleven-year-old girl with a purely hepatic form of Wilson's disease, without striking neurologic involvement. She was considered to be mildly mentally retarded. The iris was homogeneously brown, but no Kayser-Fleischer ring was identified, even by slit-lamp examination. Note the mild mongoloid slant, which was a nonrelated finding.

From a purely facial viewpoint, Wilson's disease is characterized by two common but not absolutely necessary features. One is the typical facial expression that results from involvement of the lenticular nucleus. This expression involves a characteristic open mouth and fixed smile (the so-called wilsonian risus). This facial appearance is fairly characteristic of the earlier-onset, more progressive form of the disease. Patients with the pseudosclerotic form tend to have expressionless facies more akin to those of persons with Parkinson's disease (Fig. 6-24), whereas patients with formes frustes of the disease may have no abnormality of facial expression (Fig. 6-25). The second, and perhaps most diagnostic, facial feature of Wilson's disease is the Kayser-Fleischer ring, which is an area of pigmentation that results from copper deposition in Descemet's membrane of the cornea. The ring can be seen grossly in some cases (Fig. 6-24) but in others must be viewed with oblique lighting. The Kayser-Fleischer ring is usually a smoky-brownish-greenish ring on the outer margin of the cornea, close to the limbus. (See Fig. 6-26). When typical, the ring is characteristic if not absolutely diagnostic of this disease. The Kayser-Fleischer ring is seen especially frequently in patients with the more chronic forms of Wilson's disease. It is seen in a high percentage of patients with oligosymptoms and partial symptoms but less commonly in patients with the earlier, more progressive forms. There may be some resolution of this ocular sign after treatment of the disease with chelating agents such as penicillamine. (See Fig. 6-26, B).

Recently, a few additional variations of hepatolenticular degeneration have been documented and their biochemical and clinical differences noted (Bearn, 1972).

**Corneal clouding syndromes.** Corneal clouding is a rather nonspecific finding that may be secondary to many disease processes. Trauma, secondary reactions to ocular atrophy from subluxation of the lens, cataracts, and many other conditions are associated with corneal clouding. Nevertheless, there are a few diseases that are characterized by corneal clouding that seems to be primary to the diseases.

The mucopolysaccharidoses (MPS) are now known to have many forms. A total of twelve subtypes are now clearly differentiated (Goodman and Gorlin, 1977). In addition, approximately five forms of closely related diseases called the mucolipidoses, several of which are believed to be sialase deficiencies, have been reported. Further ballooning of this previously simple group of diseases has occurred with the recognition of several phenotypically similar disorders such as fucosidosis, mannosidosis, and the generalized gangliosidosis. In the classic literature concerning the differentiation of the mucopolysaccharidoses, the presence or absence of corneal clouding was considered of great clinical importance. This facial abnormality can still be of some diagnostic use. The most common form of the mucopolysaccharidoses associated with corneal clouding is classic *Hurler's syndrome* or MPS IH. The presence of corneal clouding is a major distinguishing feature between Hurler's

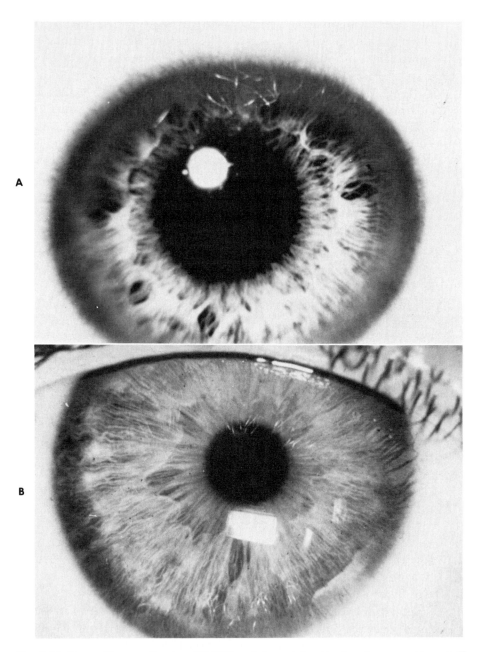

Fig. 6-26. Eyes of two patients with Wilson's hepatolenticular degeneration. A, Eye of a patient before treatment. The ring is deep brown and is distributed fairly evenly throughout the entire circumference of Descemet's membrane. B, Eye of a patient with pseudosclerotic form of Wilson's disease who had been treated with penicillamine for several months. Note the more uneven distribution of pigment in Descemet's membrane.

syndrome and the closely related *Hunter forms of mucopolysacchari-doses* (MPS IIA and IIB). In addition, *Scheie's syndrome* (MPS IS), the *Hurler-Scheie syndrome* (MPS IH/S), *Morquio's syndrome* (MPS IV), and the *Maroteaux-Lamy syndrome* (MPS VIA and VIB) are associated with definite but less dramatic corneal changes. *Sanfilippo's syndromes* (MPS IIIA and IIIB) and *β-glucuronidase deficiency* (MPS VII) are not usually associated with corneal clouding.

Many of the disorders associated with opacities of the cornea, either acquired or congenital, have been discussed in previous sections of this chapter under other headings (such as microphthalmia). These syndromes include the *Hallermann-Streiff syndrome* (Fig. 6-14), *Lenz's type of microphthalmia* (Fig. 6-15), and *Cross' syndrome*. Cloudy corneas also have been associated with trauma, congenital glaucoma (Fig. 6-27), and the *Marinesco-Sjögren syndrome* (Fig. 6-30). A variant of the Marinesco-Sjögren syndrome has been described by Garland and Moorhouse (1953).

**Megalocorneal syndromes.** *The elfin-facies syndrome with supravalvular aortic stenosis and infantile hypercalcemia (Williams' syndrome)* is associated with many facial abnormalities. The relationship between a distinctly elfin-like facies and infantile hypercalcemia was pointed out by Fanconi and associates (1952). Williams and associates (1961) called attention to the syndrome of supravalvular aortic stenosis, mental retardation, and peculiar facial features. But it was not until the work of Black and Bonharn-Carter (1963), however, that the combination of supravalvular aortic stenosis, infantile hypercalcemia, and elfin facies was recognized as a possible syndrome. Beuren (1972) pointed out more definitively that infantile hypercalcemia and supravalvular aortic stenosis—both with and without mental retardation—were the same disease. It is now accepted that the disorder is an entity of sporadic occurrence and of unknown origin, although a dysgenic defect resulting from possible hypersensitivity to vitamin D in utero is considered a possible cause (Goodman and Gorlin, 1977).

Although there are enough characteristic systemic and somatic features to establish the elfin-facies syndrome as a separate entity, the only absolutely consistent features are the abnormalities of the face. Megalocornea, one of the more prominent facial features, is characteristic of the disorder—especially when other typical facial abnormalities are also present (see Fig. 6-28). The elfin-like facies is characteristic but difficult to describe, and even this consistent feature tends to change somewhat and become less distinctive after the end of the third year of life. The most characteristic abnormalities involve the middle facial segment especially. The middle face is full, and there are shortened palpebral fissures, which tend to add to the illusion of megalocornea. The eyebrows tend to flare medially, and the eyes are wide-set. The iris shows a stellate or mosaic pattern. There tends to be a depressed nasal bridge, and the nostrils are anteverted. Epicanthal folds and esotropia may be present.

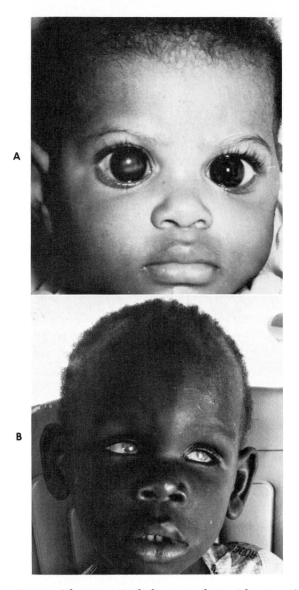

**Fig. 6-27.** Two patients with congenital glaucoma but without major neurologic or mental symptoms. **A,** Four-year-old. Note the large cornea and buphthalmos. **B,** Six-year-old blind patient who had congenital glaucoma and developed corneal clouding after operations to treat the condition. (**A,** Courtesy of Dr. John Bigger, Augusta, Georgia.)

In addition, one may encounter microcephaly, a broad forehead, a typically open and wide mouth with prominent lips (especially in older patients) and mouth angles that tilt downward, a long philtrum, dependent cheeks, a small mandible, and small teeth. Craniosynostosis has been reported. About 50% of affected patients are mentally retarded. Neither supravalvular aortic stenosis nor hypercalcemia is an absolute feature of the disorder. A variety of vascular defects, however, may occur be-

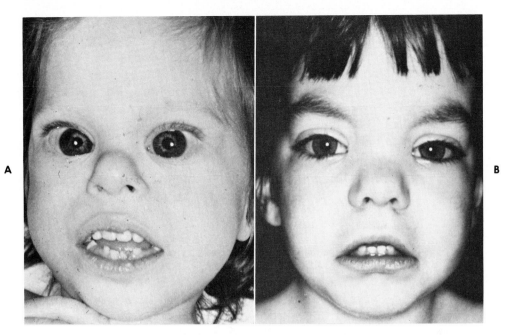

Fig. 6-28. Two patients with Williams' syndrome of elfin facies, transient idiopathic hypercalcemia, and supravalvular aortic stenosis. A, Twenty-month-old girl with typical face of this syndrome, which includes short nose, anteverted nostrils, mild mongoloid slant, long philtrum, large mouth with slightly downturned corners, mild mental retardation, supravalvular aortic stenosis, and megalocornea. Observe particularly the megalocornea, which gives the illusion of esotropia. (Patient's eyes are merely converging slightly while she looks at the photographer.) Patient also shows an extensive mosaic pattern of the irises. B, Three-year-old patient with similar facial features. Observe particularly the megalocornea. Patient also has bilateral epicanthal folds. No significant cardiac lesion was confirmed, although an innocent cardiac murmur was detected. Transient hypercalcemia was present in the early infantile period.

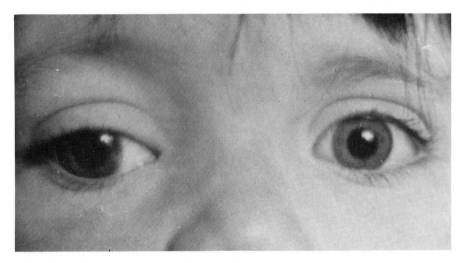

Fig. 6-29. Eyes of patient in Fig. 6-7, B. Note the characteristics of the buphthalmos, particularly the absolute, but not relative, megalocornea of the right eyeball.

sides supravalvular aortic stenosis. These include aortic, subclavian, carotid, pulmonary, and systemic vessel stenosis, often resulting from hypertrophy or proliferation of the medial and intimal segments of the arterial and valvular wall. Growth failure, other skeletal defects (such as pectus excavatum), clinodactyly, and inguinal and umbilical hernias have been reported. There may be hypoplastic nails and gonadal disturbances. X-ray films may show increased ossification of the base of the skull, the orbits, the vertebral bodies, and the metaphyseal regions of long bones.

Congenital glaucoma leading to buphthalmos, as seen in *Sturge-Weber disease*, may be associated with unilateral corneal enlargement. (See Fig. 6-29.)

## Syndromes characterized by abnormalities of the lens

**Congenital cataract syndromes.** The *Marinesco-Sjögren syndrome* is a type of hereditary spinocerebellar degeneration that was initially described by Marinesco and associates (1931) and later in more detail by Sjögren (1947). The disorder is characterized by autosomal recessive inheritance, congenital cataracts and other congenital anomalies, short stature, cerebellar ataxia, and mental retardation that ranges from mild to moderate. The ataxia becomes evident in infancy and early childhood and is associated with marked delay in psychomotor advancement. Progressive muscular paresis and atrophy have been seen in a few patients. Congenital defects are characteristic. Besides the lenticular cataract, which worsens throughout infancy, one may encounter kyphoscoliosis, alopecia, clubfoot, pes cavaus, and short digits. Adults with the syndrome are usually short, seldom being over 5½ feet tall. The patient in Fig. 6-30 had congenital cataracts. She was mildly mentally retarded, as shown by psychometric tests performed when she was 30 years old. She shows the long-term effects of bilateral cataracts—microphthalmia, marked ocular retraction, and sunken eyes.

*The oculocerebrorenal syndrome of Lowe* is also characterized by bilateral congenital cataract. This syndrome also involves severe mental retardation, small stature, muscular hypotonia, decreased muscle bulk, occasional gonadal abnormalities, hyperexcitability, and high-pitched screaming. The ears may be large in some patients (Lowe and others, 1952). (See Fig. 6-31.)

*Galactosemia* was probably first described in 1908 by von Reuss in an infant with failure to thrive and a large liver and spleen (von Reuss, 1908). It is now recognized that galactosemia, an autosomal recessive disorder, is one of the more common metabolic causes of mental retardation. Several forms of this disease are now differentiated. The classic form results from a deficiency of galactose-1-phosphate uridyl transferase (G-1-PUT). This enzyme is normally found in the liver and in leukocytes and erythrocytes. When the enzyme is absent, galactose-1-phosphate and galactose in the form of galactitol are allowed to build up in

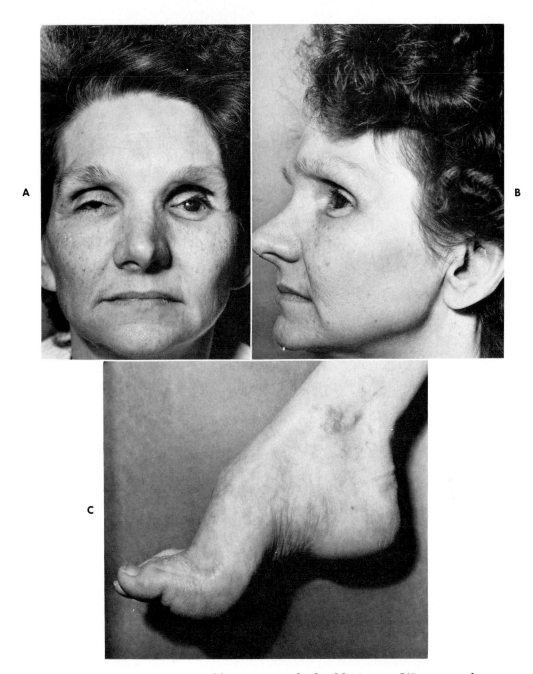

**Fig. 6-30.** Forty-three–year–old woman with the Marinesco-Sjögren syndrome associated with lenticular cataract. **A,** Frontal facial view showing enophthalmos and atrophic eyeballs related to complications resulting from the treatment of bilateral lenticular cataracts. **B,** Lateral facial view. Note atrophy of eyeball, producing pronounced retraction. **C,** Pes cavus and hammer toe deformity, which also are features of this syndrome.

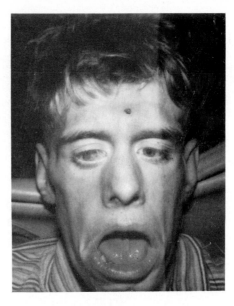

Fig. 6-31. Patient in his twenties who has unilateral congenital glaucoma with buphthalmos on the right. The left eye is normal. This patient is severely mentally retarded and hyperexcitable.

the blood and tissues. There is also a Duarte variant form. Another type of enzymatic deficiency is now known to produce galactosemia. The condition is caused by the absence of galactokinase, which is necessary for the initial phosphorylation of galactose to galactose-1-phosphate. In this type of galactosemia, there is an accumulation of galactitol, also called dulcitol, in the tissues. There are, however, no excessive amounts of galactose-1-phosphate.

Infants with galactosemia may appear normal at birth but soon develop symptoms once milk feedings begin. Early symptoms are listlessness, feeding difficulty, vomiting and weight loss, jaundice, seizures, and hypoglycemia. Later, one begins to see the characteristic lenticular cataracts, hepatosplenomegaly, emaciation, severe weakness, and hypotonia. If untreated, the transferase form of the disease often results in death or severe morbidity.

Even though the face of a sick infant has no characteristic features other than cataracts, the possibility of galactosemia should always be considered if many other features of the disease are also present.

The transferase form shows an associated aminoaciduria (due to renal tubular damage) and often is associated with severe degrees of mental retardation. This form is different from the kinase form, which is characterized by cataracts alone. It is assumed that the difference in clinical presentation between the two forms results from the fact that the galactose-1-phosphate is toxic to both the kidney and the brain, whereas dulcitol has major toxic effects only upon the lens.

**Other lenticular syndromes.** *Homocystinuria,* an uncommon inborn error of sulfur amino acid metabolism, was first recognized as a clinical entity by Gerritsen and associates (1962) and by Carson and associates (1962). This disorder is due to the absence of cystathionine synthase, which results in the formation of cystine from 3 molecules of homocysteine. Homocysteine is therefore metabolized to homocystine, which is thereafter excreted in abnormally large amounts in the urine. Homocystine, being primarily an intracellular amino acid, is usually not present in the bloodstream, since there is no renal transport system available that allows it to be reabsorbed in the renal tubule. There also is no primary absorptive mechanism for this amino acid in the gut. Because it can not be reabsorbed, almost all homocystine that reaches the tubule is excreted into the urine. In addition, however, methionine, another amino acid, is often found in abnormal amounts in both the plasma and the urine. Methionine exists one step prior to homocysteine in the metabolic pathway of the sulfur amino acids. When the level of homocysteine is elevated, a certain proportion of methionine breakdown to homocysteine is apparently inhibited. Both an absorption and a reabsorption mechanism exist for methionine, and there is also a renal clearance mechanism. Thus, after a certain blood level is reached and the reabsorption mechanism is working at its maximum rate, methionine spills over into the urine. In homocystinuria, homocystine acts as a "no-threshold" substance, whereas methionine acts as an "overflow" substance in a way similiar to the way that phenylalanine acts in phenylketonuria.

The clinical picture of homocystinuria may consist of a so-called marfanian habitus. This habitus has several dysmorphic features including dolichofacies, dolichocephaly, high-arched and narrow hard palate, excessive height, thinness, dolichostenomelia, arachnodactyly, and subluxation of the ocular lenses. In addition, talipes equinovarus, excess flexibility of the joints, kyphoscoliosis, and other orthopedic abnormalities have been reported in this disease. One feature that distinguishes it from "true" *Marfan's syndrome,* an autosomal dominant condition of uncertain biochemical basis, is the frequent presence of mental retardation. Although mental retardation is not always present in homocystinuria, it is rarely present in Marfan's syndrome. (McKusick, 1966). Patients with homocystinuria tend to be relatively hypopigmented and to have light-colored irises and blond or light brown cranial hair. Unlike the situation in phenylketonuria, there is no biochemical explanation for hypopigmentation in homocystinuria, and it is possible that this symptom simply may be a feature of the racial characteristics of the first patients reported with the disease. Of great interest to persons interested in cerebrovascular disease is the fact that patients with homocystinuria have coagulation defects that make them very susceptible to strokes, even in early life. (See Figs. 6-32 and 6-33.)

The facial features of homocystinuria tend to suggest but not to prove the presence of the disease. One feature is subluxation of the ocular lenses, which may be bilateral or unilateral, severe, mild, or even absent

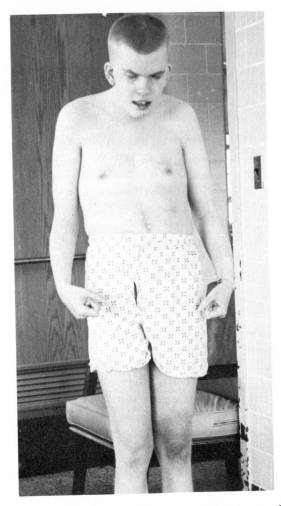

Fig. 6-32. Large 18-year-old patient with severe mental retardation, excessive aggressiveness, long extremities and digits, and bilateral subluxation of the lenses. Tests of this patient's urine indicate abnormal excretion of homocystine. He is believed to have cystathionine synthase deficiency or homocystinuria. Note the sunken eyeballs that are evident even in this full-body view.

(Fig. 6-33, *A*). Only the most severe forms of subluxation are readily evident during standard facial viewing. Iridodonesis, or a tremulous iris, is a clinical sign of an almost totally subluxed lens. However, totally subluxed lenses are not frequently encountered in homocystinuria. More common is the presence of a partially dislocated lens, the edge of which can be faintly visualized during close inspection or with a standard hand-held ophthalmoscope (Fig. 6-33, *B* and *C*). Absolute confirmation must be made by an ophthalmologist using slit-lamp examination. Occasionally, a physician may observe what would appear to be merely corneal scarring. When this feature is combined with dolichofacies and mental retardation in a hypopigmented individual, however, one should consider the possibility of homocystinuria. A person with this condition

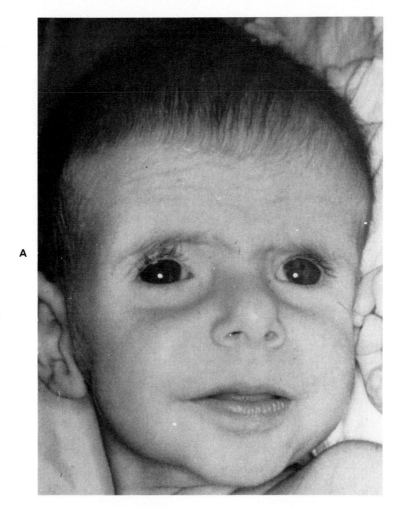

Fig. 6-33. Subluxation of the lens in three unrelated patients. A, Three-month-old infant with hypotonia, severe psychomotor retardation, and probable blindness. Note miosis, somewhat sunken eyes, and hypoexotropia on the right. Lenses were found to be mildly subluxed bilaterally. This patient was believed to have Marfan's syndrome.

*Continued.*

also may have a high-arched and narrow hard palate, but this sign is by no means specific.

## Syndromes characterized by abnormalities of the conjunctiva

Several disorders are characterized by abnormalities of the conjunctiva. Seldom, however, do any of these syndromes involve the conjunctiva alone.

**Ataxia-telangiectasia.** Ataxia-telangiectasia was first documented by Madame Louis-Barr (1934), but it was not until Shy and Magee's (1956) and Boder and Sedgewick's (1958) "rediscoveries" of the entity that it became well known to the medical profession. Although once considered

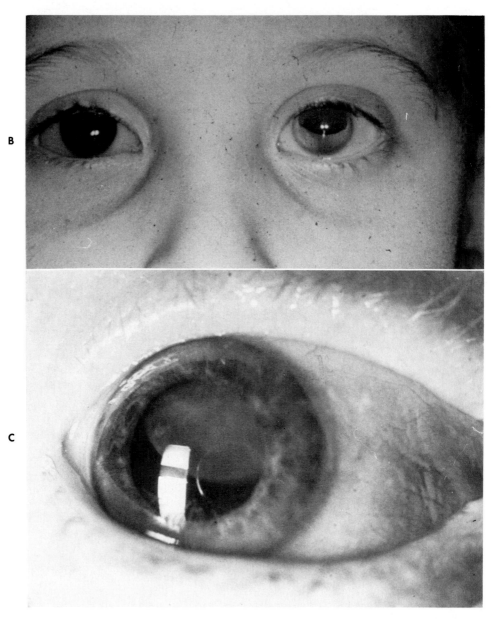

Fig. 6-33, cont'd. B, Child whose left eye displays aniridia (absence of iris) and superior subluxation of the lens. Note inferior border of lens and "red" reflection of normal retina in background. C, Close-up view of inferiorly subluxed lens in older patient with lenticular cataract. Dislocation of lens was caused by direct ocular trauma. (B and C, Courtesy of Dr. John Bigger, Augusta, Georgia.)

a very rare condition, recent experience indicates a world-wide distribution and a relatively high incidence (Goodman and Gorlin, 1977). Along with tuberous sclerosis, neurofibromatosis, Sturge-Weber disease, and von Hippel-Lindau disease, ataxia-telangiectasia is now considered one of the five major phakomatoses or neurocutaneous diseases (Dyken, 1971).

Ataxia-telangiectasia, as the name implies, is characterized by two major abnormalities, neither of which seems to be always present in all patients. The disease is inherited as an autosomal recessive trait. In typical form, it has an early onset and a fairly consistent, subacute downhill course. The ataxia is of the cerebellar type and is most often the earliest symptom or sign of the disease. However, other, nonspecific symptoms, such as mild psychomotor retardation, mild delay in attaining the usual developmental milestones, or recurrent sinopulmonary infections, may herald the neurologic symptom. Telangiectasia, ultimately present in most but not all patients, is of later onset. Sometimes telangiectasia does not appear until puberty. Even then it is sometimes only mild. The conjunctiva is usually the site of first involvement by the telangiectasia (see Fig. 6-34, A). The conjunctival involvement is soon followed by the appearance of cutaneous spider nevi. Nevus telangiectasis occurs typically on the neck, behind the ears, in the cubital and popliteal areas, and elsewhere over the body. Less characteristically, one may see these lesions in lesser numbers on the trunk, the malar area of the face, and the dorsa of the hands. The conjunctival telangiectasia characteristically develops around the age of 5 years, although earlier cases have been reported. Thus, neurologic symptoms tend to antedate the typical skin lesions. A small percentage of patients with ataxia-telangiectasia never develop typical nevus telangiectasis. (See Fig. 6-34, C.) Recurrent sinopulmonary infections, which are common in most patients, usually constitute an early sign of the disease. Infections tend to linger much longer than under ordinary circumstances. Susceptibility to recurrent infection is believed to result from an absence or a deficiency of immunoglobulins. The IgA fraction, particularly, is characteristically absent. Recent study has indicated that the alpha-fetal protein level is abnormally elevated in this disease. In typical form, ataxia-telangiectasia involves a steady deterioration in neurologic functions. So-called extrapyramidal symptoms and signs, may become one of the more dominant presentations, taking the form of tremor, masked facies, rigidity, dystonic postures, and choreoathetosis. Even in patients with pronounced, typical cerebellar ataxia and without such "extrapyramidal" signs, a fairly typical wide-eyed, masked facies is usually present. (Shy and Magee, 1956). In addition, one finds a curious immobility of the eyeballs, which is often seen when the disease has become moderately advanced. The ocular immobility has been inaccurately called oculomotor apraxia or dyspraxia (Sedgwick and Boder, 1972; Wells and Shy, 1957).

It has been pointed out that there is a very high incidence of neoplasm

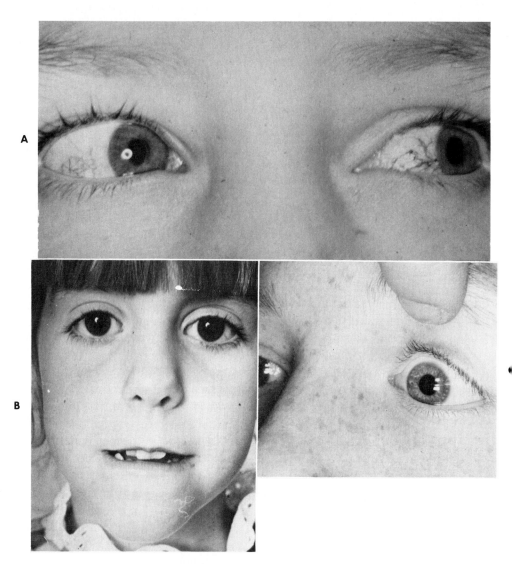

Fig. 6-34. Three patients with ataxia-telangiectasia of Louis-Barr. A, Close-up view of eyes in nine-year-old patient with well-developed ataxia-telangiectasia. Note prominent conjunctival telangiectasia on both lateral and medial sides. (See also Fig. 8-36). B, Five-year-old patient with prominent ataxia but only mild and early telangiectasia. Note the single, well-developed, obliquely oriented, dilated end artery of the left lateral conjunctiva, which is a very characteristic early feature of this syndrome. (See also Fig. 8-38.) C, Close-up view of eyes of 15-year-old patient with slowly progressive ataxia of more than 12 years' duration. He has no IgA. He shows immobility of the eyeballs and an expressionless facies but, at the time of this photograph, very little, if any telangiectasia of the conjunctiva. (See also Fig. 8-37.) He has prominent but scattered cutaneous telangiectasia. This patient has a younger sister with more characteristic features.

in patients with this disease. This fact is considered to be related in some way to the immunoglobulin deficiencies (Hecht and others, 1966).

The course of the disease is steadily downhill, and death usually occurs in the second or third decade of life. Death results from neoplasm or superimposed infections or merely from chronic neurologic debilitation and loss of vegetative functions. Postmortem examinations show widespread findings similar to those found in other spinocerebellar degenerations. No vascular lesions of the cerebellum or organs or tissues other than the skin are usually discovered.

The abnormal features of the face are very consistent for this disease and may make possible clinical diagnosis in patients with otherwise atypical courses. The typical conjunctival telangiectatic nevi, when present, are the most diagnostic. One of the earliest hallmarks of this lesion is a horizontal vascular "streak" that represents a dilated arteriole in the lateral conjunctiva. This streak usually occurs in both eyes. (See Fig. 6-34.) In addition, one characteristically observes an expressionless, wide-eyed, masked facies, which results from central nervous system probably extrapyramidal involvement. Finally, one may observe an ocular immobility that is recognizable because of slowly initiated eyeball movements, usually in horizontal planes. Eyeball movements seem to be aided by brief eyelid blinks or quick side-to-side head titubations.

**Other syndromes involving dilated conjunctival vessels.** It should be emphasized that a diagnosis of ataxia-telangiectasia should not rest solely on the presence of conjunctival telangiectasia. Such a diagnosis is merely suggested by it. Many other conditions may show conjunctival vascular abnormalities that closely resemble congenital telangiectasia. *Carotid cavernous arteriovenous fistula*, because of its more insidious and bilateral onset, may produce severely dilated conjunctival venules that look like the vascular nevi of ataxia-telangiectasia. (See Fig. 6-35.)

In 1943, Wyburn-Mason described a syndrome that had similarities to Sturge-Weber disease. This disorder was characterized by an arteriovenous angioma of the mesencephalon as well as by facial nevus flammeus (Wyburn-Mason, 1943). A person with suspected *Wyburn-Mason's syndrome*, who can be seen in Fig. 6-36, was severely mentally and physically handicapped from birth. She had a severe spastic type of quadriplegia and was totally bedridden, requiring total nursing care. Seizures were never a prominent feature of her illness. She was examined by one of us (PRD) when she was 23 years of age, when her condition was considered an atypical example of Sturge-Weber syndrome. Facial examination showed dilation of the conjunctival vessels on the right side and extremely dilated retinal vessels on this same side. Both arteries and veins were dilated. No direct arteriovenous communications or dilated angiomas were observed. She had pronounced hypoesotropia and severely contracted extremities characteristic of a severe long-standing quadriplegia. Skull roentgenograms showed, as might be expected, a thickened calvarium but no calcifications of the brain. No

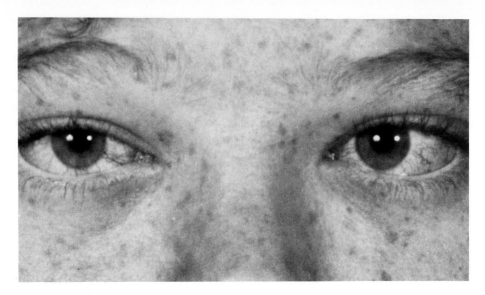

**Fig. 6-35.** Eleven-year-old boy with arteriovenous fistula between carotid artery and cavernous sinus. This close-up photograph of the eyes, which was taken 3 weeks prior to the photographs in Fig. 6-4, *A* and *B*, shows no prominent proptosis but extensive bilateral scleral vascular dilation.

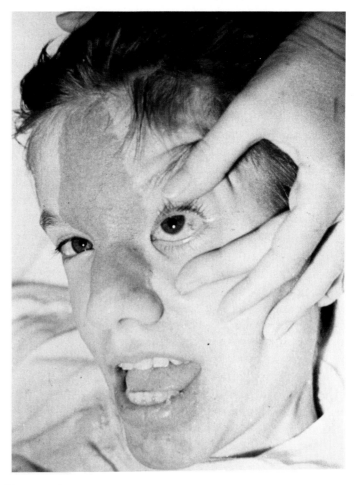

**Fig. 6-36.** Twenty-three-year-old patient with midline nevus flammeus. Note extensive episcleral hemangioma of telangiectasia that extends into the retina and probably communicates with a midbrain hemangioma. (See also Fig. 5-62.)

further investigations were performed. The final impression was that this patient had not Sturge-Weber disease, as was previously believed, but rather a variant or transitional condition between Sturge-Weber disease and Wyborn-Mason's syndrome.

**Other conjunctival syndromes.** Although *Goldenhar's syndrome*, which will be further documented in the following section, is one of the best examples of a first-arch syndrome, one also finds characteristic lesions in the conjunctiva in this disorder. Patients with this syndrome have iris colobomas, microphthalmia, malformed ear pinnae, preauricular appendages, and blind fistulas as well as other features of the first-branchial-arch syndrome. In addition, in the conjunctiva there are often dermoid tumors. These conjunctival tags probably represent persistent nests of fetal tissue derived from the first branchial arch.

## Syndromes characterized by abnormalities of the eyelids

The position of the eyelids in relationship to the eyeballs is an important facial diagnostic sign. As has been pointed out in Chapters 1 and 3, abnormalities of the eyeballs and eyelids are dependent upon a variety of nervous, muscular, and osseous factors.

**Ptosis syndromes.** An important abnormality in the shape and size of the eyelids is ptosis or "falling" of the eyelid. Severe ptosis is often associated with somatic efferent neurogenic disturbances or severe myopathic processes. Pseudoptosis, on the other hand, is seen in less severe types of myopathic processes and in visceral efferent neurogenic disturbances. A syndrome characterized by mild ptosis has been discussed in the preceding section as *Horner's syndrome*, which involves other functional deficits besides droopy eyelids. Fig. 6-18 shows a patient with congenital Horner's syndrome with anisocoria, heterochromia, and mild unilateral ptosis. Many of the other syndromes associated with bilateral ptosis are also associated with mild facial diparesis and will be discussed in more detail in Chapter 7. Yet a few diseases tend to selectively involve the eyelids more than the rest of the face. In a restricted definition, true ptosis does not always occur in these latter disorders. Contrasted to the mild ptosis of Horner's syndrome is the pronounced and almost total ptosis seen in *acute ophtathalmoplegia*. In the patient in Fig. 6-37, who suffered from acute lymphoblastic leukemia, one can see only a small amount of the eyeball and only the white portion because of the combination of long eyelashes and exotropia. If one looks closely at this photograph, one can see that the medial border of the limbus of the right eye is much more laterally placed than that of the left eye. This situation suggests exotropia of the right eye, which one would expect to accompany a total disruption of oculomotor function. This patient also had a mydriatic pupil on the right because of this oculomotor lesion. Even though lateral and internal torsion of the affected eyeball is still present because of the unopposed action of the lateral rectus and superior oblique muscles (innervated by the cranial nerves VI [abducens] and IV [trochlear], re-

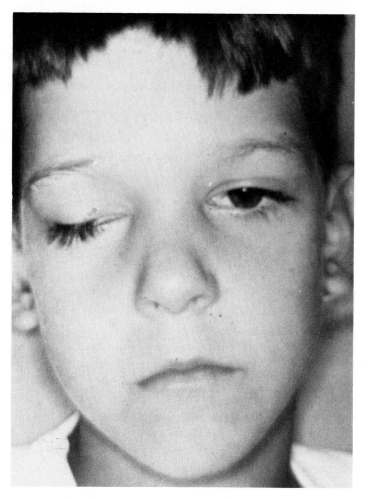

Fig. 6-37. Twelve-year-old boy with acute lymphoblastic leukemia who developed a sudden total oculomotor palsy. Note the almost total ptosis of the right eyelid. Careful observation reveals that the right eyeball is deviated externally.

spectively), findings such as those shown in Fig. 6-37 cannot properly be called "ophthalmoplegia" (that is, total paralysis of the eye). In some clinical circles it has been in vogue to refer to an "external" and an "internal" type of "ophthalmoplegia." The "external" type involves paralysis of the extraocular muscles and levator palpebri muscles, and the "internal" type involves paralysis of the fibers that innervate the pupil. Since the oculomotor fibers that, when damaged, produce "internal ophthalmoplegia" are found in the periphery of the oculomotor nerve along its intracranial course, these fibers are much more prone to injury by a wide range of intracranial lesions. An "internal" type of oculomotor lesion is in reality an external one. Therefore, "internal ophthalmoplegia" is a misnomer for two reasons. Similarly, "external ophthalmoplegia" is a manifestation of damage to fibers of the oculomotor nerve that are more centrally or internally located in the total nerve bundle. These fibers are more protected from acute trauma but perhaps are more susceptible to small-vessel vascular and metabolic disturbances. Thus, "external ophthalmoplegia" is also a misnomer. It is, however, very important to recognize a difference between selective pupillary and extraocular muscle palsy from partial oculomotor lesions. It is not uncommon to have a complete oculomotor dysfunction, as in the patient in Fig. 6-37. The deficit in this patient's case was produced by a total oculomotor nerve lesion. This patient also had mydriasis and a paralysis of the pupil on the side of the "true" ptosis. The contrast between these lesions and that in Horner's syndrome (see Fig. 6-18) is dramatic.

Acute oculomotor lesions have many causes. The most common causes are *acute head injuries* and the many varieties of intracranial vascular abnormalities, such as *aneurysms and other congenital anomalies of intracranial vessels* that characteristically insult the more peripherally placed oculomotor fibers. In addition, *brain masses* and other conditions that produce asymmetrical *herniation of the brain* contents from one intracranial compartment to the other, particularly at the incisura, are likely to affect the oculomotor nerve and thus produce oculomotor lesions. Included in the differential diagnosis of disorders that produce acute oculomotor lesions are several systemic diseases that characteristically are associated with single or multiple cranial nerve palsies. This chapter will not dwell upon the specifics of these diseases in any depth. Included in this list of disorders are the various types of *leukemia* that are particularly prevalent in childhood, metabolic disorders such as *diabetes mellitus*, endocrinologic diseases such as *thyroid and pituitary dysfunctions, other neoplasms* and *infectious diseases* at the base of the skull that cause pressure to be placed upon cranial nerves as they exit and a variety of parainfectious disorders such as *sarcoidosis, histiocytosis X*, and *collagen disease*. The eyelids and the alignment of the eyeballs are not infrequently involved by these conditions.

*Myasthenia gravis* is a disturbance in transmission of the electrical impulse at the myoneural junction. It is now recognized that there are many types of this disorder as well as a few rarer diseases that closely resemble it. Most types of true myasthenia gravis are now thought to be autoimmune diseases. For unexplained reasons, perhaps a variety of noxious insults, susceptible individuals begin to develop antibodies to receptor substance on the postsynaptic border of the myoneural junction. The antibody-receptor antigen reaction decreases the effectiveness of the postsynapsis, and the transmitter acetylcholine is not allowed to act in a normal fashion. The major deficit in myasthenia gravis is an abnormal tendency to fatigue and not the paresis or paralysis characteristic of the myopathies or the neurogenic disorders that may also be associated with ptosis. Early in the course of the disease, no constant facial stigmata may be present except during times of fatigue. Later, however, permanent facial stigmata appear. When the disease is of long standing, fibrosis may develop, particularly in the extraocular muscles. Such a condition is unresolvable by medical or surgical therapy. The extraocular muscles are particularly likely to be involved in myasthenia gravis, although all skeletal myoneural junctions may also be involved. (See Figs. 6-38 and 6-39.)

Although most instances of myasthenia gravis seem to result from an autoimmune reaction with increased amounts of antireceptor antibody, one also encounters rare congenital or familial forms of the disease that do not seem to be associated with circulating antibody. Otherwise, *congenital myasthenia gravis* is quite similar in clinical presentation to the more commonly encountered, early-onset forms of the disease. Rarely, a myasthenoid type of reaction might occur in relationship with occult neoplasms. Such a condition has been well documented in adults with the Eaton-Lambert syndrome or with polymyositis, but one of us (PRD) has also seen such a *myasthenoid syndrome* in a child who had an abdominal neuroblastoma. *Trichinosis* as well as many other diseases may produce symptoms that are very similar to myasthenia gravis. In most of these disorders, however, the face is less often primarily involved, and systemic muscular symptoms seem to predominate.

*Dystrophia myotonia or myotonic muscular dystrophy* will be discussed in more detail in other sections of this book (see Chapter 7 particularly). The ptosis that occurs in this disease is rarely the major abnor-

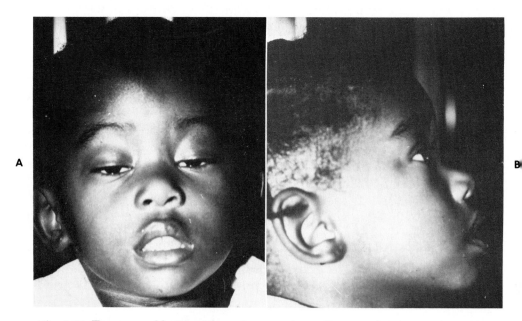

Fig. 6-38. Two-year-old girl with early-onset juvenile myasthenia gravis. A, Frontal view showing bilateral ptosis, flattened facial folds caused by facial diparesis, and mild exotropia. B, Lateral view, which allows better appreciation of ptosis.

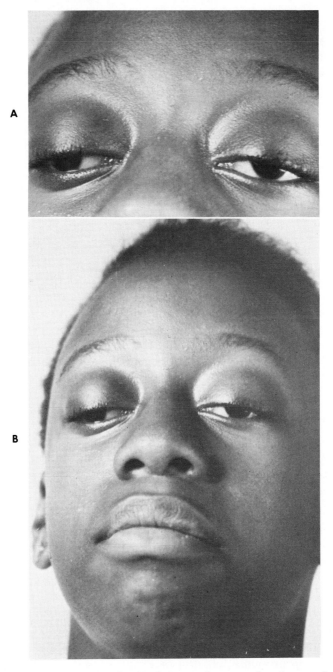

Fig. 6-39. Patient, 5½ years old, with juvenile myasthenia gravis. A, Close-up view showing bilateral ptosis, as well as exotropia on the right. B, Full facial view showing flattening caused by facial diparesis.

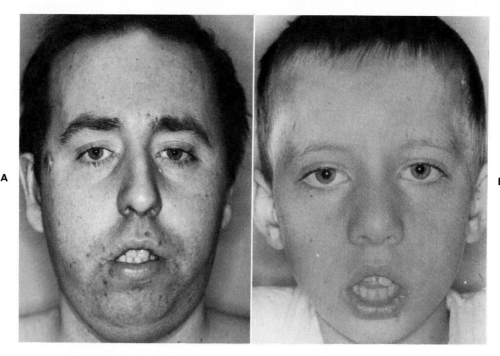

Fig. 6-40. Two patients with dystrophia myotonica. A, Patient (also seen in Fig. 5-67) with adult-onset dystrophia myotonica. Note facial flattening and mild bilateral ptosis (pseudoptosis) without ocular malalignment. B, Twelve-year-old boy with congenital dystrophia myotonica involving mild bilateral ptosis (pseudoptosis) and more severe facial and masseter diparesis. Compare the mouths of the two patients.

mal facial feature, however. (See Figs. 6-40 to 6-42.) Usually there is mild pseudoptosis rather than ptosis, although occasionally in severe forms of the disease a severe ptosis may occur.

*Facioscapulohumeral muscular dystrophy* is a form of muscular dystrophy showing primary involvement of muscles of the face and scapulae and those surrounding the humeri. The disease was first described by Landouzy and Dejerine (1885). The disorder is usually considered to be one of later onset, as compared with the more typical childhood muscular dystrophies, and to have a more protracted and less disabling course (Tyler, 1950). Recently, however, childhood and even infantile forms of the disease have been recognized (See Chapter 7.)

The essential symptoms of the disease are explained by muscular involvement in the areas of distribution suggested by the disease's name. Atrophy and weakness of all facial muscles predominate, although this is dependent upon the stage of the disease and individual characteristics. The orbicularis oculi is characteristically affected in the early stages of the disease. Sometimes its involvement is so severe as to be confused with congenital ptosis, although until late in the disease course this involvement is usually more mild and in the nature of pseu-

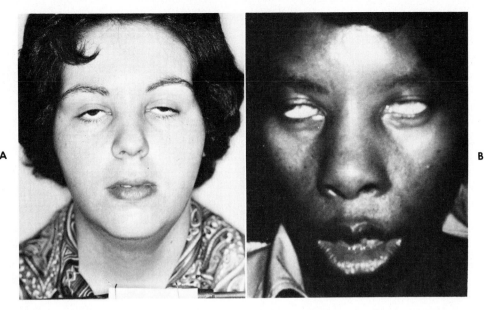

Fig. 6-41. A, Twenty-one-year-old woman with dystrophia myotonica. Her bilateral ptosis seems more obvious than the ptosis of the patients in Fig. 6-40 but actually was only slightly more severe. There is apparent severe drooping of the eyelids because the photograph was taken after the eyelids had been forcefully closed for a few seconds and a fraction of a second after the patient had been requested to open her eyelids suddenly. Myotonia evidently is affecting this patient's extraocular muscles of elevation. Thus, when the patient is asked to open the eyelids suddenly, the sustained elevation of both eyeballs causes the white sclera to be revealed. This phenomenon is called the myotonic eye sign. (See also Fig. 6-42.) B, Patient with the severe facial diplegia of Moebius' syndrome. This patient was asked to close the eyelids forcefully for this photograph. When a normal patient is asked to close the eyelids, the eyeballs simultaneously deviate upward. When there is a facial palsy and the eyelids are closed, the eyeballs elevate. At such a time the whites of the inferior sclera can be seen because the orbicularis oculi does not fully close the palpebral fissure (an occurrence known as Bell's phenomenon). Because of severe orbicularis oculi paresis in this patient, the elevation of the eyeballs, as indicated by the extensive scleral whiteness, is readily seen. Compare this example of Bell's phenomenon with the myotonic eye sign, as shown in A. Both patients have facial weakness.

doptosis. (See Figs. 6-43 and 6-44.) The muscles of the mouth, especially the orbicularis oris, are also often involved early. Inability to pucker is a common early symptom. In moderately and severely advanced cases, most of the facial muscles are involved and a "hatchet-like" facial appearance becomes typical. In advanced stages lisping and mispronouncing of words occur because of involvement of other branchially derived cranial muscles, — that is, the pterygoids, the masseters, and the temporalis masseters. Somitically derived cranial muscles, such as the extraocular muscles and the tongue, are seldom involved in this disease. Whereas the cranial musculature involvement is of particular pertinence

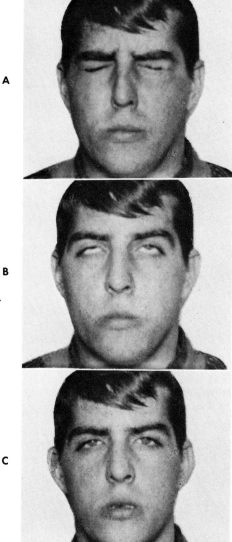

Fig. 6-42. Myotonic eye sign. A, Forced closure of eyelids. B, Sudden opening of eyelids. Observe deviation of eyeballs upward. C, Normal position of eyes. (From Dyken, P.: Neurology 16:49, 1966.)

to this book, it is important to point out that the involvement of other muscles in a rather typical distribution is very important for confirmation of a diagnosis. Typically, there is involvement of the muscle mass of the arm (the muscles around the humerus), which, in advanced cases gives a "popeye" appearance to the upper extremity. This involvement plus that of the scapulae produce an inability to raise the arms above the head. Flattening of the anterior chest (due to involvement of the pectoralis muscles) and pectus excavatum occur regularly. The neck muscles are also involved, especially those that cause flexion of the head on the neck (the sternocleidomastoid muscles). (See Fig. 6-43.) Occasionally, there is involvement of the pelvic girdle and paraspinal muscles and an

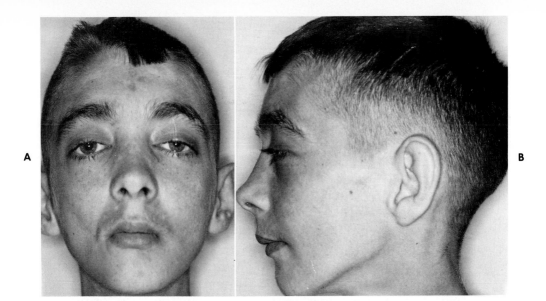

Fig. 6-43. Fifteen-year-old boy with facioscapulohumeral muscular dystrophy. A, Frontal view showing hatchet-like facies and bilateral ptosis. Facial diparesis is present, but it has not deformed the face or mouth. Observe narrow, atrophic neck muscles. Chin is tipped upward in a posture characteristic of persons with ptosis. The position apparently allows greater pupillary opening and vision. B, Lateral view. Observe that ptosis is more pronounced when chin is normally positioned. Observe also the severe wasting of the anterior nuchal musculature.

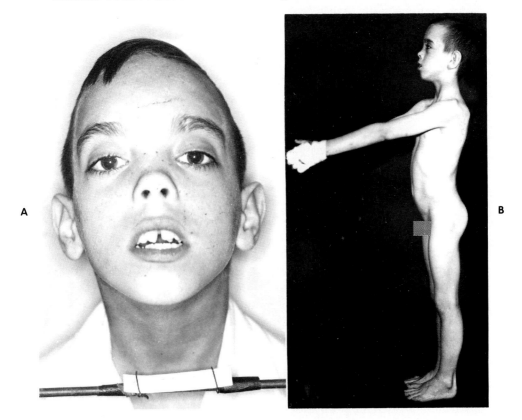

Fig. 6-44. Ten-year-old brother of patient in Fig. 6-43. A, Facial view showing milder ptosis than in brother and less severe atrophic features of face and neck. The chin is tipped upward, suggesting that the ptosis is nevertheless a significant disability. B, Lateral body view. Ptosis was an acquired and progressive problem in both brothers.

associated lordosis. The lower extremity may also be involved, but this is usually a late feature.

Because the disease is inherited as an autosomal dominant trait, a high percentage of individuals in a given family are affected.

Laboratory findings in this disease are not diagnostic. The creatine phosphokinase level may be normal or only slightly elevated. There may be minor electrocardiographic abnormalities. Muscle biopsy and electromyography usually show abnormalities, but they are not diagnostic.

The facial features in this disease are characteristic but are similar to those found in many disorders including dystrophia myotonica and nemaline myopathy. Late myasthenia gravis may show similar facial abnormalities, but involvement of somitically derived cranial musculature is a characteristic of myasthenia gravis, whereas it does not occur in facioscapulohumeral muscular dystrophy. The absence of ophthalmoplegia also distinguishes the syndrome from the many forms of the "ophthalmoplegia-plus" syndromes such as the Kearns-Sayre syndrome and the mitochondrial myopathies.

*The Kearns-Sayre syndrome* is a disorder (Kearns and Sayre, 1958) that is now grouped in a larger category of diseases called the mitochondrial myopathies and the "ophthalmoplegia-plus" syndrome. The cardinal features of the disorder as it was originally delineated include ophthalmoplegia, facial and somatic weakness, retinitis pigmentosa sine pigment, and conduction defects of the heart. Endocrinopathies, mental retardation, growth retardation, and other features, subsequently have been added to the original list of disabilities. The disorders now listed under this category include congenital or childhood-onset muscle diseases, all of which are characterized by abnormalities in the mitochondria of skeletal muscle. These myopathic abnormalities consist of giant pleomorphic mitochondria that oil-red-O and PAS staining may show as "ragged-red" muscle fibers. The muscle changes are probably not the primary source of abnormalitity in these diseases, however. Recent reports have related the muscle abnormality to other, as yet uncertain, neurologic disorders such as *Leigh's subacute necrotizing encephalomyelopathy* (Jabbour and others, 1976).

Early in the disease process there may be few facial stigmata. Affected patients soon show evidence of facial weakness and mild ptosis coexistent often with mild skeletal muscle weakness. Visual problems, signs suggesting cardiac difficulties, recurrent infections, seizures, and mentation problems may be associated. The only facial stigmata displayed by the patient in Fig. 6-45, when she was first evaluated for recurrent seizures at age 5 years, were mild facial weakness with bilateral ptosis. The patient showed mild somatic hypotonia and paresis, mainly of proximal musculature, and a very blond-appearing retina, which on later study displayed patchy areas of atrophy with prominent choroid vessels but without pigmentary changes. Electrocardiographic studies showed abnormalities in cardiac conduction. Muscle biopsy showed numerous

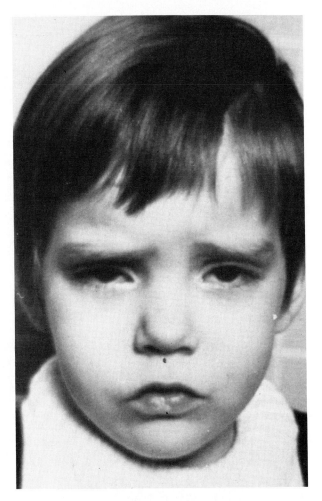

**Fig. 6-45.** Six-year-old girl with mild bilateral ptosis and intermittent diplopia who also had seizures, retinitis pigmentosa sine pigment, and cardiac conduction defect. Appropriate testing showed no evidence of myoneural junction dysfunction. She was believed to have the Kearns-Sayre syndrome. Observe mild ptosis in addition to scrawling quality of eyebrows, which was not a constant feature of the facial appearance at the time of the photograph. She also shows mild bilateral facial weakness.

ragged-red changes in muscle fibers. The patient had continued facial as well as somatic weakness over a follow-up period of only 1½ years. The patient in Fig. 6-46 was believed to have a variety of the "ophthalmoplegia-plus" syndrome. She had severe facial and somatic stigmata at the age of 32, when the photograph was taken, and she also showed a retinitis pigmentosa. This patient seems properly classified as having the Kearns-Sayre syndrome.

There are other syndromes characterized by ptosis. *Leprosy* typically presents as a partial, bilateral facial paresis (see Fig. 7-12). This disease may show bilateral or unilateral ptosis. Many other congenital myopa-

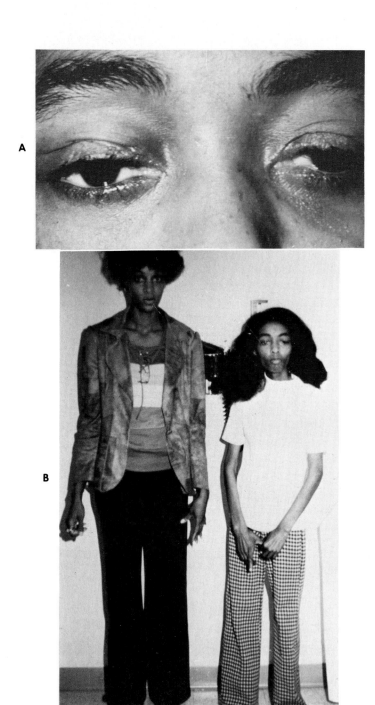

Fig. 6-46. Twenty-eight-year-old woman with typical features of well-advanced Kearns-Sayre syndrome. A, Close-up view of eyes showing bilateral ptosis and exotropia. B, Full-body view of patient with normal-sized and neurologically intact sister. Very small stature is a feature of the syndrome. Patient also had cardiac and retinal abnormalities typical of this syndrome.

thies, such as *nemaline myopathy,* also may be associated with varying degrees of ptosis.

**Other eyelid syndromes.** There are many other syndromes characterized by abnormalities of the eyelids. One of the more frequently occurring syndromes that has been recognized only recently is the *fetal alcohol syndrome,* which is characterized by short palpebral fissures. It seems established that maternal alcohol ingestion has a direct effect in producing the condition. The syndrome is characterized by a wide range of congenital malformations, one of the most characteristic of which is shortened palpebral fissures. This may give the illusion of wide-set eyes and may be associated with epicanthal folds. (See Fig. 6-47.)

*Waardenburg's syndrome* involves abnormalities in the relationship of the eyelids to the eyeballs. This syndrome (Fig. 6-48) creates the impression of wide-set eyes or hypertelorism because of the dystopic canthorum that typically exists. (In contrast, see Fig. 6-49.) The dystopia canthorum persists into juvenile and adult periods of life, although it may be less obvious in early childhood, when there is normally a relative dystopia canthorum. The cardinal features of Waardenburg's syndrome have been discussed previously.

*The Schwartz-Jampel syndrome* may be characterized by a peculiar

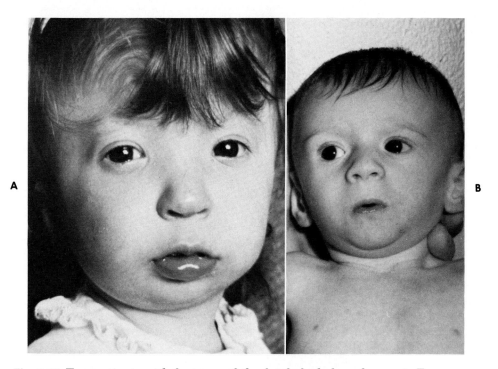

Fig. 6-47. Two patients with features of the fetal alcohol syndrome. **A,** Four-year-old girl who is mildly mentally retarded. Note the short palpebral fissures. Patient also has mild midface retraction, long philtrum, and small nose. **B,** Six-month-old infant with short palpebral fissures, small nose, long philtrum, and small mouth. (**B,** Courtesy of Dr. Charles Linder, Medical College of Georgia.)

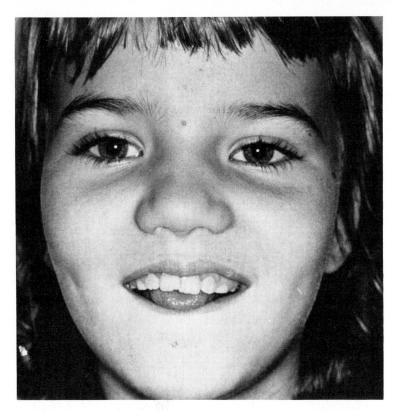

Fig. 6-48. Fifteen-year-old girl with sensorineural deafness believed to be associated with Waardenburg's syndrome. Note dystopia canthorum, mild hypertelorism, and medial hyperplasia of eyebrows.

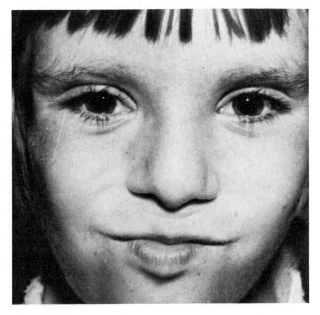

Fig. 6-49. Thirteen-year-old girl with Turner's syndrome. Note mild illusory hypertelorism. The pterygium colli is barely discernable in this photograph. (Courtesy of Dr. Charles Linder, Medical College of Georgia.)

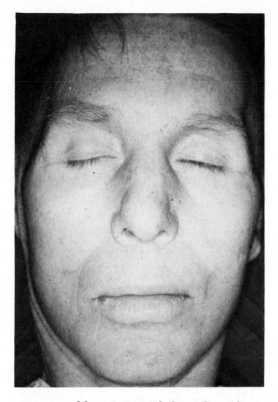

**Fig. 6-50.** Thirty-seven-year-old patient with hypothyroidism, ataxia, and opso-clonia. Note thickened skin around eyebrows, nose, and eyelids.

eyelid abnormality as well as other facial abnormalities (see Fig. 7-18) (Schwartz and Jampel, 1962). The peculiar abnormality, called bleph-arophimosis, is also rarely reported in *dystonia musculorum defor-mans* (Zeman and Dyken, 1967) and the *cerebrooculofacioskeletal (COFS) syndrome* (Preus and Fraser, 1974), a rare disorder that also may involve microphthalmia.

Simple thickening of the eyelids as well as other areas of the face is a characteristic of hypothyroidism, especially the acquired forms. (See Fig. 6-50.)

Xanthomata of the eyelids are characteristic of an uncommon syn-drome called cerebrotendinous xanthomatosis. (See Fig. 6-51.)

Other rare syndromes characterized by shortened or small palpebral fissures are the *10 q + syndrome* and the *4 p + syndrome* (Goodman and Gorlin, 1977).

## Syndromes characterized by abnormalities in orbital slant

The slant of the orbital structures is an important diagnostic facial feature that is reflected in part by the intercanthal line. In mongoloid syndromes the intercanthal line is slanted downward medially to form a

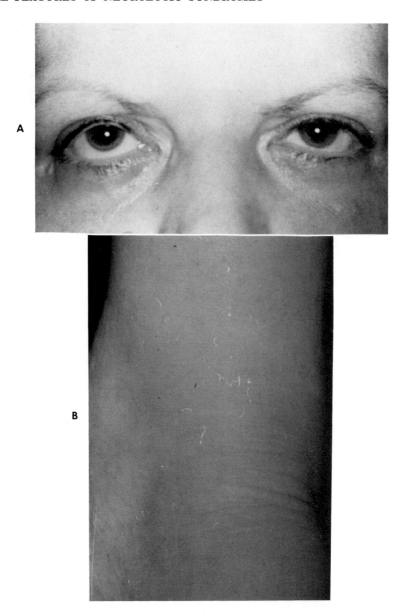

Fig. 6-51. Fifty-one-year-old woman with cerebrotendinous xanthomatosis. This patient, who had had several psychiatric disturbances, showed thickened tendons and multiple xanthomata over the body but especially around the eyes. A, Close-up view of face. Note the two xanthomata near the eyelids close to the lateral canthi. B, Close-up view of thickened Achilles tendon.

V. The converse of this type of slant is represented by many of the first-branchial-arch syndromes. In such a situation, because of hypoplasia of the structures that compose the lateral and inferior aspects of the bony orbit, the intercanthal line is slanted downward laterally, giving an impression of an A or a tent. Under normal situations, as discussed in Chapters 1 and 3, the intercanthal line is parallel to the other horizontal facial lines or at least does not vary considerably from this presumed norm.

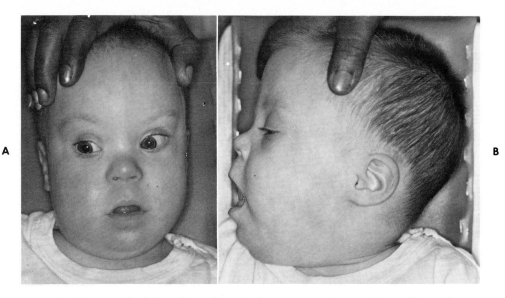

Fig. 6-52. Six-month-old male infant with proven trisomy 21. A, Frontal view showing mongoloid slant and Brushfield spots. Observe other facial stigmata of Down's syndrome as well. B, Lateral view.

**Mongoloid syndromes.** Langdon Down (1866) first described the syndrome later recognized by Lejeune and associates (1959) to be caused by a chromosomal abnormality. This condition is now identified as *Down's syndrome* or *trisomy 21*. In about 95% of the cases, the disorder results from a total trisomy of the twenty-first chromosome. In the balance of instances, the defect is a translocation (familial type of Down's syndrome) or a mosaicism (a mixture of cell lines). (See Fig. 6-52.) The most prominent clinical feature of Down's syndrome is the slant of the palpebral fissures that bears the name "mongoloid" slant. This facial feature was one of the earliest recognized abnormalities of the syndrome and accounts for the less-preferred name for the condition—mongolism. Unfortunately, mongolism is still used in both medical and nonmedical circles to refer to the disorder. The syndrome has many distinctive features, which are particularly predominant in the trisomy form. These include somatic smallness (especially reduction in height), mental retardation (usually at the trainable mentally retarded level—intelligence quotients between 25 and 70), delayed bone age, clinodactyly of the fifth finger, simian crease (especially unilateral), muscular hypotonia, congenital malformations of the heart (especially atrioventricular defects), relative hypotrichosis, duodenal atresia, umbilical hernia, underdeveloped male genitalia, and short, broad neck with cervical-occipital abnormalities. In addition, afflicted persons frequently have brachycephaly, middle facial hypoplasia with underdevelopment of maxillary and nasal bones, flattening of nasal bridge, mild ocular hypotelorism, small oral cavity with short palates (see Chapter 7), protruding tongues with hypertrophied papillae (see Chapter 7), delayed dentition with reduced dental caries, epicanthal folds, Brushfield spots, a mosaic pattern of the iris,

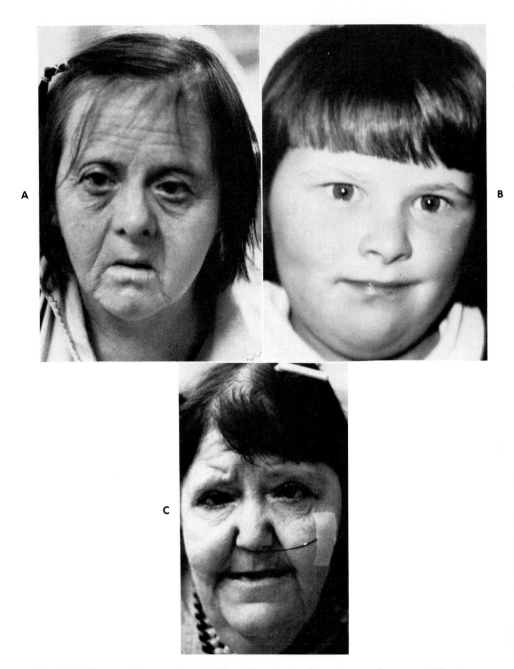

Fig. 6-53. Two adults and a child with proven Down's syndrome. A, Forty-one-year-old patient with trisomy 21. Observe mild mongoloid slant, small rounded facies, and small mouth. B, Eight-year-old girl with mongoloid slant, Brushfield spots, and rounded, delicate facies. Patient has a mosaicism of trisomy 21. C, Thirty-two-year-old patient with trisomy 21 showing similar facial features. The microcephaly is more obvious in this patient.

lenticular cataracts, heterotropias, and small, rounded, "shell-like" ears with small lobules. (See Fig. 6-53.)

The clinical features are quite suggestive, but confirmation of the chromosomal defect is necessary for several pertinent reasons. First, the varieties of the chromosomal defect are important to characterize, particularly the familial form, which may be predicted and eradicated. Second, there are forms of phenotypical Down's syndrome that do not involve a chromosomal defect and that do not have the usual prognostic implications. Some of these conditions may involve mosaicisms rather than trisomy or may be caused by other closely related chromosomal disturbances that are as yet undiscovered. True Down's syndrome, on a chromosomal basis, is associated with several features that decrease the life expectancy of affected persons. These mortality threats are susceptibility to (1) respiratory infections such as tuberculosis, (2) blood dyscrasias (especially lymphoblastic leukemia), (3) cervical-occipital dislocations and sudden neurologic symptoms due to transection of the cervical spinal cord, (4) cardiac failure, and, more recently recognized, (5) seizure disorders in infancy, childhood, and adulthood. A definite trend toward infantile spasms has been recently pointed out (Zellweger and others, 1976). All of these complications in true Down's syndrome favor an accurate clinical and chromosomal diagnosis. In the days before more accurate chromosomal identification with banding techniques, uncertainty existed as to whether the triplication involved the twenty-first or the twenty-second chromosome. *Trisomy 22* or the *cat's-eye syndrome* is now recognized as a definite clinicogenetic syndrome with features quite different from those in Down's syndrome (Crawford, 1961). (See Fig. 6-54.)

Mongoloid slanting of the palpebral fissures occurs in several other syndromes as well. Some of these, like the holoprosencephalies, have been discussed in this book in other sections. Others characterized by mongoloid slant are *familial recurrent brachial plexus neuritis* (also called the *Dreschfield-Taylor-Erickson syndrome*), *the C syndrome* (also called the *Opitz trigonocephaly syndrome*), *chondrodysplasia punctata* (also called *Conradi's syndrome*), the *5 p+ syndrome* (referred to as the antithesis of the cri-du-chat syndrome), and the *9 p− syndrome*. These rare syndromes are completely discussed in Goodman and Gorlin (1977).

**First-branchial-arch syndromes.** The first branchial arch supplies what in the mature being becomes the lateral bony orbit, the zygomatic arches, and the ears (see Chapter 7 for further details). In direct facial viewing, the slant of the palpebral fissures is determined by these important embryogenic structures. Because of hypoplastic bony support, the palpebral fissures can be slanted downward in the reverse direction of what is seen in Down's syndrome or trisomy 21. When this situation occurs, it is said that an antimongoloid slant exists. A variety of early fetal insults or noxious agents may influence the development of first-branchial-arch

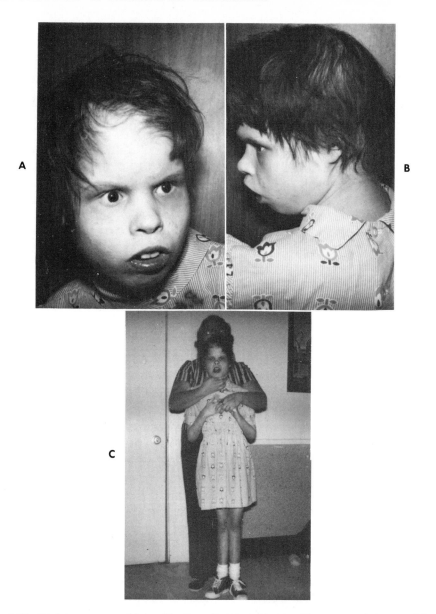

**Fig. 6-54.** Eighteen-year-old institutionalized patient with proven trisomy 22. A, Frontal facial view showing *no* stigmata of trisomy 21. There is mild midfacial retroaction and frontal bossing. B, Lateral facial view. C, Full-body view. Note size of patient in comparison to normal woman. The patient is severely mentally retarded and extremely hyperexcitable. She ruminates and self-mutilates constantly.

derivatives. In addition, cytogenic disturbances appear to influence the development of these structures. There is a large number of first-arch syndromes associated with neurologic dysfunction.

One of the most important first-arch syndromes is the *Rubinstein-Taybi syndrome,* also known sometimes as the *broad thumbs syndrome*

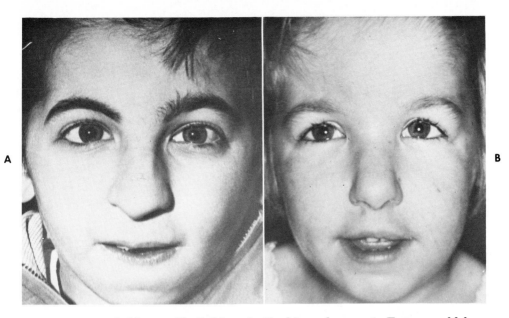

Fig. 6-55. Two children with Rubinstein-Taybi syndrome. A, Ten-year-old boy. Note the mild antimongoloid slant resulting from zygomatic hypoplasia, hypoplasia of mandible, micrognathia, and long beak-like nose. Patient is moderately retarded and has seizures. B, Eight-year-old girl who has recurrent seizures and is mildly mentally retarded. She shows antimongoloid slanting, a long, somewhat beaked nose, and hypoplasia of first-branchial-arch derivatives.

(Rubinstein and Taybi, 1963). The syndrome consists of a rather characteristic first arch–derivative hypoplasia. Antimongoloid slant of the palpebral fissures is usually pronounced. In addition, one sees a high-arched and narrow palate, a beak-like nose, relative micrognathia, low-set and sometimes malformed ears, and zygomatic hypoplasia. Other associated craniofacial features are seen as well, including microcephaly, prominent forehead, heavy eyebrows, long eyelashes, and heterotropia. Nevus flammeus of the forehead has been reported. Low birth weight and, later, short stature are common. Mental functioning is usually moderately deficient. Another constant feature of this syndrome is big and widened thumbs or halluces. Somatically, one sees a wide variety of orthopedic abnormalities irregularly associated with this syndrome. These include medial angulation of the thumbs and big toes, polydactyly, hyperextensible joints, kyphoscoliosis, and stiff-legged gait. Of vital importance to the neurologist is the heightened incidence of mixed-seizure disorders in persons with this syndrome. The disorder is quite characteristic facially and can be distinguished from other first-arch syndromes by the combination of relative hirsutism, beaked nose, and prominent antimongoloid slant (Rubinstein and Taybi, 1963). Fig. 6-55 shows two mild to moderately mentally deficient children with facial features characteristic of the Rubinstein-Taybi syndrome. Observe the prominent antimongoloid slanting, the long and narrowed noses with tendency of the tip to be beaked, the relative hirsutism (even in the light-complexioned child), and the relatively small chins that suggest a degree of micrognathia. Fig. 6-56, *A*, shows the associated broad thumbs in the more mildly affected patient seen in Fig. 6-55, *B*, and Fig. 6-56, *B*, shows an even more strikingly broad hallux in the same patient. Fig. 6-57 shows yet another severely retarded and institutionalized patient with the syndrome. This patient has even more pronounced features of the first-arch syndrome. He is quite hirsute, as is evident especially in Fig. 6-57, *B*. Each of these patients had recurrent seizures in addition to the other features of the syndrome.

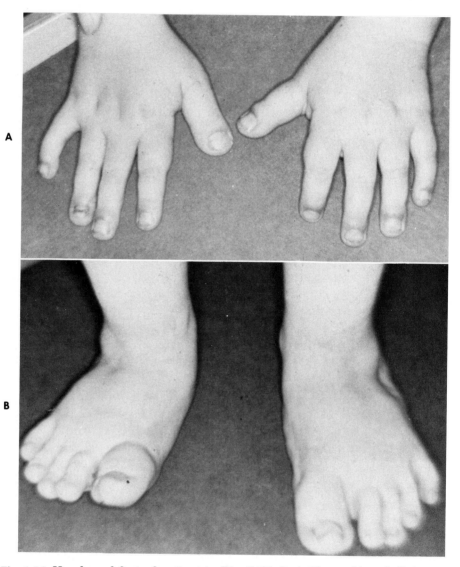

Fig. 6-56. Hands and feet of patient in Fig. 6-55, *B*. **A**, Note widened digits, especially the thumbs. **B**, Note extremely widened halluces.

*The Hallermann-Streiff syndrome* is a slightly different first-arch syndrome. This condition was described by Aubry (1893) but was clarified by Hallermann (1948) and Streiff (1950). It has been discussed in the section on abnormalities in ocular size earlier in this chapter (see Fig. 6-10, *B*). Typically, patients show the following features of the first-branchial-arch syndrome: (1) mandibular hypoplasia, (2) micrognathia, (3) mild antimongoloid slant of the palpebral fissures, (4) mild symmetrical hypoplasia of the zygomatic arches, (5) occasional deafness, (6) high-

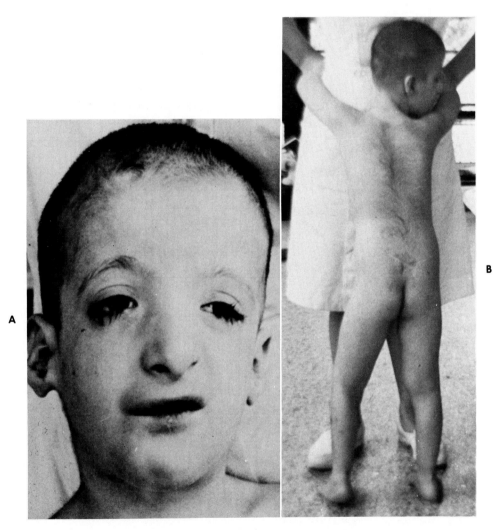

Fig. 6-57. Patient with Rubinstein-Taybi syndrome who was severely mentally retarded and showed resistant, recurrent seizures. A, Frontal facial view showing severe antimongoloid slanting, long and beak-like nose, zygomatic and mandibular hypoplasia, micrognathia, and deformed lobules of the right ear. B, Posterior body view showing pes planus and marked hirsutism. Close observation reveals a broadened right big toe. Also, the features of the first-arch syndrome can be appreciated in the lateral view of the face.

arched and narrow palate, and (7) small mouth. In addition, patients have a long and beaked nose, hypotrichosis, frontal bossing and delay in suture closure, and ocular abnormalities such as microphthalmia and cataracts.

According to the recent mammoth reference book *The Face in Genetic Disorders*, by Goodman and Gorlin (1977), there is a total of twenty-six syndromes characterized by antimongoloid slanting of the palpebral fissures. In addition, we have selected four more syndromes that we believe involve antimongoloid slants. (In comparison, Goodman and Gorlin list only eleven conditions characterized by mongoloid slant of the palpebral fissures [see the table on p. 553]. Interestingly, trisomy 21 is not included, but four conditions—Noonan's syndrome, trisomy 22, the 22 q+ syndrome, and the cloverleaf skull anomalad, which, in our experience, are usually associated with antimongoloid slants—are included.) Many of the thirty or so conditions reported as showing antimongoloid slanting are extremely rare or do not have major neurologic symptoms. Others involve major abnormal facial features that allow them to be discussed more appropriately in other sections of this book. Examples of this latter group are *Goldenhar's syndrome* (see this chapter's section on conjunctival syndromes), *Treacher Collins' syndrome* (see Chapter 7), *Apert's syndrome* (see Chapter 5), the *whistling face syndrome* or *craniocarpotarsal dysplasia* (Chapter 7), the *OPD syndrome* (Chapter 7), Turner's syndrome (Chapter 7), *Noonan's syndrome* (later in this section and in Chapter 7), and *Sotos' syndrome* (Chapter 7). (See Fig. 6-58.)

Several cytogenic disturbances are characterized by partial first-arch syndromes. For example, the *9 p+ syndrome*, the *10 q+ syndrome*, the *11 p+ syndrome*, the *monosomy 21 and 21 q— syndrome*, the *trisomy 22 syndrome*, and the *XXXXY syndrome* are associated with antimongoloid slanting. One of the more severe and distinctive chromosome syndromes associated with features of a disturbance in the first branchial arch is *Edwards' syndrome* or *trisomy 18*. This syndrome involves low-set ears, micrognathia, and narrow palatal arch. *The Lejeune syndrome* or monosomy 21 was first described by Lejeune as the antithesis of Down's syndrome (Goodman and Gorlin, 1977). It is characterized by first-arch signs consisting of antimongoloid slant, micrognathia, and large low-set and malformed ears. Additional symptoms include microcephaly, deep-set eyes, blepharochalasis, Brushfield spots, cleft lip and palate, prominent nasal base, hypertelorism, severe mental retardation, severe neonatal hypotonia, low birth weight, congenital heart disease, hypospadias, renal defects, cryptorchidism, various orthopedic deformities, and pyloric stenosis. Similar features are seen in the *21 q—syndrome*. The *cat's-eye syndrome* or trisomy 22 is also characterized by features of the first-arch syndrome, including antimongoloid slant; beaked and prominent nose; low-set and malformed ears; preauricular skin tags, appendages, and/or pits; atresia of the external ear canals, and micrognathia. Colobomas of the iris, microcephaly, craniofacial asymmetry, microphthalmia, cata-

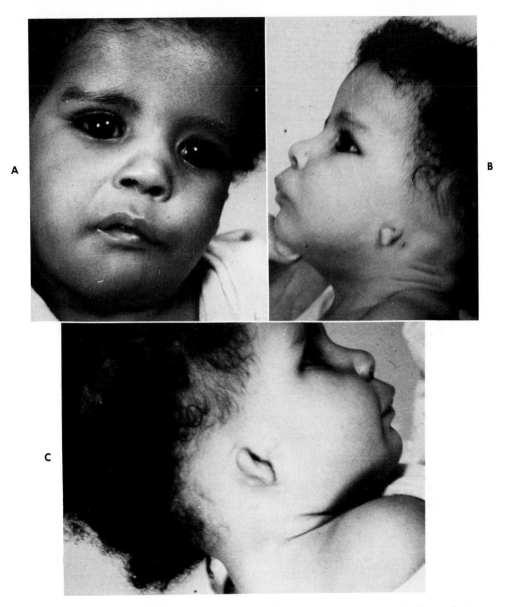

Fig. 6-58. Eight-month-old patient with Goldenhar's syndrome. A, Frontal view showing mild antimongoloid slanting, left facial palsy, bilateral zygomatic hypoplasia, and abnormally formed ears. B, Left lateral view demonstrating absent ear formation with rudimentary ear tags and more severe zygomatic hypoplasia. Note especially the puffiness and flattening of the face on this side. C, Right lateral view showing similar but less severe features. (Courtesy of Dr. Patricia Hartlage, Medical College of Georgia.)

racts, hypertelorism, heterotropia, long philtrum, cleft palate, growth retardation, mental retardation, hypotonia, underdeveloped musculature, hernia, congenital heart disease, arachnodactyly, congenital hip dislocation, cryptorchidism, imperforate anus, and renal agenesis are seen in this syndrome and in the similar 22 q+ syndrome, or partial trisomy of the long arm of chromosome 22. (See Fig. 6-54.)

## Syndromes characterized by abnormal ocular alignment

Precise alignment of the eyes is necessary for three-dimensional binocular vision without diplopia. The term heterotropia is synonomous with the terms squint or strabismus, as mentioned in Chapter 3. Many diseases are associated with heterotropia of ocular, neurogenic, or myopathic basis.

**Multiple sclerosis and other dissociative eyeball syndromes.** Multiple, or disseminated, sclerosis was first described by Charcot in the 1870s (Dejong, 1970). This disease is an acute or chronic, remittent or progressive disease of unknown etiology that affects primarily the white matter of the central nervous system. It is thus considered a prototype example of a demyelinating disease. The diagnosis of multiple sclerosis is based upon clinical grounds primarily, although certain laboratory investigations recently have been shown to produce characteristic if not pathognomonic evidence. These investigations include measurement of immunoglobulin levels in the cerebrospinal fluid, evoked potential patterns, computer-assisted tomography of the brain and spinal cord, and tests for the presence of myelinoclastic substances in the cerebrospinal fluid. The hallmark to the diagnosis, however, still is the characteristic course of the disease and the disseminated clinical findings. Dissemination of the plaques of demyelination, which are characteristic of the disease, throughout the central nervous system over a period of time produces the characteristic clinical features of remissions and exacerbations. In other words, typical multiple sclerosis is a disease involving dissemination of lesions in both time and space.

The disorder affects both sexes equally. The onset of symptoms usually occurs in young to middle-aged adults. Rarely, if ever, does the typical disease affect prepubescent children. The number of cases beginning before age 15 or after age 50 is almost negligible. The incidence is usually believed to be much higher in temperate zones, with some exceptions.

One of three modes of onset usually occurs. The first type is most common and includes a mild single symptom or sign, such as blurring of vision in one eye, a frank retrobulbar optic neuritis, clumsiness, or a paresthesia limited to one part of the body. This initial symptom may last for only a short time and be followed by apparent full recovery. Weeks, months, or even years may pass with no further symptoms or recurrence of the original symptom. It is thought that occasionally no further symptomatology might develop at all, such as in instances of unexplained nonrecurrent retrobulbar neuritis. Usually, however, a second exacerbation begins within weeks or months of the initial one. Thereafter, the course is one of recurrence with periods of relative normality in between. A second type of onset and course begins as an acute, fulminating, inca-

pacitating illness with paralysis, blindness, mental clouding, inconti-
nence, and/or severe sensory disturbance. Such a type may lead to death
or to severe disability, and periods of exacerbation may be longer. Complete recovery may seem to occur, followed by recurrences, or partial
recovery may take place and be characterized by residual symptoms and
subsequent exacerbations. The last mode of onset involves an insidious
and gradually developing disability that persists over several years and
that shows less tendency toward fluctuations and remissions. Such later-
onset types of multiple sclerosis could very well represent other disorders; many resemble other sporadic diseases of unknown nature, such
as nonhereditary spinocerebellar degeneration, progressive spastic para-
paresis, and lateral sclerosis.

The most common symptoms and signs of multiple sclerosis are (1)
visual impairment with paracentral and central scotomas with and
without frank optic atrophy but usually with at least mild temporal pallor; (2) ocular motility defects, such as jerk nystagmus in all directions
and diplopia, especially associated with conjugate gaze dissociation; (3)
pyramidal tract dysfunction; (4) paresthesias and other sensory defects;
(5) ataxia; (6) dysarthria; (7) personality and mood deviation, especially
in the direction of facetiousness, unconcern for illness, and emotional
instability; and (8) autonomic dysfunctions, with bladder disturbances
predominating.

From a facial viewpoint, the disease should be considered if two major findings are present. (They are not necessarily discussed in order of
decreasing frequency.) The first major finding is conjugate gaze disso-
cation, which is due to the presence of plaques of demyelinization in the
medial longitudinal fasciculus (MLF) of the brainstem between the
sixth and the third cranial nerve nuclei. These lesions produce what is
called internuclear ophthalmoplegia. The presence of such ocular motility deficits is best demonstrated by having the patient follow an object
laterally. When this is done, there is a deficiency of adduction of one eye,
with the poorly adducting eye pointing to the side of MLF involvement.
At rest, no obvious eyeball malalignment is necessarily seen. When the
MLF lesion is close to the oculomotor nuclei, however, abduction at rest
may be seen in one or both eyeballs because of abnormalities in the adducting muscles of the eye innervated by the third cranial nerve. (See
Fig. 6-59.) Internuclear ophthalmoplegia is a very useful clinical sign of
multiple sclerosis that indicates fairly specifically the presence of a lesion in the medial longitudinal fasciculus on the same side as the lag-
ging adducting eye. A second important facial feature that is helpful in
the diagnosis of multiple sclerosis is a wide-eyed, nonconcerned facial
appearance with mild eyelid retraction. This appearance will be further
discussed in Chapter 8. This feature is difficult to explain in pathophys-
iologic terms but seems to be directly correlated with the mental status
of the patient and is perhaps related to disruption of supranuclear fron-
tomesencephalic and frontopontine fibers.

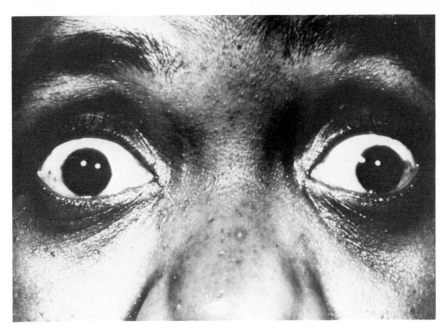

Fig. 6-59. Close-up view of face of 43-year-old patient with multiple sclerosis. Eyelids are artificially retracted. Observe exotropia, which was associated with an internuclearis ophthalmoplegia. (See also Fig. 8-41, *A*.)

Dissociations of the eyeballs are seen in other brainstem disorders as well, but these diseases are of a type different from that of the diseases already described. It has been claimed that a variety of disorders characterized by vasculitis, such as *systemic lupus erythematosus*, may be associated with internuclear ophthalmoplegia. Other disorders also are sometimes associated with such ocular disturbances.

**Pontine glioma, Leigh's disease, and other syndromes of progressive esotropia.** One of the more ominous signs in neurology is the development over a few days or weeks of a gradually worsening esotropia in a child. A wide variety of neural diseases may be responsible, including neoplasms of the pons and several degenerative diseases.

*Pontine glioma* is one of the more common brain tumors of childhood. Histologically, it may be a rather benign-appearing neoplasm. It usually begins in the pons and tends to show its maximum effects in this area. Medullary gliomas, either as secondary or primary sites, also occur, but the midbrain is a very rare location for pathology, either primary or secondary. When the midbrain is involved with glioma, the involvement tends to be from above and to be associated with optic nerve tract lesions. These latter neoplasms (discussed briefly with proptosis earlier in this chapter) have a more benign and therefore favorable outlook. The onset of symptoms depends, to a great extent, on the initial site of the tumor. Such tumors usually arise in the pons, somewhat asymmetrically in an area close to the abducens or sixth cranial nerve nucleus or fiber.

As the tumor progresses, there is usually involvement of the corticospinal tract, first on the same side and then on the other. Soon thereafter, involvement of the opposite abducens nuclei, and often of the facial nuclei and fibers as well, occurs. These new symptoms and signs develop slowly over weeks and are progressive. The biologic characteristics of pontine gliomas allow them to spread throughout the neuraxis, following fiber directions. The growth is longitudinal rather than horizontal, which probably accounts for the reasonably slow development of symptoms. Soon, however, other dysfunctions become evident, such as dysphagia, dysphonia, and ataxia. Ultimately, the clinical picture – unfortunately – is characterized by severe motor disability with losses of vegetative functions and by decerebrate and decorticate rigidity in the face of reasonably well-preserved mental functioning. The diagnosis can almost be suggested by the characteristic clinical picture, although confirmation by CT scanning or other neuroradiologic procedures is mandatory. Even so, surgical intervention may be indicated for palliation if, as is rarely the case, increased intracranial pressure develops. Rarely, one may encounter a large cystic cavity within the tumor mass that can be relieved transiently by puncture and drainage. No treatment is totally satisfactory. Corticoids, radiation, and chemotherapy have been used but with little lasting results.

The facial appearance, of course, changes depending upon the stage of the disease process. The patient seen in Fig. 6-60 is at a terminal stage. Observe the severe degree of bilateral esotropia, the lack of facial expression, and the absence of a significant external degree of hydrocephalus. Note also the nasogastric tube for feeding purposes.

*Leigh's disease* or *subacute necrotizing encephalomyelopathy* was originally delineated by Leigh in 1951. The onset of symptoms begins in early infancy or childhood and includes signs of brainstem dysfunction such as swallowing and feeding difficulty, incoordination, unexplained vomiting, episodes of intermittent hyperventilation or sobbing, ophthalmoplegia, and other cranial nerve dysfunctions. In addition, affected persons are paretic and hypotonic and may show loss of vision and convulsions or signs of peripheral neuropathy. Although gross examination of the brain is frequently normal, serial sections may show small irregular areas of gray discoloration suggesting necrosis, particularly in paraventricular areas and in the midbrain and pontine tectum and tegmentum (Farmer, 1968). Microcysts and spongiform changes are seen especially in the brainstem (Richter, 1957). It is believed that Leigh's disease is a result of an inhibitory factor found in urine, blood, cerebrospinal fluid, and the brain that affects the ability of thiamine pyrophosphate ATP phosphoryl transferase to catalyze the formation of thiamine triphosphate (TTP) from thiamine pyrophosphate (TPP) (Pincus, 1972). From a facial viewpoint, patients with Leigh's disease typically show a picture of estropia. Facial paresis as well as other cranial nerve defects also may be encountered.

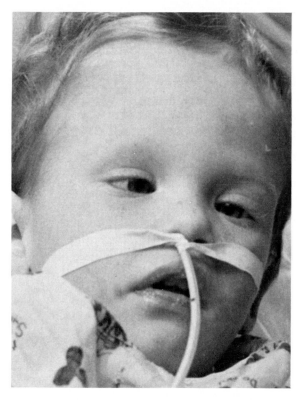

Fig. 6-60. Twenty-seven-month-old child with an extensive pontine glioma. Patient is terminal at this stage but has normal mental capabilities. Observe bilateral esotropia and facial diparesis. Bulbar function failure required nasogastric feedings. There is no evidence of macrocephaly or increased intracranial pressure. The esotropia results from bilateral abducens nerve nuclear destruction. Patient also showed intermittent signs of decerebration and severe corticospinal tract dysfunction.

Closely related to Leigh's disease but without apparent disturbance in thiamine metabolism is the syndrome called *myoclonic ataxia with multiple cranial nerve palsies* (Dyken, 1971). The original patient with this diagnosis is seen in Fig. 6-61, *A*, early in the development of the disease. At this time, when 5 years old, she was irritable and ataxic and showed a constant myoclonia with only a mild degree of esotropia and facial diparesis. Subsequently, these latter symptoms began to predominate. In the early stages of the disease, the symptoms were such that a pontine glioma was considered to be the most likely diagnosis, but repeated pneumoencephalography and arteriography over several years failed to reveal any mass, and she was living—although disabled—at 17 years of age. In the early stages, when her condition was followed closely, the myoclonic ataxia seemed to worsen at times. During one of these exacerbations, corticoids were given, which seemed to temporarily relieve the ataxia and myoclonia but not the cranial nerve palsies, which were slowly but relentlessly progressive. It has been reported that a

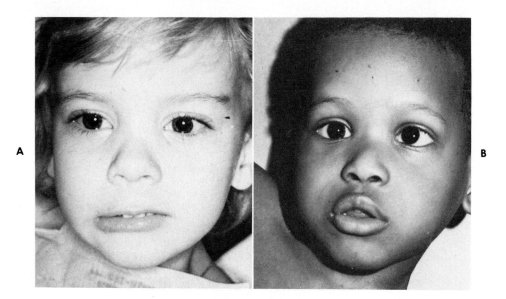

Fig. 6-61. Two patients with progressive myoclonic ataxia and multiple cranial nerve palsies (that is, myoclonic ataxia–plus). A, Five-year-old with two-year history of myoclonic ataxia showing mild facial diparesis and irritability. Photograph was taken a few weeks before development of progressive esotropia. This patient's condition was followed for several years, and numerous studies were done to demonstrate pontine neoplasm. None, however, was revealed. Ataxia and somatic myoclonus continued, with no causal agents ever being demonstrated. Transient remissions in slowly downhill course were brought about through glucocorticoid therapy. The disease appeared to involve subclinical inflammation. Cytomorphologic studies of cerebrospinal fluid showed lymphocytic-plasmacytic reactions, which seemed to support this contention. This patient's condition was followed until he was about 18 years of age. (The case was followed subsequently by Dr. Les Drew, Indiana University School of Medicine.) A younger sister showed a similar clinical picture. B, Two-year-old boy with slowly progressive myoclonia and ataxia. This patient also developed generalized myoclonic seizures. Note bilateral esotropia. He had an 8-year-old brother with an identical clinical picture. In the cases of both siblings, extensive–and unsuccessful–studies were done to exclude neoplastic, infectious, and metabolic causes for the syndrome. Observe facial diparesis.

younger sister of this patient developed a similar problem. Leigh's disease was considered to be the most likely diagnosis but was never proved by biochemical studies. Another similar patient and his older brother were recently examined. (See Fig. 6-61, B.) These siblings had an earlier onset of the disorder, with seizures also being a more serious problem. Each sibling showed a striking myoclonic ataxia and cranial nerve palsies with esotropia predominating.

Another syndrome closely related to Leigh's disease has been called the myoclonic ataxia-plus syndrome, which is perhaps identical to the syndrome just described. Affected infants have a sudden onset of ataxia of a myoclonic type and extraocular involvement with heterotropia and abnormal eyeball movements (see Fig. 6-62).

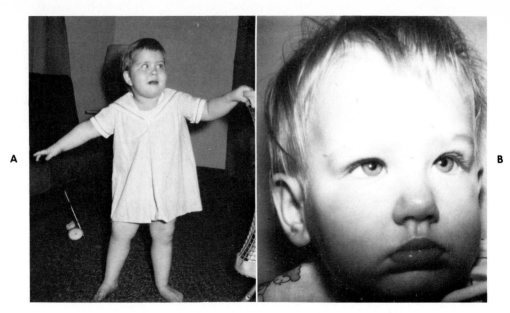

Fig. 6-62. Two infants with the myoclonic ataxia–plus syndrome. A, Full-body view of 19-month-old patient showing ataxia, esotropia, and Cushingoid facies and soma. Treatment with glucocorticoids resulted in temporary remissions in an otherwise downhill course. B, Close-up view of face and eyes of 7-month-old patient with slowly progressive myoclonic ataxia and mild, though worsening, esotropia.

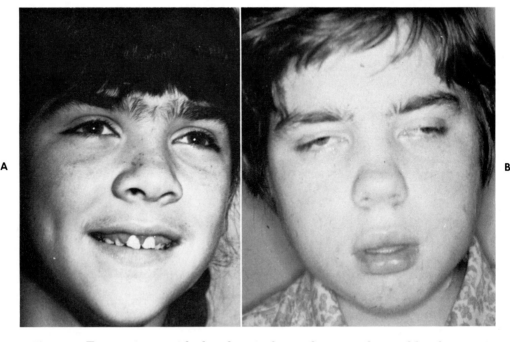

Fig. 6-63. Two patients with the chronic form of neuronal ceroid-lipofuscinosis (juvenile amaurotic idiocy). A, Thirteen-year-old girl with dementia and moderately advanced case of the disease. Note right exotropia, facial hirsutism (from phenytoin treatment), gum hyperplasia (also from phenytoin), and silly facial expression. (See also Fig. 8-32, B.) B, Eighteen-year-old girl with advanced case of the disease. Note dull and demented facial expression and left exotropia. Also observe facial hirsutism and thickened lips. Both features probably result from phenytoin ingestion. Patient also shows poliosis. (See also Fig. 8-32, C.)

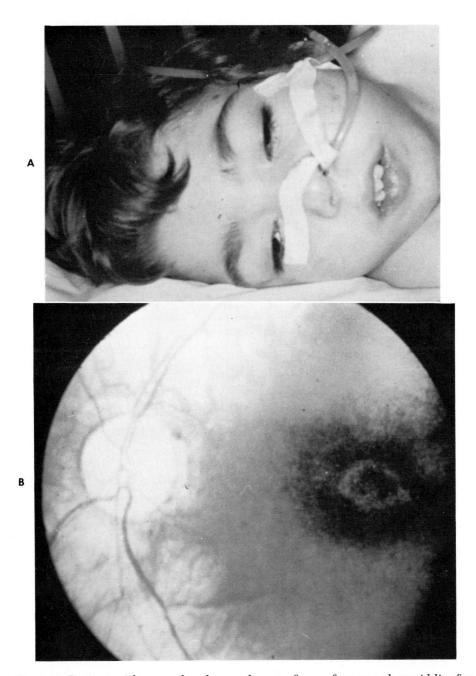

Fig. 6-64. Patient with severely advanced acute form of neuronal ceroid-lipofuscinosis (late infantile amaurotic idiocy). A, Facial view showing severe dementia, puffiness and edema of face and lips, eczema, and right exotropia. Patient was terminally ill and required nasogastric feedings. (See also Fig. 8-31, C.) B, Fundus photograph showing typical retina of neuronal ceroid-lipofuscinosis. Note optic atrophy of waxy type, attenuation of retinal vessels, patchy retinal atrophy, and granular pigmentary degeneration, particularly of the macular region.

**Other degenerative diseases associated with exotropia.** *The neuronal ceroidlipofuscinoses* are particularly prone to show a variety of heterotropias, usually exotropia types. (See Figs. 6-63 and 6-64, *B*.) Another disorder, called *opticocochleodentatic degeneration*, is characterized by early onset and slow degeneration that is associated with optic atrophy, cochlear and dentate nucleus degeneration, and exotropia. Many other neurologic defects also occur in this rare degeneration. (See Fig. 6-65.) Other neurologic degenerative diseases, such as Pelizaeus-Merzbacher disease, are characterized by exotropia. (See Fig. 6-66.)

**Nonprogressive heterotropias.** It is doubtful whether an isolated extraocular muscle weakness is always a sign of neurologic dysfunction. We have seen nonprogressive squints associated with *dystrophia myotonica* (Fig. 6-67); the *hereditary hemiplegia-hemihypoplasia-hemiathetosis syndrome* (Fig. 6-68), also called hereditary athetoid hemiplegia (see Chapter 7); phenylketonuria (Fig. 6-69); and other diseases.

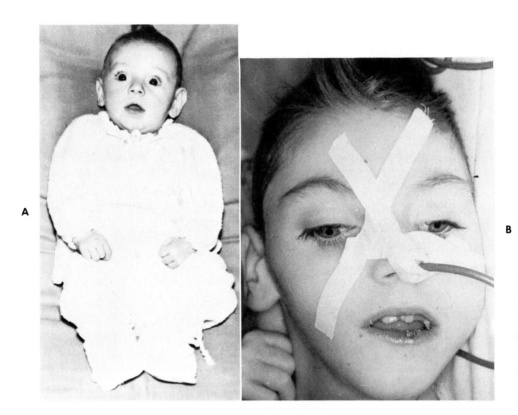

**Fig. 6-65.** Longitudinal photographic study of patient with opticocochleodentatic degeneration. **A,** Full-body view at 6 months of age. Observe wide-open expression (caused by eyelid retraction) but otherwise normal facial features. There is no heterotropia. **B,** Facial view soon before death at 8 years of age. Note right exotropia and forced eyeball deviation downward. Patient required nasogastric feeding at this stage. (Same patient is shown in Fig. 5-48. His older brother is shown in Fig. 8-33.)

## Syndromes characterized by hypotelorism, hypertelorism, and other abnormalities of the central middle face

Hypotelorism and hypertelorism already have been defined in Chapter 3. A number of syndromes are characterized by either abnormally close-set or wide-set eyes. In addition, there are a few diseases that show either hypoplasia or hyperplasia of the central middle face and that are not associated with either hypotelorism or hypertelorism but that are probably closely related. These disorders will be discussed here.

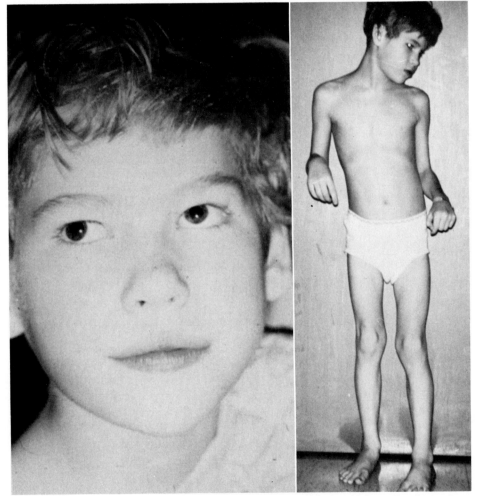

A       B

Fig. 6-66. Twelve-year-old patient with Pelizaeus-Merzbacher disease. A, Facial view showing dull but pleasant expression. Observe mild exotropia on the right and poor photographic reproduction of eyeballs because of the constant rotary-type nystagmus characteristic of this disease. Patient also shows mild microcephaly and is mentally retarded. B, Full-body view showing incoordination and abnormal postures. Glassy ocular appearance is possibly related to photography. The poor focus in the area of the eyes results from the patient's constant ocular movement.

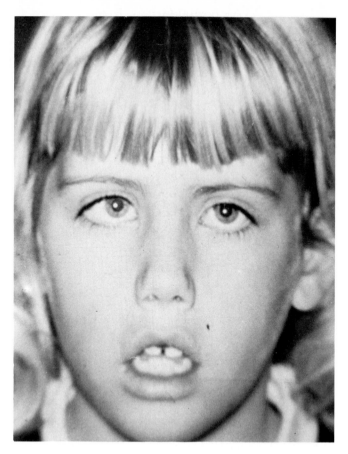

Fig. 6-67. Ten-year-old girl with congenital dystrophia myotonica. Note the mild right esotropia. Extraocular dysfunctions occur frequently in patients with dystrophia myotonica and in their nonaffected relatives. Observe also the flattened face and the mildly tented upper lip characteristic of congenital dystrophia myotonica. The patient is mildly mentally deficient.

Holoprosencephalies. The term holoprosencephaly was used by De-Myer and Zeman (1963) to include a group of anomalies in which there is only one cerebral ventricle and either no cleavage or incomplete cleavage of the cerebral hemispheres. In this anomalad, one may find abnormalities of the corpus callosum, hippocampus, and/or basal ganglion. Many of the diseases within this group of anomalies have also been called arhinencephalia because of the common but not consistent association of cleavage malformations with defective evagination of olfactory and optic structures. The term holotelencephaly has also been used to refer to the holoprosencephalic anomalad. Specific syndromes of this group of disorders are cyclopia, ethmocephaly, cebocephaly, alobar holoprosencephaly, semilobar holoprosencephaly, and lobar holoprosencephaly. Each of these craniofacial anomalies is characterized by varying degrees of hypotelorism and other characteristic middle facial and lower facial abnormalities. (See Chapter 7.)

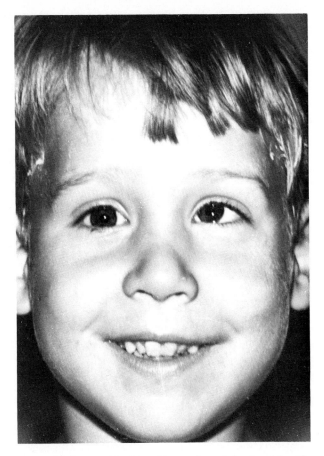

Fig. 6-68. Five-year-old boy with hereditary hemiplegia, hemihypoplasia, and hemiathetosis. (His disorder is also known as hereditary nonprogressive athetotic hemiplegia.) Note hyperesotropia on the left. Patient is mildly mentally retarded and hyperactive. (From Haar, F., and Dyken, P.: Neurology 27:849, 1977.)

It is helpful to think of a spectrum of defects, with the most severe being the cyclopic monster. This anomaly is rarely associated with a viable birth and is incompatible with life for longer than a few hours. Cyclopia is characterized by a midline single eye, rudimentary eyelids, and a proboscis (rather than a nose), which is usually placed above the completely or partially fused eyeballs. The proboscis is a tubular appendage with a single cavity that ends blindly at the base of the skull and does not communicate with the nasopharynx. *Ethmocephaly*, which is the next most severe craniofacial defect, is distinguished from cyclopia by the fact that two separate orbits exist. A proboscis is present and again is located above the orbits, a feature that distinguishes it from *cebocephaly*, in which the proboscis is situated below the orbits. Both ethmocephaly and cebocephaly are severe anomalies not only of the cranioface but also of the brain. Patients with ethmocephaly and cebocephaly, however, live longer than cyclopic monsters. There are many examples of persons

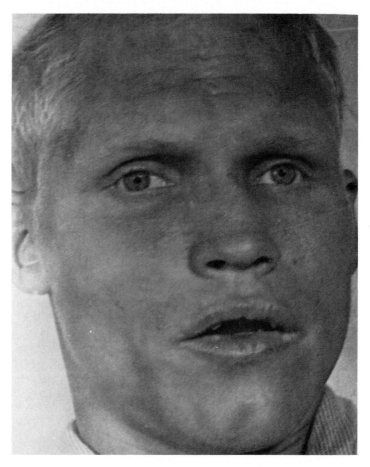

**Fig. 6-69.** Twenty-three-year-old institutionalized patient with untreated classical phenylketonuria. Note pronounced right exotropia. Observe also the vacant, dull facial expression and the hypopigmentation, which was not found in other family members. Extraocular dysfunctions are seen only rarely in this disease. Patient was profoundly mentally deficient, had other nonspecific neurologic abnormalities, and was autistic as well as extremely excitable when disturbed.

with the latter two defects surviving past the neonatal period. *Alobar holoprosencephaly* is less severe than any of the last three conditions. In the syndrome there is severe hypotelorism, but the eyeballs and bony orbits are definitely separated. Usually there is a formed nose with a midline septum and two nares rather than a proboscis. This form of holoprosencephaly is usually associated with a midline cleft lip and palate with absence of a median philtrum-premaxillary anlage (see Chapter 7). The brain has the severe midline defects that characterize the holoprosencephalies (DeMyer and others, 1964). Life may continue throughout infancy. (One of us [PRD] has observed a typical alobar holoprosencephalic child who lived for 4 years.) *Semilobar holoprosencephaly* has a less severe clinical course and less severe facial and brain defects. There is usually no "pancake" type of brain defect, and the cleft lip and palate is often of the bilateral lateral type (see Chapter 7). The *lobar holoprosen-cephalies* represent not a distinct syndrome but rather a heterogeneous group of malformations ranging from severe midline defects to defects as mild as partial agenesis of the corpus callosum with and without facial anomaly. Rarely, no facial defect may be seen, even in the more severe central nervous system malformations. According to DeMyer (1975), this may be true in as many as 5% of cases. Some forms of anencephaly (see Chapter 5) may fit into this group. The converse is not true, however. When the face is typical, there is invariably a midline brain defect.

Holoprosencephaly with cleft lip and palate and severe hypotelorism may be associated with chromosome abnormalities. Trisomy 13 may show both facial and brain features of holoprosencephaly. Other malformations, however, are also characteristic (Goodman and Gorlin, 1977).

There is usually a cleft lip and palate, either purely midline or bilateral lateral, in the alobar and semilobar types. The nasal bridge and base are usually defective, and the nasal septum is small or absent entirely. The orbits are characteristically close together but separated. Because of pronounced hypoplasia of the nasal base, one obtains the impression of larger than normal eyes. The eyes are, however, of normal size if not somewhat small. Ocular colobomas may be present, as well as other ocular and retinal anomalies. The palpebral fissures usually have a mongoloid slant. The eyebrows often meet in the midline. The ears are usually of normal size but appear large because of relative hypoplasia of the face and sometimes the cranium. (See Fig. 6-70.)

Abnormal transillumination of the cranium may be present. This has been shown to outline the associated "pancake" deformity of the cerebral hemispheres seen in the alobar type. The diagnosis may be confirmed by CT scan or pneumoencephalogram, which shows a single cerebral ventricle. It is doubtful whether the CT scan alone can distinguish all the necessary anatomic features well enough to act as a substitute for final autopsy confirmation.

**Other hypotelorism syndromes.** Hypotelorism occurs in other less severe neurologic conditions that are sometimes associated with severe hypoplasia of the entire central middle face (midface "retraction"). A fairly typical example of midface retraction is the *18 q− syndrome* or *de Grouchy's syndrome.* This disorder is characterized by multiple anomalies and a deletion of the short arm of the chromosome 18. (de Grouchy and others, 1964). Persons affected usually are severely retarded and have severe hypotonia and seizures, gonadal and somatic orthopedic abnormalities, and (often) congenital heart disease. Facially, there is hypotelorism but, more prominently, a characteristic retraction of the central middle face. The nose is small and short, and the chin is prominent. There may be a variety of congenital ocular defects, including glaucoma, heterotropia, nystagmus, optic atrophy, and retinal degeneration. Cleft lip and palate has been reported.

One is struck with the similarity of the de Grouchy syndrome to what

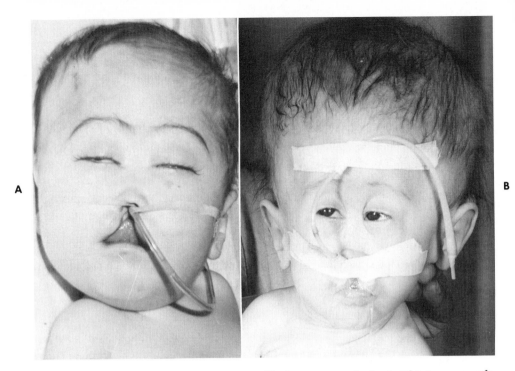

Fig. 6-70. Two patients with alobar type of holoprosencephaly. A, Thirteen-month-old patient with typical facial features of alobar holoprosencephaly—midline cleft lip and palate, hypoplastic nose, and severe hypotelorism. B, Seven-month-old patient with similar facial features, with hypotelorism being prominent. This patient also has a complicating hydrocephalus. (See Fig. 5-25.)

we describe in Chapter 7 as the *MMM syndrome*, which consists of severe mental retardation, midface retraction, and macrosomatia but no chromosomal abnormality. In this syndrome there are less severe somatic anomalies, if they occur at all in a consistent fashion.

Occasionally, one encounters relatively normal individuals with hypotelorism. Fig. 6-71, *A*, shows one patient—to our knowledge, normal in every other fashion—who was evaluated for mild developmental delay. This patient was said to have facies arhinoides by Dr. William DeMyer several years ago (DeMyer, personal communication).

Additionally, patients sometimes are seen who have midface hypoplasia with other (nonspecific and probably unrelated) anomalies. The patient in Fig. 6-72 was dwarfed and mildly mentally retarded. Further classification of her dysplastic syndrome was not made. She also had large ears and a constantly pleasant, unconcerned facial expression that probably represented her character rather than unusual proptoplasm. The patient in Fig. 6-72, *B*, had a Klippel-Feil deformity of the neck (which, to our knowledge, is not related to midface retraction) and a small, hypoplastic nose. It was very probable in this instance that the facial appearance represented a familial constitutional factor, since this

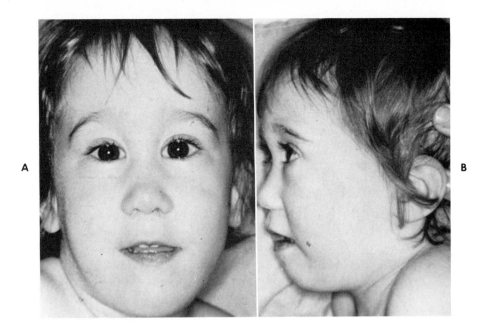

Fig. 6-71. Patient of three years of age with facies arhinoides. Patient is normal neurologically. A, Frontal view showing long facies with long, depressed nose and marked hypotelorism. B, Lateral view showing depressed nasal base and bridge and midface retraction.

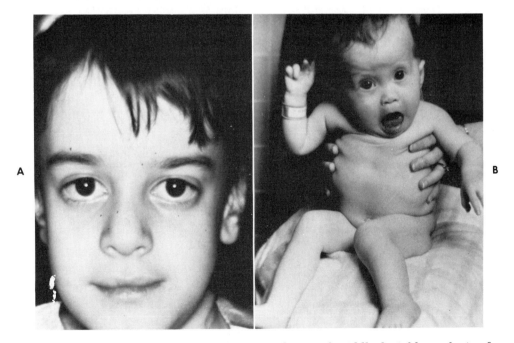

Fig. 6-72. Two patients with hypotelorism and central middle facial hypoplasia of uncertain significance. A, Eight-year-old moderately retarded girl with depressed nasal base, midface retraction, and mild hypotelorism. B, Eight-month-old infant with Klippel-Feil deformity, pronounced central middle facial hypoplasia, and hypotelorism.

patient's father, who was normal, as an infant had a similar facial appearance.

Hypotelorism may occur in several other syndromes as well, including *trisomy 21, craniotelencephalic dysplasia* (Holmes and others, 1972), *Meckel's syndrome* (Hsia, and others, 1971), *the N syndrome* (Hess, 1974), and *familial brachial plexus neuritis* (Taylor, 1960).

**Hypertelorism syndromes.** The term hypertelorism merely means a condition of excessive distance (see Chapter 3). Yet when the word is used, one is usually referring to ocular hypertelorism. Specifically, this condition involves an excessive distance between the medial borders of the eyeballs or bony orbits. Many syndromes are associated with ocular hypertelorism. Goodman and Gorlin's text (1977) lists fully seventy syndromes that are associated with this abnormal facial feature. We will discuss mainly some typical hypertelorism syndromes in this section, but many will be omitted here because we believe they are more appropriately discussed in other chapters. We also have omitted some of the rarer and, we believe, less important syndromes associated with hypertelorism. Hyperplasia of the middle face is associated intimately with hypertelorism, and brief mention of some of these syndromes will be incorporated in this section as well.

Noonan and Ehmke (1963) described individuals who had phenotypic features of *Turner's XO syndrome* but who had normal chromosomes. Since then, it has been recognized that these signs and symptoms are distinct from Turner's syndrome and represent a separate genetically determined entity that is usually identified as *Noonan's syndrome* (see Chapter 7). The syndrome consists of small stature (below the tenth percentile), mental retardation, webbing of the neck, and short neck, with low posterior hairline, congenital heart disease (valvular pulmonary stenosis is the most common cardiac finding), many osseous deformities (including pectus carinatum et excavatum, kyphoscoliosis, clinodactyly, cubitus valgus), and gonadal abnormalities (cryptorchidism, delayed pubescence). Patients have prominent hypertelorism with a broad forehead and flat nasal base and bridge. Sometimes one finds a slight antimongoloid slant to palpebral fissures, epicanthal folds, ptosis, coarse hair, receding chin, high-arched palate, low-set ears, and dental anomalies. (See Fig. 6-73.) These same facial features may be seen in the XO females with *Turner's syndrome,* but in Noonan's disease they may be even more prominent. In Turner's syndrome mental retardation is not as prominent, whereas in Noonan's syndrome affected persons are characteristically mentally retarded, sometimes in profound degrees. The cardiac picture in Turner's syndrome is also less commonly abnormal. If a cardiovascular lesion is present, it often takes the form of coarctation of the aorta.

Larsen and associates (1950) recognized the essential features of the syndrome now bearing his name. *Larsen's syndrome* includes pronounced ocular hypertelorism and peculiar facies, multiple congenital

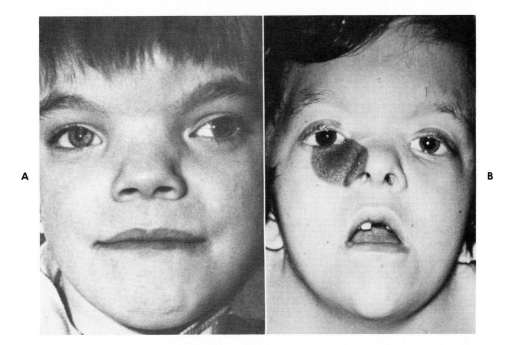

Fig. 6-73. Hypertelorism in two patients with similar facies but different clinical problems. A, Severely retarded 12-year-old girl with Noonan's syndrome. Patient has pterygium colli and dwarfism. Observe severe hypertelorism and left exotropia. B, Mildly mentally retarded patient of 14 years of age who has less severe hypertelorism, mildly antimongoloid slanting, and bilateral pterygium colli. Patient has Turner's syndrome. Observe low-set ears in relationship to webbed neck.

joint dislocations, foot deformities, and cleft palate. Patients with Larsen's syndrome may have bilateral anterior dislocation of the tibia on the femur, with displaced patellae, bilateral elbow and hip dislocation, subluxation of the shoulders, talipes equinovarus or equinovalgus, and short metacarpals and nails. There is usually severe ocular hypertelorism, prominent forehead, flattened midface, and depressed nasal bridge. (See Fig. 6-74.) Cleft palate is seen in only about half of reported cases. Micrognathia has also been observed.

*Waardenburg's syndrome* was fully described by Waardenburg in 1951, although it is probable that Mende (1926) had recognized it many years before. The syndrome is mentioned here because it is associated with dystopia canthorum, which is often confused with true ocular hypertelorism. As has been pointed out before, there is usually a lateral displacement of the medial canthi of the eyelids, which gives the illusion that the eyes are widely spaced. In some instances of Waardenburg's syndrome, however, true ocular hypertelorism is believed to exist. The syndrome has several distinctive features that allow differentiation and systemically from the other syndromes discussed in this section. These features include heterochromia, hypopigmentation of hair and irides,

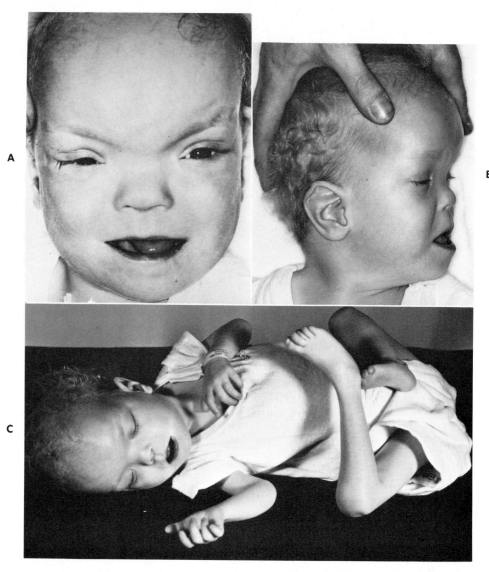

Fig. 6-74. Ten-month-old girl with Larsen's syndrome. **A.** Frontal facial view showing nasal base hypoplasia and severe hypertelorism. Patient shows psychomotor retardation. **B,** Lateral facial view. Note nasal base hypoplasia, small nose, and slightly deformed ear. Patient also shows mild prognathism. **C,** Full-body view showing congenitally dislocated hips with contractures of many joints.

sensorineural deafness, medial whorling, and prominence of eyebrows and other features.

In 1926 Greig used the term oxycephaly to describe the condition of a mother and a daughter with craniofacial anomalies and polydactyly (Greig, 1926). Two years before, he had discussed hypertelorism in the same journal (Greig, 1924). Thus, some persons use the term *Greig's syndrome* to refer to hypertelorism. This is an error because it is obvious that hypertelorism represents a symptom or a sign and not a syndrome.

*Greig's syndrome* actually is the syndrome of cephalopolysyndactyly, often also associated with ocular hypertelorism, which subsequently has been described by several other authors (Marshall and Smith, 1970; Temtamy and McKusick, 1969).

The *cri-du-chat syndrome*, also called the *cat-cry syndrome*, was first described by Jejeune and associates (1963). This disorder results from a deletion of the short arm of the fifth chromosome. A characteristic feature of the facial appearance affected patients is ocular hypertelorism. (See Fig. 6-75.) They have rounded facies, oblique palpebral fissures, low-set and angulated ears, and microcephaly. On occasion, facial asymmetry, preauricular tags, and epicanthal folds have been reported. Affected persons are often severely mentally retarded and have growth failure, muscular hypotonia, various orthopedic deformities, and a variety of other congenital defects. A striking feature of this syndrome is a low, throaty, somewhat weakened cry resembling that of a cat in heat. This cry occurs transiently in the neonatal and early infantile periods. (See Fig. 6-75.) Patients are known to survive to adulthood (Berg and others, 1965).

*Frontonasal dysplasia*, perhaps better known as the *median cleft face syndrome* (DeMyer, 1975), involves a striking degree of ocular hypertelorism. This syndrome shows a broad nasal base, a flattened and widened nose, preauricular tags, and occasional anterior encephalocele. Mental retardation may be present.

The mucopolysaccharidoses are all characterized by some degree of ocular hypertelorism, but this facial finding is especially characteristic of the two varieties of *Hunter's syndrome* (MPS IIA [the severe form] and MPS IIB [the mild form]). Both forms are sex-linked and characterized by dermatan sulfate and heparan sulfate excretion in the urine. Each form is thought to represent a deficiency in the enzyme sulfoiduronide sulfatase (Goodman and Gorlin, 1977). The milder form (Fig. 6-76, *A*) is not incompatible with survival to the fifties and with fair intelligence. The more severe form involves coarser facial features, more skeletal defects, more severe mental deficiency, and shorter survival.

## Other central middle facial syndromes

This section represents a miscellaneous grouping of syndromes developed to allow a discussion of some disorders that are difficult to classify but that show characteristic abnormalities in the central middle face.

It is believed that Brachmann first described this syndrome in 1916, but it was not until Madame Cornelia de Lange's work in 1933 that the entity was fully delineated (Brachmann, 1916; de Lange, 1933). The characteristic features of what is now commonly referred to as *de Lange's syndrome* are many. Affected patients are usually severely to profoundly mentally retarded. They are dwarfed in later life but also are considered quite small even at birth. In infancy they are very hypertonic and show excessive body as well as facial hair. The skin is coarse and

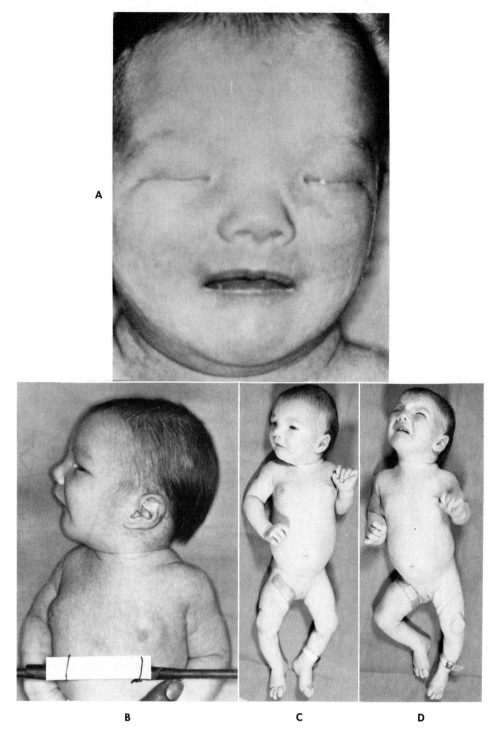

Fig. 6-75. Two-month-old patient with cytogenically proved deletion of short arm of fifth chromosome, or cri-du-chat syndrome. A, Frontal facial view showing shield-like forehead and hypertelorism. B, Lateral facial view showing shield forehead and mild hypognathia. Note livedo reticularis of skin. C, Frontal body view of patient resting and undisturbed. D, Patient crying after having been disturbed. Cry is low, throaty, and repetitive, resembling the cry of a female cat in heat.

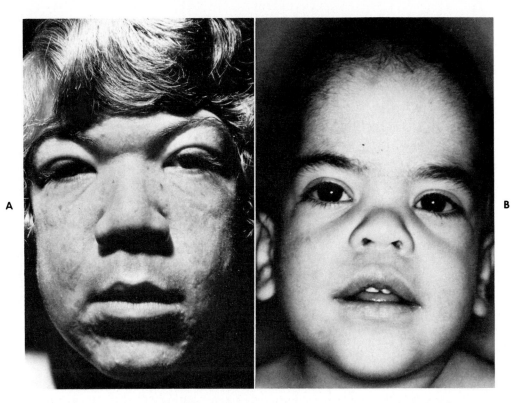

Fig. 6-76. Hypertelorism and superciliary hyperplasia in two patients with muco-polysaccharidosis. A, Eighteen-year-old patient with the mild form of Hunter's syndrome (MPS IIB). Observe superciliary hyperplasia, midline eyebrow, and hypertelorism, as well as other facial stigmata suggesting this syndrome. (A, from Dyken, P.: Neurology 16:49, 1966.) B, Seven-year-old patient with the severe form of Hunter's syndrome (MPS IIA). Observe the superciliary hyperplasia, facial hirsutism, coarser facial features, and ocular hypertelorism. Notice the large ear lobules as well. (See also Fig. 6-92, C.)

dry, and cutis marmorata is usually present in infancy as well as adulthood. They may have recurrent convulsions. There are frequently multiple anomalies of the extremities. Micromelia, oligodactyly, clinodactyly, ectrodactyly, short and proximal thumbs, and simian creases are common. Persons with de Lange's syndrome have small nipples, umbilicuses, and genitalia, with occasionally cryptorchidism and hypospadias occurring in males. Cardiac malformations also are reported.

Affected patients have microcephaly, sometimes even out of proportion to their extremely small bodies. The most characteristic facial feature consists of a narrow, "pinched-up" central middle face with prominent midline eyebrows ofer a small, narrow, slightly depressed nasal base. (See Fig. 6-77, A.) The nose is small, and anteverted nostrils are usually prominent. The eyelashes are long and sometimes curly. There may be multiple ocular abnormalities including nystagmus, microphthalmia, ptosis, and optic atrophy. The philtrum of the upper lip is

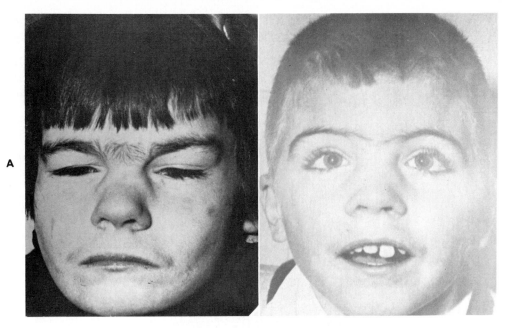

Fig. 6-77. Two patients of differing degrees of disability resulting from the De Lange or DeLange-Brachmann syndrome. A, Twenty-two-year-old severely mentally retarded and dwarfed patient. Note characteristic pinched facial features with prominent midline eyebrow, hypotelorism, small upturned nose, thin lips, wide mouth with downturned corners, and microcephaly. B, Nine-year-old, relatively normal-appearing youngster with only moderate mental retardation. Note midline eyebrows, mild antimongoloid slanting, small upturned nose, broad mouth with downturned corners and narrow lips, and facial hirsutism. Observe large incisor to left of midline. Patient is small but not dwarfed.

long, and affected persons typically have thin lips and oral lines that slope downward at the lateral corners. The teeth are small and widely spaced. Cleft palate has been reported in some cases, as has micrognathia. The ears are low-set. Fig. 6-77 shows two patients with the syndrome. The patient in Fig. 6-77, A, is quite dwarfed. The patient in Fig. 6-77, B, is only mildly to moderately mentally retarded and is small but not dwarfed.

The *trisomy 18 syndrome* shows many somatic as well as facial abnormalities. Besides having mild first-branchial-arch features, affected patients also have a somewhat prominent, shield-like upper central face. In addition to these features, the *13 q− syndrome* also involves microcephaly, trigonocephaly (see Chapter 5), mild hypertelorism, and a peculiar broad nasal base.

*Coup de sabre*, a variety of Parry-Romberg disease or hemifacial atrophy, is associated with congenital or acquired linear depressed atrophic lesions of the skin of the upper and middle face. This condition may be associated with mild hyperpigmentation and with progressive atrophy of skin and underlying subcutaneous tissue, cartilage, or bone. The

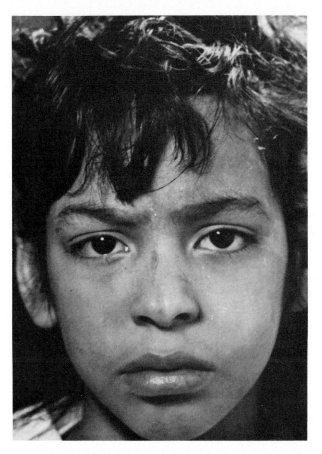

**Fig. 6-78.** Patient with coup de sabre or Parry-Romberg disease. Observe linear, scarred, slightly hyperpigmented lesion on the right of the nose close to the midline. (Same patient is shown in Fig. 5-65.)

progressive atrophy may remit spontaneously or be unrelenting. Fig. 6-78 shows a 12-year-old patient who, in addition to coup de sabre, suffered from systemic lupus erythematosus. (See Chapters 5 and 7.)

## SYNDROMES OF THE LATERAL MIDDLE FACE

When skin blemishes are discussed, the distinction between the central and the lateral middle face is arbitrary and perhaps meaningless, but we find it useful to continue our segmental approach. We have placed many of the neurocutaneous diseases in this section because most neurocutaneous conditions that affect the middle face extend to the lateral aspects.

### Syndromes characterized by laterally extending skin blemishes

**Tuberous sclerosis (Bourneville's disease).** Bourneville (1880) first recognized tuberous sclerosis as a clinicopathologic entity. His work extended over several years and has been refined by a number of early as well as recent authors (Bloom, 1963.) The term tuberous sclerosis, which literally means "hard potato," refers to the paraependymal lesions that surround the ventricular surfaces of the brain. The term was coined because a cut surface of these brain lesions looked like that of a freshly cut potato. Vogt in 1908 pointed out the characteristic clinical triad of mental deficiency, epilepsy, and adenoma sebaceum. More recent authors have emphasized the presentation in earlier life of another typical triad: psychomotor retardation, infantile spasms, and depigmented spots or nevus anemicus (Wilkins and Broder, 1970).

The clinical features of tuberous sclerosis are many. Most patients are mentally deficient, although in mild instances this is not always recognized as the primary feature of the disease. Mental deficiency seems to be proportional to the severity and difficulty involved in controlling associated seizures. Psychological testing may show relatively normal intelligence scores, particularly in childhood. Seldom, however, does careful and extensive psychological testing not indicate at least some learning defects or frank intellectual deficiency of mild degree. Some adults have been reported with normal intelligence. If one tested all family members of patients with typical tuberous sclerosis, it is probable that many of them would be basically normal mentally because they would have only fragments of the syndrome.

Seizures, which are almost always present in the full syndrome, are of various types and degrees of severity, including particularly the myoclonic varieties such as spasms in infancy and minor seizures in early childhood. In adulthood, generalized tonic-clonic convulsions are more common. Absence and psychomotor seizure types are less common. The frequency of seizures covers a spectrum ranging from rare convulsions, which are easily controlled by standard anticonvulsant medication, to very refractive types, which occur daily and are uncontrolled by even the most modern drugs. As mentioned previously, the degree to which seizures have been controlled during the course of the disease seems to determine the degree of mental deficiency encountered.

Cutaneous involvement in typical cases of the disease is constant, although the type and distribution vary between individuals. The classic adenoma sebaceum (this term is really a misnomer; it is preferable to refer to the lesions as angiofibromas) is of two basic types, neither of which develops early in life. One type is maculopapular and erythematous. Typically, this lesion is distributed rather evenly over the bridge of the nose and in the malar area in a butterfly pattern that, when well developed, extends into the lateral face. (See Fig. 6-79, A.) This skin lesion is typical and is important in predicting brain involvement with tubers. A second type of adenoma sebaceum is also maculopapular but rather than being reddened has an avascular, pale appearance. This second type, which is simply a fibromatous lesion rather than an angiofibroma, is less regularly distributed and tends to cluster at the nostril and to be less extensive (see Fig. 6-79, B). The skin blemish is of less significance

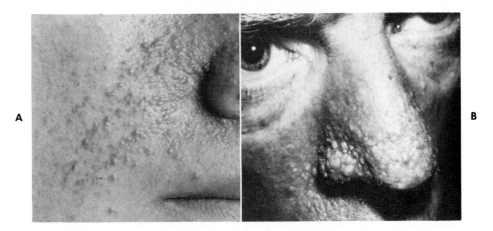

Fig. 6-79. Close-up views of two types of adenoma sebaceum. A, Adenoma seba-ceum of Pringle, or angiofibromatosis, which is diagnostic of tuberous sclerosis. Observe regular, maculopapular distribution of lesions over the malar region. The lesions are reddened. B, Adenoma sebaceum of Balzer. These lesions are also seen in patients with tuberous sclerosis but are not nearly as specific for the dis-ease. Notice that the distribution of these skin lesions is more irregular and that they tend to be clustered at the nares rather than on the malar region. The lesions are pale and show less, if any, vascular component.

in predicting central nervous system involvement or tuberous sclero-sis and, in fact, can be seen in persons who have no other cutaneous or systemic features of the syndrome. Yet both lesions are seen in the dis-ease and are useful as markers for the gene for tuberous sclerosis. In addition, white, ash-leaf shaped, depigmented spots are usually distrib-uted somatically, although they may be seen over the face as well (see Fig. 6-80). They vary from pinhead sized to several centimeters across and are flattened, with a slightly irregular border. Cafe-au-lait spots are uncommon. Shagreen or sharkskin-like patches classically occur in this disease. They usually occur asymmetrically in the flank and may seem to follow a dermatome distribution. Similar "leather" patch lesions are seen elsewhere on the body and even on the cranium. Classic shagreen patches represent thickened epidermal and dermal hamartomas of slightly different histology than angiofibromas. They are hyperpig-mented. Subungal or epiungal fibromas are seen in a much smaller percentage of cases. These lesions emerge from the nail bed and early in development may resemble simple hangnails. Soft polypoid fibroma-tous and lipomatous masses on the face, scalp, and body also are seen (see Chapter 5). Flat plaques occur infrequently on the mucous mem-branes of the gingiva and lips (see Chapter 7). Many organs are involved with hamartomas in tuberous sclerosis. The retina shows the so-called phakoma or birthmark, as described by Van Der Hoeve (1920), which is really of three types. One is a flattened peripheral lesion that has an areolar appearing surface similar in a fashion to the tuber in the brain. This type of retinal lesion is diagnostic of tuberous sclerosis. A second

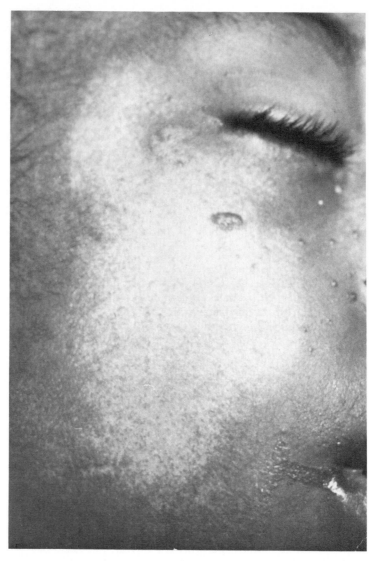

Fig. 6-80. Close-up view of 4-year-old black patient with tuberous sclerosis. Adenoma sebaceum, although not well developed, is seen irregularly in the malar region. In blacks these lesions are not reddened; they simply are more deeply pigmented. Note the extensive area of facial leukoderma, which involves most of the central and lateral middle face. Facial leukoderma is seen in tuberous sclerosis and usually involves the middle face. It is not, however, specific for tuberous sclerosis. (See also Fig. 8-44.)

type of retinal phakoma is located closer to the papilla or disc and is usually elevated. This lesion usually has a smoother and more irregular surface appearance and may resemble a tumor. The third type is a combination of the peripheral and papillar lesions.

The inner table of the skull is characteristically thickened in tuberous sclerosis. Rarely, one sees localized osseous hypertrophy of the outer lay-

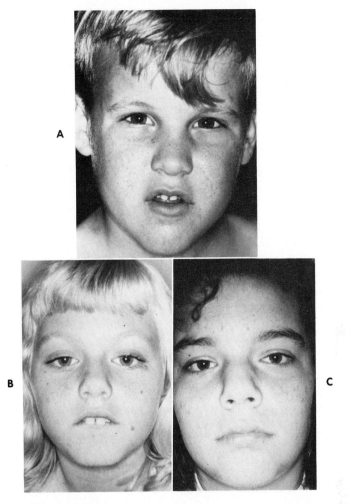

Fig. 6-81. Variations of angiofibromatosis in patients with tuberous sclerosis. A, Five-year-old boy with many depigmented spots, seizures, and mild mental retardation who shows early evidence of angiofibromas on the malar region. Note small macular lesions scattered irregularly and intermixed with lentigines. B, Eight-year-old girl with mental retardation, recurrent seizures, epiungal fibroma, depigmented spots, and early adenoma sebaceum of Pringle. Note the irregular distribution of the skin lesions. There is a sharkskin leather patch on the neck, as well as other pigmented fibroma on the face. C, Fifteen-year-old mildly retarded patient. Note irregular, dirty-appearing lesions on the face, mainly in the malar area. Patient also has lentigines and acne vulgaris that may be related to the angiofibromas.

er of the skull, as well as of other bones, which resembles the bony changes in fibrous dysplasia. X-ray film may show small, punched-out cystic lesions of the phalanges. These lesions probably represent fibrous replacement of bone. The kidney is involved in an estimated 40% of cases (Kissel and Schmitt, 1963) (a figure that, in our experience with over 150 patients, seems excessively high). Renal hamartomas are the most common type of involvement. Cardiac rhabdomyomas usually, but not always, are of benign nature. There is a heightened incidence of all types of nervous system neoplasms in this disorder, but gliomas and meningiomas are particularly predominant. Other systemic neoplasms are also seen, including pheochromocytoma.

The facial abnormalities, of course, are the hallmark features of the disease. One typically sees regularly distributed angiofibromas that, when fully developed, extend into the lateral face. It is important to point out that facial angiofibromas develop slowly and are not fully developed until the mid-juvenile period (around ages 10 to 15). In younger patients the angiofibromas are sparse and irregular and can easily be overlooked, even though they usually are present in some degree by 3 to 5 years of age. Fig. 6-81 shows the development of these lesions. In addition, one may see small depigmented spots, larger plaques of leukoderma (Fig. 6-82), fleshy lipofibromas, and leather patches (Figs. 6-82 and 6-83). Fibrous dysplasia may also occur on the forehead (See Chapter 5.)

**Other skin blemish syndromes of the lateral middle face.** Sugarman and Reed (1969) described a patient with congenital leukoderma involving one side of the middle face. This skin lesion was associated with psychomotor retardation and seizure disorder but with no other features suggesting other commonly known hypopigmentation syndromes. Review of the incidence of facial cutaneous plaques of congenital hypopigmentation among persons with neurologic defects and mental retardation has revealed six other examples of congenital leukoderma with dis-

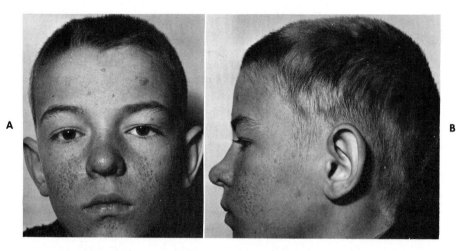

A

B

Fig. 6-82. Fairly typical malar area angiofibromatosis in a patient of 12 years of age who has all the features of tuberous sclerosis. A, Frontal view showing evenly distributed reddened adenoma sebaceum in the malar region as well as on the chin. Note that lesions spare bridge of nose, nasal base, and forehead as well as lateral areas of cheeks. A few forehead fibromas and leather patches are present. B, Lateral view showing lateral extent of adenoma sebaceum as well as cranial white hair growing out of leukoderma of depigmented spots behind the cranial hairline.

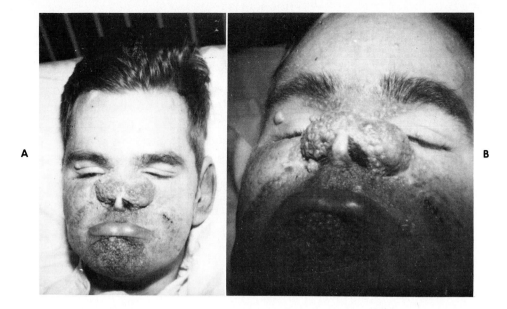

Fig. 6-83. Facial deformity caused by severe tuberous sclerosis in institutionalized patient in his twenties. Patient has refractive seizures and is profoundly mentally retarded. A, Full facial view. Note the cauliflower-like involvement of the nose resulting from coalescent angiofibroma. Forehead is essentially spared. B, Close-up view of nose.

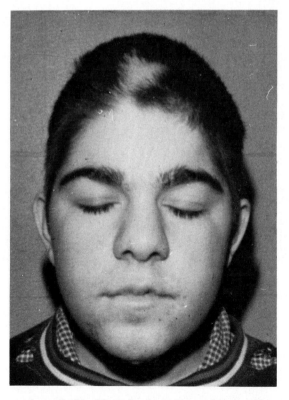

Fig. 6-84. Patient with probable Waardenburg's syndrome. Note medial eyebrow hyperplasia and white forelock of hair associated with leukoderma. Patient also had mild dystopia canthorum (which is not visible in this photograph because the eyes are closed.) He had no hearing defect, but he was moderately mentally retarded, and he had had seizures in early infancy. (See also Fig. 5-59, B.)

tribution over the cranioface (Dyken and others, 1972). Two of these patients had clinical stigmata of trisomy 21 and were shown to have chromosomal confirmation of this condition. They were considered to have dysmigration syndromes. In these two patients, the leukoderma was distributed on the cranium in back of the hairline. Another patient was found to have a large facial leukodermal patch that turned out to be associated with tuberous sclerosis (see Fig. 6-80). One patient had a white lock of hair and may have had other atypical features of Waardenburg's syndrome (Fig. 6-84). Two patients had symptoms very similar to those of the patient described by Sugarman and Reed. It was later discovered that three more patients also had these symptoms (see Figs. 7-20 and 6-85). In only the patient observed in Fig. 6-85 was the lesion confined to the middle face. *Craniofacial leukoderma of Sugarman-Reed* was suggested as the preferred name for this condition. Such skin lesions are always congenital, nonprogressive, and asymmetrical, usually with unilateral distribution. Mental retardation, hyperactivity, learning disability, or visual perceptual defects are usually present in persons with this syndrome. Seizures may or may not occur but were present in

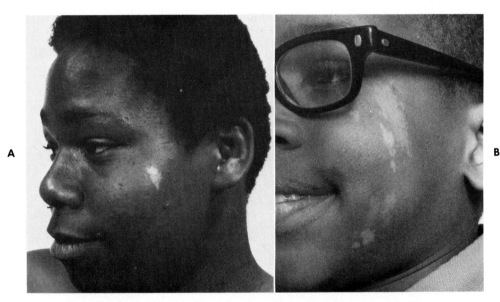

A

B

Fig. 6-85. Two patients with craniofacial leukoderma similar to that described by Sugarman and Reed. A, Nineteen-year-old moderately retarded patient with recurrent psychomotor seizures. Note small patch of leukoderma in lateral middle face on left that had been present since birth. Electroencephalographic study showed epileptogenic activity arising from the left hemisphere—mostly in the left temporal lobe. B, Nine-year-old boy who, according to psychometric testing, had normal intelligence but intertest scatter. The scatter in Wechsler scale subtests was especially evident in verbal functions. Note the "tear-streaked" irregular patch of congenital leukoderma involving mainly the lateral middle face but extending into the lower face as well.

Sugarman and Reed's patients and in three out of five of ours. Leukoderma over the body has not been seen in our cases, except for one patient with a Waardenburg-like syndrome who we do not consider to have the syndrome of Sugarman-Reed (see Fig. 6-84). One should always be cautious in making a diagnosis of this syndrome in early life, since patients who appear to have the syndrome may later develop typical features of tuberous sclerosis. Such a patient is shown in Fig. 6-80.

Herpes zoster infections may be associated with a variety of neurologic presentations including radiculitis, myelitis, and amyotrophia. In one instance a herpes zoster infection of the lateral aspects of the middle facial segment was associated with the hallmark symptoms of *Devic's neuromyelitis optica*. This syndrome is believed to be one childhood expression of multiple sclerosis. It is characterized by the onset of a retrobulbar neuritis within days of rapidly developing catastrophic transverse myelitis. In the variation of this syndrome seen in Fig. 6-86, a typical herpes zoster vesicular rash in the area of the middle face preceded the neurologic symptoms by several weeks.

*The teardrop pigment syndrome* has recently been seen in one infant of 5 months of age. At the third month of gestation, the mother developed a sudden total unilateral peripheral facial palsy that persisted to the time of examination of the infant. The infant was born after an arm-presentation but otherwise nontraumatic birth that left him with an Erb's palsy from which, however, he was rapidly recovering. Delay in the attainment of psychomotor milestones was evident. Microcephaly and a developmental level judged to be 3 months when the child was 5 months of age were the neurologic manifestations of this neurocutaneous syndrome. (See Fig. 6-87.)

*Sturge-Weber disease* has been discussed in prior sections of this chapter as well as in Chapters 5 and 7. In this syndrome a port wine nevus flammeus type of capillary hemangioma usually is observed to extensively involve the face in unilateral trigeminal distribution. In the patient in Fig. 6-88, the port wine stain, as viewed directly, was quite small and seemed to involve only a small area on the lateral and upper aspects of the lateral canthus (Fig. 6-88, *A*). A more extensive hemangioma could be observed on the side of the face in the area lateral to the vertical outer canthal line (Fig. 6-88, *B*). This laterally placed hemangioma extended to the midline in the cervical-occipital area (Fig. 6-88, *C*) and over the rest of the body (Fig. 6-88, *D*). No intracranial calcifications were observed. Yet there was mild mental retardation, recurrent focal motor seizures, and moderate contralateral hemiplegia and hemihypoplasia, as seen in Fig. 6-88, *D*.

## Syndromes characterized by abnormal ears

**Syndromes of low-set ears.** The *first-arch syndromes* are often characterized by abnormally low-set ears as a result of the zygomatic arch and the mandible being hypoplastic. As has been pointed out by Goodman

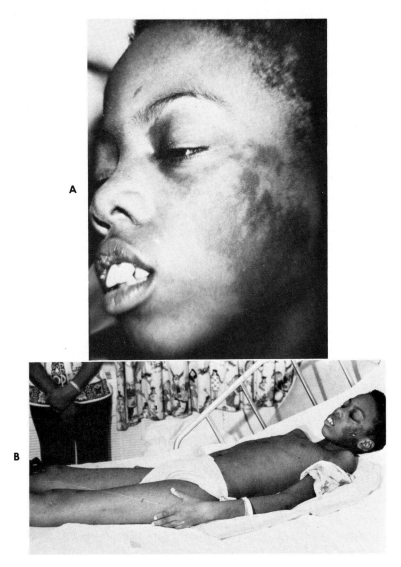

Fig. 6-86. Twelve-year-old boy who was normal neurologically and cutaneously until several weeks before this photograph was taken. He then developed a streaky vesicular rash over the side of the face that was diagnosed as being compatible with herpes zoster. Soon thereafter, in the period of recovery from this skin erruption, hyperpigmentation occurred, and he suddenly developed profound neurologic symptoms that included a rapidly developing transverse myelitis and a cord transection at the C-4 level. Retrobulbar neuritis developed soon afterward, and he became blind. He was diagnosed as having Devic's neuromyelitis optica. Cerebrospinal fluid findings were compatible with this syndrome, which, to our knowledge, has not been associated with herpes infection. Repeated attempts to culture a virus from many body fluids and tissues were unsuccessful. A, Oblique facial view showing dull expression and extensive hyperpigmented lesion of the lateral middle face, where the herpes-like eruption had started. B, Lateral body view showing severe quadriparesis and facial lesions.

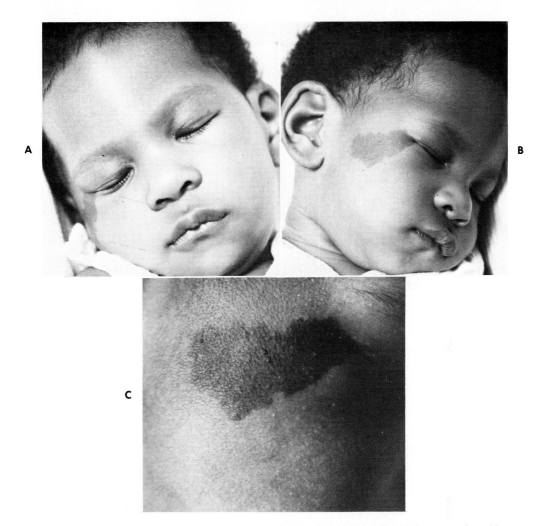

Fig. 6-87. Four-month-old boy who was born with a brachial plexus palsy. His mother suffered from idiopathic Bell's palsy during the third trimester of pregnancy. At birth (the delivery was not traumatic) an unusual chocolate spot was observed on the face. This patient had mild psychomotor retardation and recurrent generalized seizures. A, Frontal facial view of a teardrop band of hyperpigmentation, the color of bittersweet chocolate, in the right lateral middle face. The lesion extended from the lateral canthus to the nasal line. B, Lateral view of teardrop lesion. C, Close-up view of lesion.

and Gorlin (1977), low-set ears are often an optical illusion, and many of the enormous number of references to syndromes associated with them result from totally subjective observations. In the first-arch syndromes associated with hypoplastic mandibles and zygomatic arches, there is often posterior rotation of the auricles, which tends to make the ears seem low-set. In the patient in Fig. 6-89, another optical illusion would appear to be acting to make the ears appear to be dramatically low-set. This patient has tilted his head upward, which causes the ears to be

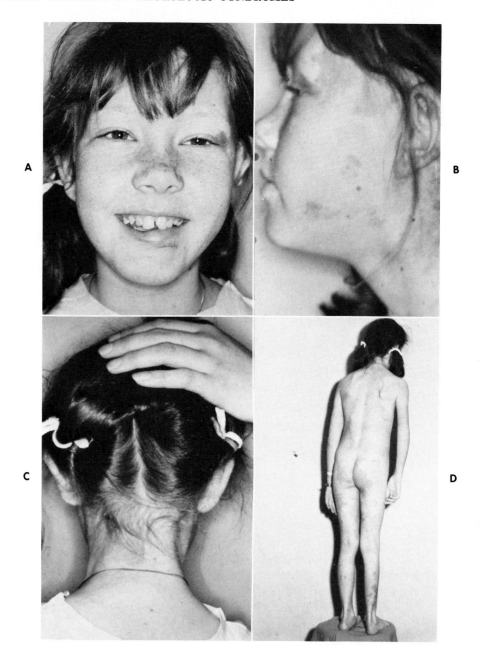

Fig. 6-88. Eleven-year-old girl with atypical Sturge-Weber syndrome. A, Frontal facial view showing small port wine nevus flammeus just lateral and superior to the left lateral canthus. A small hemangioma also is seen on lower left lip. Face is slightly asymmetrical. B, Left lateral facial view showing more extensive but spotty distribution of the nevus flammeus. Lesion involves the entire left ear and is even more extensive on the left neck. C, Posterior view of head showing extent of nevus flammeus on left posterior neck. Nevus extended to the exact midline and to C-6 level. D, Posterior body view showing extensive spotty distribution of nevus flammeus over the body and extremities. Observe the relative hypoplasia of the right side. The patient was mildly retarded, had a hemiparesis on the right, and suffered from recurrent seizures.

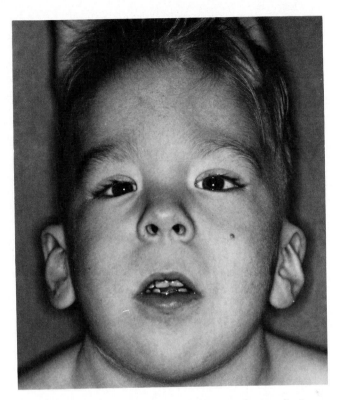

Fig. 6-89. Four-year-old patient in whom mild mental retardation was suspected. This full facial photograph shows several artifactitous facial abnormalities caused by improper cranial posturing for the photograph. The chin is elevated, causing the ears to be posteriorly rotated and tilted so that, from a full frontal view, they appear to be very low-set. In actuality, the rostral part of the left ear is poorly formed and there is a prominent anthelix, but the ears are not low-set. The tilting back of the head also gives a false impression of anteverted nostrils. The nose and nostrils actually are entirely normal. In addition, there is an illusion of wide-set eyes or hypertelorism. This impression results from the presence of mild bilateral epicanthal folds. Finally, since the head is tilted backward in this photograph, one views the bifrontal diameter of the cranium rather than the more usually viewed biparietal diameter. Thus the cranium also appears to be small or microcephalic. The head circumference of this patient is, in reality, slightly large for sex and age. The photograph was taken originally to show the unruly tufts of cranial hair seen occasionally in persons with mental retardation. Since a hand was used to keep the patient still, this feature is not demonstrated well.

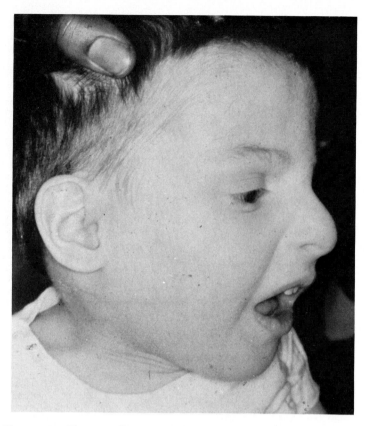

Fig. 6-90. Two-year-old mentally retarded youngster with low-set and posteriorly tilted ears. This patient also had a long, beaked nose and a mild first-branchial-arch syndrome. There was severe body ichthyosis and mild hypotrichosis.

tilted backward. When he is observed from below, as the camera has done, the chin and the ears seem much lower than in direct frontal viewing. This patient did, however, have a mild first-arch syndrome and did have rostrally limited helices and prominent anthelices. The patient in Fig. 6-90 also had a mild first-arch syndrome, with a beak-like nose best viewed laterally. The ears are normally formed and are not posteriorly tilted; yet they are low-set in terms of the rules we presented in Chapters 1 and 3.

**Syndromes of large and floppy ears.** Large and floppy ears are a characteristic of many *congenital neuromuscular diseases.* This feature is believed to result from congenital weakness, hypoplasia, or atrophy of the muscle that holds the cartilaginous ear close to the cranium. (See Fig. 6-91.)

*Sotos' syndrome* of cerebral giantism is characterized by large, pendulous ears in addition to mental retardation, macrocephaly, frontal

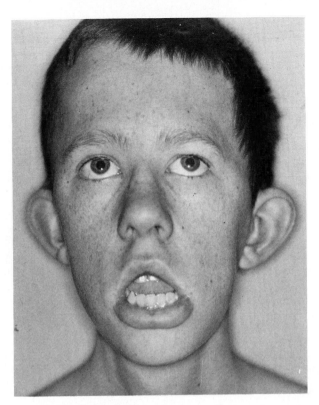

**Fig. 6-91.** Fifteen-year-old patient with congenital dystrophia myotonica. The ears are quite large and protruding, a feature that recently has been pointed out to be characteristic of patients with congenital neuromuscular disorders. It is believed that this feature often results from the congenital absence or dysfunction of the muscles that hold the ears close to the cranium. Observe also the moderately severe facial diparesis, the masseter diparesis causing the jaw and mouth to be held open, and the "tented" upper lip and shortened philtrum.

bossing, dolichocephaly, recessive frontal hairline, ocular hypertelorism, anteverted nostrils, antimongoloid slant, precocious dentition, prognathism of the mandible, large birth size, increased rate of somatic growth, clumsiness, large hands and feet, large arm span, seizure disorders, kyphoscoliosis, and respiratory and feeding problems (Sotos and others, 1964).

The *Hurler-Hunter varieties of the mucopolysaccharidoses* involve a very characteristic ear lobule. This lobule is large and pendulous and seems to be distended. Other types of mucopolysaccharidosis do not show this characteristic feature as frequently. Each of the patients in Fig. 6-92 has MPS IIA, or the severe form of Hunter's syndrome. (See also Fig. 6-55, *B*.)

**Other ear syndromes.** Many first-arch syndromes also are characterized by abnormally formed ears—especially *Treacher Collins' syndrome* and *Goldenhar's syndrome*, both of which show a wide variety of abnor-

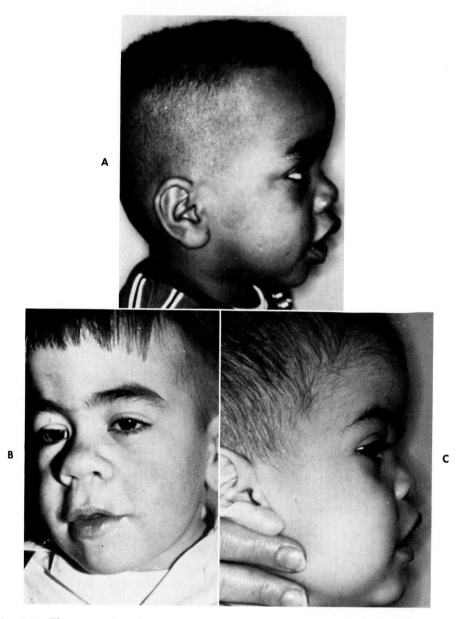

Fig. 6-92. Three unrelated patients with the severe form of Hunter's syndrome (MPS IIA). A, Lateral view of five-year-old showing many characteristic facial features—particularly the enlarged ear lobules which are characteristic of this syndrome as well as of Hurler's syndrome. (See also Fig. 8-9, C.) B, Oblique view of eight-year-old patient with Hunter's syndrome showing characteristic facial features and large ear lobules. C, Lateral view of patient Fig. 6-76, B, who has Hunter's syndrome. Note greatly enlarged ear lobules.

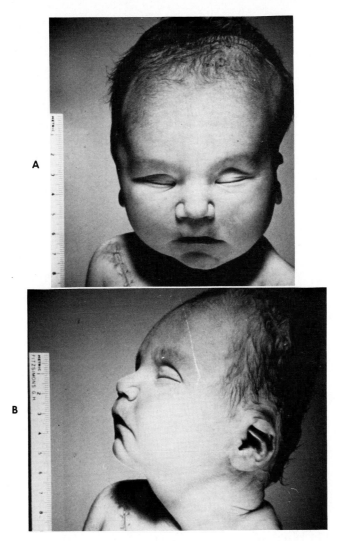

Fig. 6-93. Postmortem photographs of patient who died in the first week of life from Potter's syndrome associated with renal agenesis. A, Frontal view showing mongoloid slanting and abnormally formed ears. B, Lateral view of same patient showing abnormally formed ears. (Courtesy of Dr. Charles Linder, Medical College of Georgia.)

malities in ear formation including poorly demarcated and bifurcated ears, absence of the pinnae, preauricular ear tags, and malformed traguses (Goldenhar, 1952; Treacher Collins, 1900). Such abnormalities are often associated with a variety of hearing deficits.

*Potter's syndrome* of renal agenesis, unusual facies, and abnormal ears (Fig. 6-93) and the *OPD syndrome* may show external as well as internal malformations of the ear (Smith, 1970).

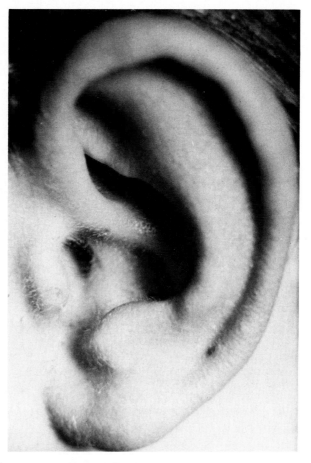

**Fig. 6-94.** Close-up view of normally formed ear showing residual scarring from herpetic-like eruption in the concha associated with a total facial palsy on the same side as the ear eruption. This disorder, which is called Ramsay Hunt's syndrome, is often associated with geniculate neuralgia.

*Ramsay Hunt's syndrome* of geniculate ganglion neuralgia (Fig. 6-94) is characterized by a vesicular herpetic-like rash in the anterior portion of the external auditory canal and sometimes in the neighboring face. This lesion may be quite mild and only erythematous rather than vesicular. Associated is neuralgic pain in the ear and the face. A facial palsy on the side of the rash may be present.

# CHAPTER SEVEN

# Syndromes of the lower facial segment and neck

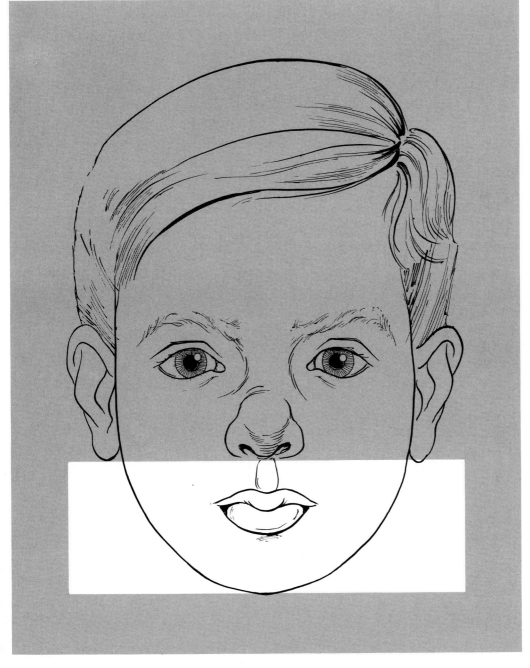

In this chapter syndromes that are characterized primarily by abnormalities in the lower face and neck will be discussed. The normal structures of the lower facial segment and the abnormalities of this segment have been discussed in Chapters 1 and 4.

# SYNDROMES OF THE CENTRAL LOWER FACE
## Syndromes characterized by cleft lip and palate

Cleft lip and palate represents a significant abnormality in medical practice. Often this abnormality exists without other congenital malformations or neurologic symptoms (see Chapter 4). Animal studies have shown that a variety of insults at critical periods of organogenesis in utero may produce cleft defects. These critical periods are also important periods in brain development. Consequently, certain types of cleft lip and cleft palate are prone to be associated with deficits of the central nervous system.

It has been suggested that the type and extent of clefting may predict the neurologic status of the patient. Cleft lip alone in most instances does not suggest a high likelihood of neurological impairment. Similarly, a pure cleft palate is usually not associated with neurologic syndromes. A greater risk of accompanying neurologic or brain dysfunction occurs in those persons who have both cleft lip and cleft palate. The location of the cleft lip and palate also is related to a likelihood of brain malformation. Such malformation is least likely in cases of unilateral cleft lip and palate and most likely in cases of purely midline cleft lip and palate.

**The holoprosencephalies.** The general principles concerning cleft lip and palate hold true particularly in the spectrum of syndromes usually grouped under the term holoprosencephaly, which literally means whole or undivided prosencephalon or fore-brain. This term is considered preferable to previous designations such as arhinencephalia and holotelencephaly (DeMyer, 1975). In the holoprosencephalies an insult in organogenesis interferes with the normal cleaving of the prosencephalon. This insult occurs in the early periods of embryonic life. The defect ranges in degree from very mild (having no obvious facial consequences) to very severe (causing serious brain and facial midline abnormalities). DeMyer has suggested that a spectrum of midline abnormalities exists, ranging from the most severe, the cyclopic monster, who is seldom viable at birth, to the ethmocephalic and cebocephalic deformities, which are characterized by severe ocular hypotelorism with or without cleft lip and palate, to the alobar type of holoprosencephaly with purely midline cleft lip and palate (see Fig. 7-1, A), to the semilobar type with bilateral lateral cleft lip and palate (Fig. 7-1, B), to persons without major facial defects. It is possible that what DeMyer calls the lobar type of holoprosencephaly exists only as a partial midline defect of the central nervous system. Partial agenesis of the corpus callosum might be one example.

The disorders of holoprosencephaly that are associated with facial abnormalities produce a very characteristic appearance in an affected

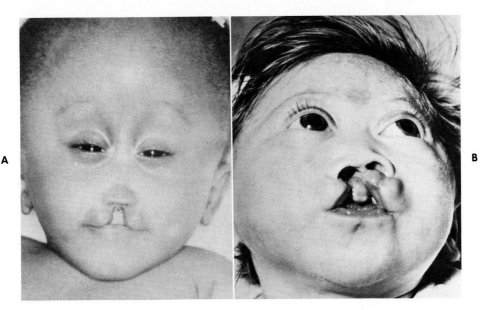

Fig. 7-1. Midline and bilateral lateral cleft lip and palate in two patients with holoprosencephaly. **A,** Six-month-old with alobar type of holoprosencephaly. Note midline cleft lip and palate and severely hypoplastic prolabium. Observe also other features of holoprosencephaly, including hypoplastic nose with separated nares, midfacial hypoplasia, hypotelorism, depressed nasal base, hydrocephalic contour of cranium, and mild mongoloid slanting. **B,** Three-month-old with semilobar type of holoprosencephaly. Note bilateral lateral cleft lip and palate with rudimentary prolabium. Observe other facial features of holoprosencephaly, including deformed nares, hypoplastic nasal bridge and base, midfacial hypoplasia, and hypotelorism.

person because of multiple midline facial defects, not all of which are limited to the lower facial segment. Abnormalities of the middle facial segment (see Chapters 3 and 6) also occur. These include hypotelorism, abnormalities of the nasal base, bridge, and tip, and abnormalities of the central middle face and maxilla. The lower face is also characteristically involved in these defects. Although the cyclopic monster and the ethmocephalic and cebocephalic malformations may not be associated with cleft lip and palate, the central lower face is always abnormal even in these anomalads. There is always a relative hypoplasia of central lower facial structures. The mouth line is usually short, and the oral cavity may be extremely small, giving the illusion of a relatively large tongue. The alobar holoprosencephalic anomalad is almost always associated with a cleft lip and palate, usually of the midline variety. The extent of the brain abnormality seems to be directly related to the type and extent of the clefting. Patients with more extensive brain malformation generally have the purely midline cleft lip and palate (see Fig. 7-1, *A*). Patients with less extensive brain malformation generally have the bilateral or double-lateral cleft lip and palate (Fig. 7-1, *B*). This type of clefting is also seen in the semilobar type of holoprosencephaly. On the other hand, less severe brain defects, such as those found in the lobar types, tend to be associated with more irregular or even unilateral cleft lip and palate. In some very rare cases, no major clefting abnormalities are witnessed. Nevertheless, the type and the extent of the clefting usually are good indicators of the condition of the brain and thus of the neurologic prognosis.

The defects mentioned may be produced by a wide range of in utero insults or result from chromosomal abnormalities. Trisomy 13 has been associated not only with holoprosencephaly but also with cleft lip and palate. In trisomy 13 there are usually other severe somatic defects as well, particularly digital, urologic, and cardiac abnormalities. In a newborn the presence of these severe somatic defects helps in distinguishing trisomy 13 from the nonchromosomal types of holoprosencephaly.

**Other clefting syndromes.** The *otopalatodigital (OPD) syndrome* was initially described by Taybi in 1962. It is possibly related to some of the milder forms of holoprosencephaly and is characterized by abnormalities of the ears, palate, and digits (Taybi, 1962). Dudding and associates specifically delineated the syndrome in 1967 and called it the otopalatodigital syndrome. This constellation of dysplastic abnormalities is reasonably common in clinical practice. The syndrome consists of cleft lip and palate, deafness, dwarfism, pugilistic facies, and a variety of bony dysplasias. The syndrome usually is seen in males, although females do have the disorder, perhaps in milder form. Roentgenograms show hypoplastic facial bones and distinctive changes of the hands and feet, with secondary ossification centers existing at the base of the second metacarpal and the base of the second metatarsal. The big toes and thumbs are shorter than normal because of this growth characteristic. There is usually mental retardation, and speech development is slow. There may be pectus excavatum, syndactyly of the toes, limited wrist supination, limited elbow extension (due to subluxation of the head of the radius), clinodactyly of the fifth finger, shortened terminal phalanges with rather square distal parts, short fingernails, irregularly positioned toes, and deafness of a conductive type (Dudding and others, 1967).

There may be occipital bossing, a broad forehead with lateral extension of the eyebrows, ocular hypertelorism, unusual slant to the palpebral fissures, and broad nasal base. The nasal bridge is short, sometimes saddled, and slightly broadened. The nasal tip may be flat, broad, and deformed. The most distinctive facial feature is the pugilistic appearance that results mainly from the cleft lip and palate, relative hyperplasia of the chin and jaw, and a small, but flattened nose (see Fig. 7-2).

There are a number of neurogenic syndromes associated with cleft defects. These include the *first-branchial-arch syndromes* (Tessier, 1976) (see Chapter 6), some of *the craniodysostoses* (Forland, 1962) (see Chapter 5), and other nonchromosomal syndromes and anomalads such as the *EEC syndrome* (Pries and others, 1974), the *OFD II syndrome*

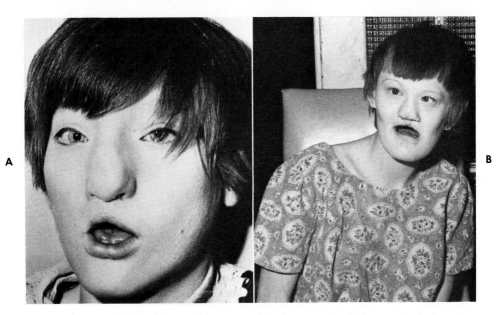

Fig. 7-2. Two patients with the otopalatodigital (OPD) syndrome. A, Moderately retarded 12-year-old with corrected cleft lip and palate. Observe deformed upper lip with shortened philtrum, deformed nose with protruding nasal base, mild mongoloid slanting, and relative prognathism. This patient is deaf. B, Severely retarded 18-year-old. Note surgically corrected cleft lip and palate with deformed upper lip and shortened philtrum. Nasal tip is broad and somewhat deformed, whereas nasal base is protruding, rather than retracted, resulting in the "pugilistic" facial appearance characteristic of this syndrome. Mild prognathism is also present. This patient is probably deaf.

(Rimoin and Edgerton, 1967), the *Pierre Robin anomalad* (Hanson and Smith, 1975), *Roberts' syndrome* (Freeman and others, 1974), *Larsen's syndrome* (Larsen and others, 1950) (see Chapter 6), *Stickler's syndrome* (Stickler and others, 1965), the *multiple pterygium syndrome* (Aarskog, 1971), *Meckel's syndrome* (Opitz and Howe, 1969), *diastrophic dwarfism* (Taybi, 1963), and a host of other even more rare syndromes (Goodman and Gorlin, 1977).

Many cytogenic disorders besides the trisomy 13 syndrome have been associated with cleft defects. Other chromosomopathies associated with cleft defects are the *4p− syndrome* (Johnson and others, 1976), *11 p+ syndrome* (Falk and others, 1973), the *18 q− syndrome* (de Grouchy, 1969), and the *XXXXY syndrome* (Zaleski and others, 1966).

## Syndromes characterized by facial palsy or facial diparesis

The distinction between unilateral facial palsy and bilateral facial weakness is important diagnostically, as was stressed in Chapter 4. Unilateral facial palsy usually is caused by a neurogenic lesion, whether it be nuclear, peripheral, or supranuclear, whereas bilateral facial muscular weakness most often is associated with myopathic processes as well as with nuclear, peripheral, or supranuclear neurogenic disturbances.

**Unilateral facial palsy.** Idiopathic paralysis of one side of the face has been known since ancient times but was first discussed as an entity by Charles Bell in the 1820's (Swaiman and Wright, 1975, p. 903). This very common neurologic dysfunction is presumed to have many causes. Nevertheless, a diagnosis of *Bell's palsy* should be reserved for instances of unilateral paralysis without known cause. Typically, the patient experiences the onset of a total unilateral facial paralysis after awakening from a night's sleep. This paralysis persists for weeks to months and then gradually improves even without treatment. In a sizable proportion of persons, however, the palsy never completely disappears and is replaced by other facial phenomena — hypoplasia of the facial muscles and facial hemispasm. Bell's palsy is presumed to have an as-yet-undiscovered infectious basis. The affected person is usually a young adult who is healthy in other respects. Often a history is obtained of a possible contact with infectious agents and of other constitutional signs of viral diseases that appeared several days or weeks prior to the onset of the symptoms. Some investigators believe Bell's palsy is caused by a hypersensitivity reaction to these noxious agents. Various studies have indicated that the site of the lesion is the periphearl nerve, in the facial canal. Surgical procedures to relieve bony pressure on the edematous facial nerve have been recommended as a possible early treatment of the disorder. In addition, it has been suggested that corticoids are useful in the medical treatment to relieve the edema.

In the acute phase of the disorder, the face at rest may appear to be relatively normal (see Fig. 7-3, *A*). A mild asymmetry may be noticed, accompanied by mild flattening of the nasolabial fold on the side of the palsy. The cheek may appear full and floppy, and the mouth line may be tilted to the side of the facial weakness. The palpebral fissure is also usually wider on the side of the weakness, and the forehead wrinkles may be less prominent because of involvement of the upper face as well. Drooling may be present. The true extent of the involvement is best appreciated after mild effort on the part of the patients to show the teeth and to close the eyes. Severely affected patients cannot perform these actions (Fig. 7-3, *B*). Through further testing of facial nerve function (lacrimation, taste, somatic afferent sensory loss, sensitivity to loud noises), one often can locate the site of facial nerve involvement fairly accurately.

Sudden unilateral facial palsy also may be seen in a host of other diseases. Facial palsy characteristically occurs in *sarcoidosis.* In this disease there usually are other characteristic features that allow for differential diagnosis, including an associated respiratory disorder, signs of systemic disease such as weight loss, iridocyclitis, and myalgia, and other symptoms or signs. Other disorders associated typically with facial palsies include *diabetes mellitus, mumps,* and other infectious diseases (Kunstadter, 1965). The *Melkersson-Rosenthal* syndrome is character-

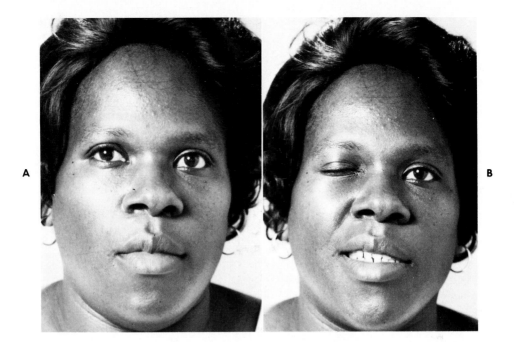

Fig. 7-3. Patient in her late twenties who developed total unilateral facial palsy several months before these photographs were taken. She was pregnant at the time. A, Appearance when at rest. Note mild flattening of facial wrinkles on the left, mild enlargement of left palpebral fissure, and fullness of left cheek. B, Appearance when asked to show teeth and close eyelids. Observe lack of movement of left face and absence of nasolabial fold. Eyelid is not closed. Because of the absence of eyeball elevation (Bell's phenomenon), it was evident that the patient was not actively closing the eyelids. (See also Figs. 6-42 and 6-43.)

ized by facial palsy, edematous tongue, and lingua plicata (furrowed or folded tongue). (See Fig. 7-4.)

**Bilateral facial paresis.** Batten and Gibbs (1909) and Steinert (1909) independently distinguished myotonic dystrophy from Thomsen's myotonia congenita because of the consistent association of myotonia, muscular wasting, and other dystrophic features in affected patients. The term myotonia literally means "a condition of tension in the muscle." The term dystrophy refers not only to skeletal muscle wasting but also to degenerative changes of cardiac muscle, smooth muscle, eyes (particularly the optic lens), endocrine glands, hair, skin, bones, and blood. Almost all tissue systems have been reported to be involved in this disease—a fact that has caused speculation that the basic defect is related to diffuse abnormalities in membranes rather than to abnormalities of specific tissues (Renwick and others, 1971). The genetic picture in myotonic dystrophy is important for diagnosis of the condition. Not only is myotonic dystrophy inherited as an autosomal dominant trait but also there is a curious maternal effect that accounts for the slightly different presentation in young children (Harper and Dyken, 1972; Dyken and Harper, 1973). Typically, the disease manifests itself in the late juvenile

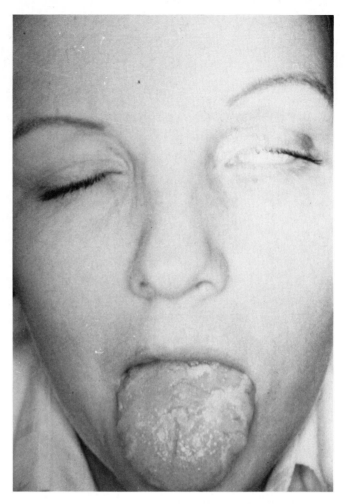

Fig. 7-4. Twenty-year-old female patient with the Melkersson-Rosenthal syndrome. Note left facial palsy and enlarged edematous tongue with lingua plicata (folded tongue). (See also Fig. 7-42.) (Courtesy of Dr. Thomas Swift, Medical College of Georgia.)

and early adult periods, except in children of affected mothers, who have characteristic symptoms in the neonatal period. Antecedents of persons with typical myotonic dystrophy of usual onset may have only fragments of the disease, such as isolated endocrinopathy, frontal baldness, lenticular cataracts, or mildly unusual facial and somatic stigmata (see Fig. 7-5).

The facial stigmata depend upon the onset of facial muscular involvement. In the typical form, which occurs after the maximum growth of the face, one sees characteristic facial features that have been likened to those of a tapir. The face is narrow and seemingly long, with narrowed jaw angles (Fig. 7-6). The muscular process affects the muscles of mastication as well as those of facial expression, and the jaw thus tends to droop open, giving an appearance of length. The temporal fossae appear

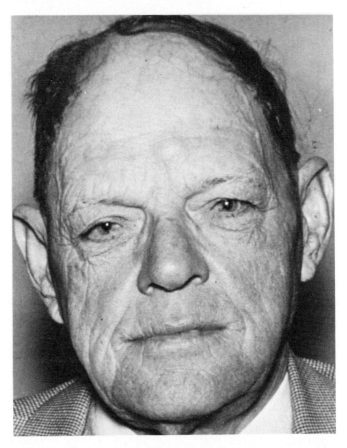

Fig. 7-5. Sixty-two-year-old father of patient with classic dystrophia myotonica. This man had frontal baldness, presenile lenticular cataracts, and diabetes mellitus. No pronounced myotonia was present, but he showed mild paresis of the distal somatic musculature. He has normal facial wrinkling for his age, with exception of lack of prominence of nasolabial folds. Observe mildly apathetic facies, sagging anterior neck, and mild atrophy of temporal fossae.

scooped out because of atrophy of the temporal muscles. Males frequently have frontal baldness. There is usually mild ptosis, and wrinkling of the forehead occasionally occurs as a compensatory mechanism (Fig. 7-6, *B*). There is a dulled facial expression with a sneering quality that is believed to result partially from an effort of the patient to close the lips over the opened orifice to prevent drooling. In addition, the mouth appears slightly puckered or pursed, which may be a result of mild myotonia of the orbicularis oris muscles. The mouth line is horizontal but may seem to be short for the reasons mentioned. The characteristic facial appearance of the patients in Fig. 7-6 is quite typical and represents one of the best clues to early diagnosis of the disease. Little is added to the diagnostic process by having the patient forcibly close his eyes and show his teeth (Fig. 7-7). Even patients severely affected with facial diparesis

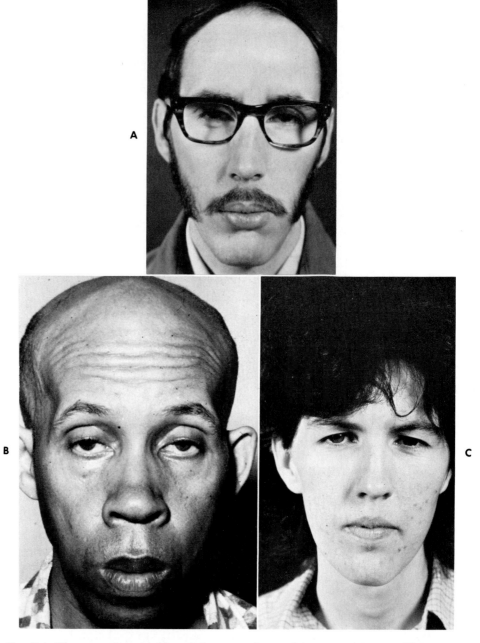

Fig. 7-6. Three patients with adult-onset dystrophia myotonica. **A,** Thirty-one-year-old male who had onset of muscular symptoms during his twenties. Note long lower face resulting from masseter diparesis, which causes the jaw to be held open slightly. Lips are protruded over the open mouth to control saliva. Observe narrowed angles of jaw, absence of nasolabial folds, mild ptosis, frontal baldness, temporal atrophy, narrow neck, and narrow face in general. **B,** Twenty-five-year-old male who had onset of muscular symptoms of dystrophia myotonica in teenage period. He has facial features similar to those of patient in **A.** There is even greater ptosis and a greater tendency to pucker the lips over the open jaws. (This patient is also shown in Fig. 5-54, *A.*) **C,** Twenty-eight-year-old female with facial features similar to those of patients in **A** and **B** but with less extensive involvement. There is no frontal baldness. Note again the narrow-angled jaw, the long lower face, the narrow neck, and especially the puckered or pursed lips.

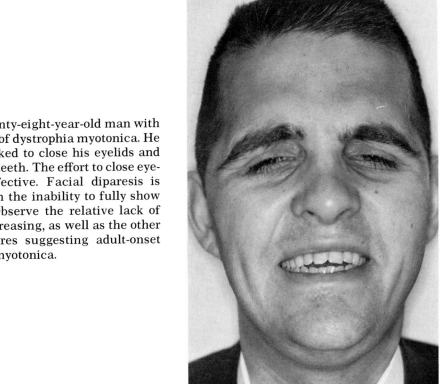

Fig. 7-7. Twenty-eight-year-old man with a mild form of dystrophia myotonica. He has been asked to close his eyelids and to show his teeth. The effort to close eyelids is ineffective. Facial diparesis is evident from the inability to fully show the teeth. Observe the relative lack of nasolabial creasing, as well as the other facial features suggesting adult-onset dystrophia myotonica.

can accomplish these tasks. The neck muscles typically are involved in dystrophia myotonica. The sternocleidomastoid muscles, which are especially affected (usually bilaterally), may be seen in frontal facial viewing to be wasted. The neck, which in general is quite thin, can be best appreciated by lateral viewing (Burian and Burns, 1967; Caughey, 1963; Dodge and others, 1965).

In the severe early-onset form of dystrophia myotonica, one sees distinct differences from the signs described above. These differences result from the early onset and the long-standing nature of the disease. Rather than the puckered lips that are so characteristic of the other, later-onset, types of this disorder, one sees a "tented" upper lip (Figs. 7-8 and 7-9). This abnormality results from long-standing congenital facial diparesis, which causes severe weakness and wasting of the facial, masseter, and pterygoid muscles and also of neighboring soft tissues and bones. The ears may be large and drooping. These lower facial abnormalities persist throughout adult life and provide a means of recognizing the congenital form of the disease. Compare the photograph of a patient

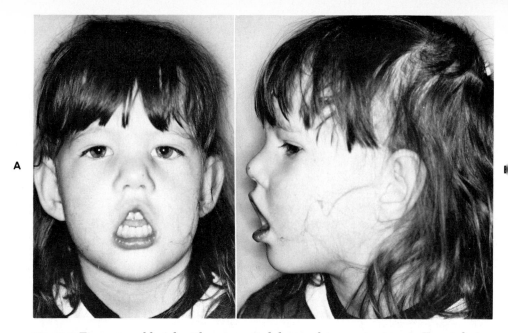

**Fig. 7-8.** Five-year-old girl with congenital dystrophia myotonica. **A,** Frontal view showing characteristic features when patient is at rest. Observe "tented" upper lip with shortened philtrum resulting from long-standing facial diparesis. The jaw is held open because of masseter and pterygoid diparesis. The teeth are poorly positioned. Observe other facial features of congenital dystrophia myotonica including mild ptosis, temporal wasting, narrow anterior neck, and small nose. **B,** Lateral view. (Same patient is shown in Fig. 7-10.)

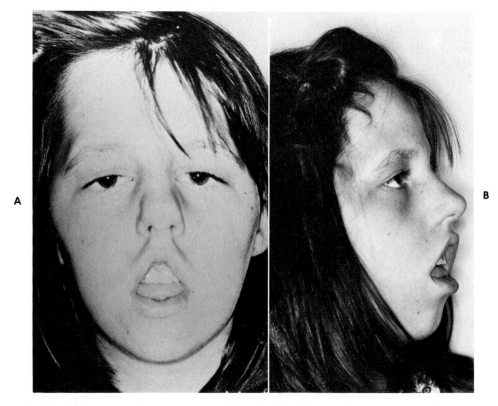

**Fig. 7-9.** Nine-year-old girl with congenital dystrophia myotonica. **A,** Frontal view showing tented upper lip, short philtrum, small nose, maloccluded teeth, narrow lower face with narrow jaw angles, bilateral ptosis, narrow neck, and temporal wasting. **B,** Lateral view.

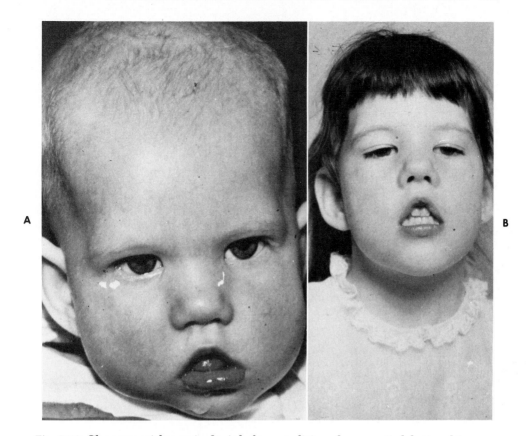

Fig. 7-10. Changes with age in facial abnormalities of congenital dystrophia myotonica. A, Three-month-old baby with congenital dystrophia myotonica. Note dull facial appearance, drooling as a result of masseter/pterygoid and facial diparesis, mild ptosis (pseudoptosis), temporal wasting, and slightly bulging cheeks. B, Same patient at 8 years of age. Note similar lower facial abnormalities, with tented upper lip, short philtrum, small nose, temporal wasting, and narrow neck. Ptosis is still present and has become slightly worse. Same patient is shown in Fig. 7-8. (From Dyken, P., and Harper, P.: Neurology 23:465, 1973.)

at 3 months of age (Fig. 7-10, A) with the photograph of the same patient at 8 years of age (Fig. 7-10, B). Patients with the severe congenital form of dystrophia myotonica usually have a more severe muscular problem and are usually mentally retarded or at least have much more pronounced mental deficiency than persons with the other forms of the disease. They also show a multitude of physical birth defects, such as clubfoot, multiple arthrogryposis (Fig. 7-11), congenital heart defects, inguinal hernia, osteoporosis, and congenital cataracts. Such patients have pathologic fractures and recurrent infections that are sometimes refractory to standard forms of treatment.

Moebius (1888) recognized a symptom constellation consisting of congenital facial diplegia, bilateral abducens nerve palsy, and skeletal

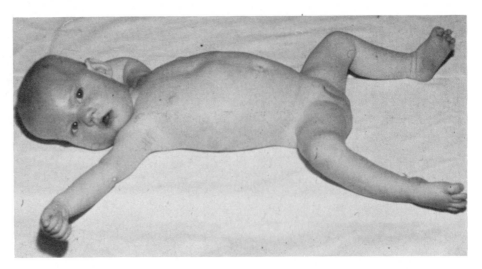

Fig. 7-11. Full-body view of patient in Fig. 7-10, *A*. Note bilateral talipes equinovarus and dislocation of the hips. (From Dyken, P., and Harper, P.: Neurology 23: 465, 1973.)

and muscle defects. This constellation was accepted immediately as an independent syndrome. Since the original description, many other cases have been reported, some of which correspond to the original cases and some of which do not. The diagnosis of *Moebius' syndrome* is still essentially a clinical one. The characteristic features are present at birth and result from paralysis of the muscles supplied by the sixth and seventh cranial nerves and, less often, the twelfth, ninth, and tenth cranial nerves. In several autopsy examinations nuclear hypoplasia has accounted for the lack of cranial nerve innervation. In autopsies of other persons whose conditions have also corresponded to the typical clinical picture, no neural pathology centrally or peripherally has been seen. In one autopsy described by Pitner and associates (1965), a 48-day-old child showed almost total absence of the facial muscles. The facial nucleus and nerve, however, were normal. Electromyographic studies of persons with Moebius' syndrome may show abnormalities, with few, if any, motor unit potentials.

One occasionally finds mental retardation in persons with this syndrome. Skeletal and muscle deformities occur in about 30% of cases. Poland's anomaly of unilateral hypoplasia of the pectoralis muscle is a common associated abnormality. One sees talipes, camptodactyly, clinodactyly, hypoplasia of the hand, fingers, or nails, and syndactyly much more frequently than in the general population.

There is usually bilateral facial palsy with expressionless facies, drooling, and open eyes while sleeping. Esotropia is frequently present. One may also see ptosis, atrophy of the tongue, and external ear abnormalities. The ears may be large and protruding. Occasionally, there is

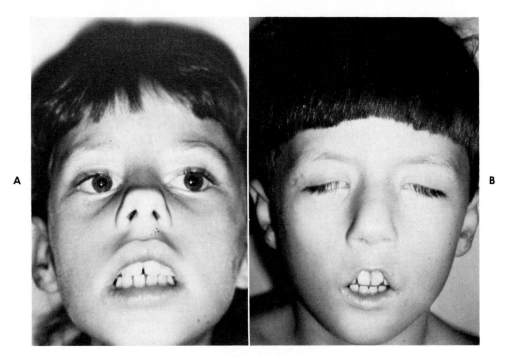

Fig. 7-12. Two juvenile patients with congenital facial diplegia or diparesis. **A,** Eight-year-old girl who had had immobile facies from birth. Her condition later progressively worsened and became associated with skeletal musculature involvement of face, scapula, and humerus. Her disorder thus was believed to be an unusual form of facioscapulohumeral muscular dystrophy without family involvement. View at rest shows flattening of nasolabial folds and an expressionless facies but no tented upper lip (as in dystrophia myotonica) even though the philtrum is shortened. **B,** Ten-year-old boy with Moebius' syndrome. Patient was asked to close eyes and to show teeth. Observe the shortened philtrum, mild tenting of upper lip, and absence of nasolabial folds. Patient shows Bell's phenomenon as well. (**B,** Courtesy of Dr. Patricia Hartlage, Medical College of Georgia.)

hearing loss. As would be expected, attempts to close the eyelids and show the teeth are unsuccessful. (See Fig. 7-12.)

The diagnosis of Moebius' syndrome involves differentiation from neonatal myasthenia gravis, dystrophia myotonica, and other disorders. *Duane's retraction syndrome* is associated with limitation of abduction of the eye but not facial diplegia, tongue atrophy, or the other skeletal and muscular defects. *Poland's anomaly* of an absent or deficient pectoralis major and a small, syndactylous hand on the same side actually may be a part of Moebius' syndrome. A number of ocular and facial myopathies are seldom associated with problems from birth. Facioscapulohumeral muscular dystrophy (a discussion of which follows) has been reported to be associated with congenital facial diplegia.

As pointed out by Goodman and Gorlin (1977), Moebius' syndrome may be part of a larger spectrum of disorders that includes, among others, the *hypoglossia-hypodactylia syndrome,* the *oromandibular-limb hypogenesis syndrome, Hanhart's syndrome,* the *ankyloglossum superius syndrome,* and *dysgenesis of the nucleus ambiguus of Plott.*

*Facioscapulohumeral muscular dystrophy* is another entity that typically involves facial diparesis and that can be easily confused with

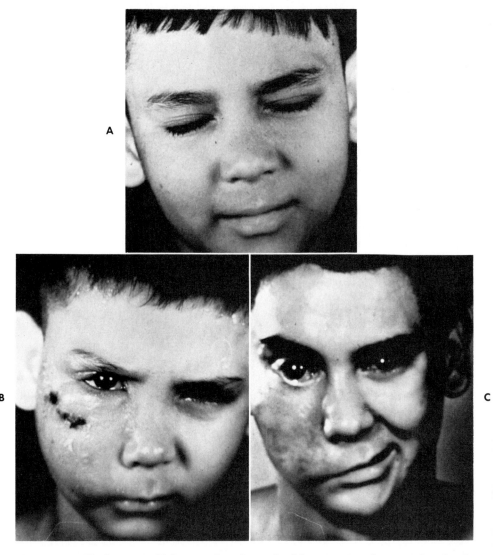

Fig. 7-13. **A,** Eight-year-old boy with tuberculoid leprosy involving right cheek, lower lid, and upper lip. Underlying facial nerve branches were involved, but no weakness was apparent. **B,** Same patient developed tuberculoid reaction during chemotherapy with sodium sulfoxone (Diasone). The tuberculoid lesion became inflamed, and right facial weakness ensued (note widened right palpebral fissure and drooping of right corner of mouth). **C,** Same patient years later. Permanent right facial weakness is present because of involvement of nerve branches underlying the tuberculoid lesion. (Courtesy of United States Public Health Service Hospital, Carville, La., and Dr. Thomas Swift, Medical College of Georgia.)

both dystrophia myotonica and Moebius' syndrome. Facioscapulohumeral muscular dystrophy, which is a rare disease, usually begins in the juvenile period. The disorder is inherited usually as an autosomal dominant trait, but there appears to be no maternal effect, and congenital cases are extremely uncommon. Involvement of the face is typical, but in addition, the scapular and humeral muscles are also involved. The ocular muscles are never involved. Associated congenital physical defects are seldom present, and myotonia is never present. From a facial viewpoint alone (Fig. 7-12), one does not see severe facial diparesis, and the mastication muscles seem relatively spared. There is no temporal atrophy, no squint, and no tented or pursed lips. Only rarely is ptosis present, and then quite late in the disease (Tyler and Steners, 1950).

**Partial facial palsy.** It once was believed that leprosy was a rare disease in the United States, even though it was one of the more frequently encountered diseases in the world. It has been estimated, however, that leprosy is encountered more frequently in the United States than was once commonly publicized. Reasons for this increase in the number of cases reported include improved worldwide travel and altered immigration characteristics, as well as a diminution in the social stigma associated with this so-called dread disease.

Leprosy is believed to be caused by a bacillus that attacks the peripheral nervous system. In the lepromatous form of the disease, granulomas appear on cranial nerves at random intervals—perhaps in a pattern related to physical and temperature characteristics of the face and body (Swift, 1974). This characteristic random involvement of the face, and of the cranial nerves in particular, produces an unusual partial facial paresis, neither purely unilateral or symmetrically bilateral. The cranial nerve involvement is not limited to the facial nerve; other cranial nerves may also be affected, although less commonly. In addition to the effects of facial and cranial nerve deficits, the patient with lepromatous leprosy has many other facial stigmata that relate to larger granuloma accumulation within the skin. These accumulations produce lumpy areas and streaks of localized atrophy of the skin and the subcutaneous tissues, hypertrophy of the skin, and flocking skin lesions. The so-called leonine facies characteristic of this disease results from a combination of these neural and nonneural granulomas (see Fig. 7-13).

## Syndromes characterized by hemihyperplasia and birthmarks of the lower face

The phakomatoses or neurocutaneous diseases diffusely affect the face as well as other structures of the body and are not limited to any one facial segment. Since the lower face is affected in many of these conditions, a section in this chapter will be devoted to these disorders. Further discussions are found in other chapters of this book.

*Sturge-Weber disease* is a disorder that involves many facial stigmata that are not limited to the lower face. Further discussion of this syndrome can be found in Chapters 5, 6, and 8. When a port wine nevus flammeus is present, the involvement of the upper face is probably the most consistent and the involvement of the middle face is probably the most important for management (that is, the lesion there is associated with buphthalmos and congenital glaucoma, which may need special treatment). Yet in patients with extensive port wine hemangiomas, particularly those distributed bilaterally, there is often extensive involvement of the lower face as well (Fig. 7-14). One may find hemangiomatous involvement of the cheeks, lips, gums, tongue, and throat (Fig. 7-14, *A*), resulting in extensive lower facial deformity. The port wine hemangioma is composed of weakened tissue that is more susceptible to injury. Since the associated hemangiomatosis of the pia-arachnoid produces severe seizure disorders and mental retardation by indirectly producing ischemia in the neighboring brain, persons with Sturge-Weber

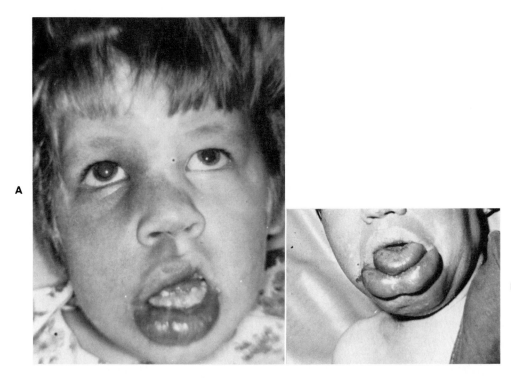

Fig. 7-14. Hypertrophy of the lower face and lips in patients with Sturge-Weber syndrome. **A,** Seven-year-old with prominent right-sided port wine nevus flammeus. Note pronounced hypertrophy of the right lower face and lips. Chronic phenytoin ingestion may account for some of the gingival hyperplasia. **B,** Forty-three-year-old patient with severe bilateral nevus flammeus. Observe enlarged lower face, lips, and tongue. These abnormalities resulted from the nevus itself, changes associated with phenytoin use, and traumatic hemorrhage. Patient had a seizure immediately before this photograph was taken, and, while falling, struck lower face, producing a subcutaneous hematoma. Hematoma continued to worsen, ultimately requiring a tracheotomy. (See also Fig. 8-48.) (From Dyken and others: Pediatr. Basics 6:10, 1972.)

disease tend to fall and to have increased susceptibility to injury. Injuries to the face in the area of the hemangioma itself can produce extensive hemorrhage into the surrounding tissue, which can be a threat to life, as in the instance of the patient in Fig. 7-14, *B*. This patient sustained an injury during a seizure, resulting in the development of an extensive hematoma of the lips, tongue, lower face, and upper neck. A tracheotomy was required to maintain an open airway. Contrast the patients in Fig. 7-14 to the patient in Fig. 7-15, who is black and who has a milder form of the syndrome.

Closely related to Sturge-Weber disease is a syndrome identified as *angioosteohypertrophy of Klippel-Trénaunay-Weber*, which is characterized by hypertrophy of the extremities and by other somatic features. This syndrome is known to be associated with the port wine type of nevus flammeus, which is usually distributed irregularly in the area of the

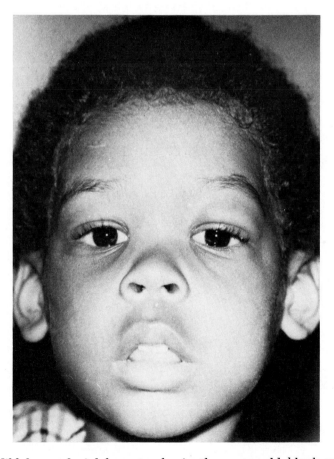

Fig. 7-15. Mild lower facial hypertrophy in three-year-old black patient with Sturge-Weber syndrome. Note port wine nevus flammeus on the left. Observe demarcation of nevus from normal skin at midline of the philtrum of the upper lip. There is mild hypertrophy of the left upper eyelid and resultant mild narrowing of the palpebral fissure.

second and third division of the trigeminal nerve, in contrast to typical Sturge-Weber disease. Angiomatosis of the lower face, tongue, palate, pharynx, and gums and hypertrophy of the mandible may be seen. Persons with this disorder also have accelerated growth and premature eruption of teeth on the involved side. (The hemangioma is unilateral). This syndrome is not as likely to be related to hemangiomatosis of the piaarachnoid as Sturge-Weber disease, and there is therefore less likelihood of mental retardation, seizures, and hemiplegia. An exception to this rule was found in the patient in Fig. 7-16, who was severely retarded. He did not have prominent facial involvement of the port wine stain but did show marked angioosteohypertrophy of one lower extremity (Fig. 7-16, *B*). This patient had a variety of nonspecific facial abnormalities in addition to an irregular, mottled-appearing capillary hemangioma of both sides of his lower face. Contrast this patient with the patient in Fig. 7-16, who has a mild form of the syndrome.

Another neurocutaneous disease that may be associated with hypertrophy of the lower face particularly is *von Recklinghausen's disease*, or neurofibromatosis. Von Recklinghausen's disease has many forms, some of which do not involve the face. The facial hemihyperplastic form

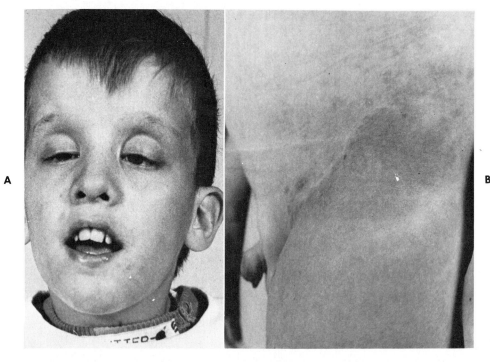

A B

**Fig. 7-16.** Sixteen-year-old severely retarded patient with Klippel-Trénaunay syndrome. **A**, Frontal facial view showing a mild, flat irregular nevus flammeus of lower lip and mouth. Observe also dull facial expression and epicanthal folds. **B**, Lateral view of left hip and groin showing extensive cavernous hemangioma of lower left extremity. The hemangioma was associated with bluish color and hypertrophy of the extremity. (**B**, From Dyken and others: Pediatr. Basics 6:10, 1972.)

of von Recklinghausen's disease (Fig. 7-17), which characteristically is present at birth and therefore is of special interest to pediatricians, is believed to result from a combination of lymphedema and local tissue dysplasia. Occasionally, this form of neurofibromatosis involves the upper and middle face more extensively than the lower face and may be associated with proptosis and buphthalmos of the eyeball. The form of the disease present in such a case is probably more closely related to bony abnormalities of the sphenoid wing and is characterized by a heightened incidence of optic nerve glioma. Facial hemihypertrophy with von Recklinghausen's disease not only may be a cosmetic tragedy but also involves a slightly greater incidence of generalized tissue dysplasia and thus a poor prognosis because of the presence of mental retardation, epilepsy, dwarfism, and a variety of neoplasms.

*Tuberous sclerosis*, which is also discussed in Chapters 5, 6, and 8, characteristically affects the middle facial segment. The lower facial segment, especially the chin, may be a primary site of adenoma sebaceum

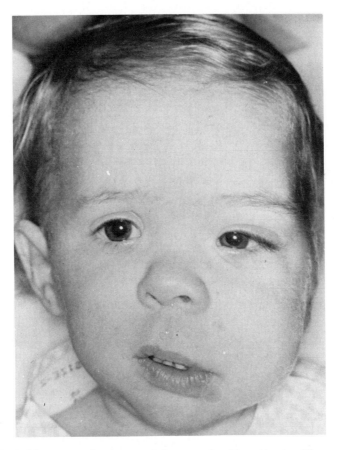

Fig. 7-17. Facial hypertrophy in an eight-month-old patient with von Recklinghausen's disease. Note tissue hyperplasia of the left lower face particularly. Observe distortion of the mouth and lips and narrowing of the left palpebral fissure. An illusion of esotropia exists because of the distortion — no deviation of the eye is shown by the corneal reflection.

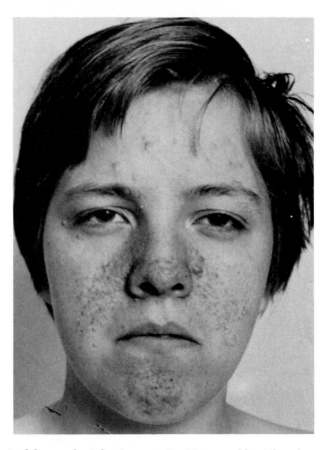

Fig. 7-18. Typical lower facial stigmata in 15-year-old with tuberous sclerosis. Note distribution of angiofibromas of tuberous sclerosis on the chin. This chin distribution of adnoma sebaceum seems to develop later in tuberous sclerosis. Observe also the distribution of the lesion on the tip of the nose, which is another late feature.

(see Fig. 7-18). In one young patient with tuberous sclerosis in a stage prior to the development of adenoma sebaceum, a cellulitis of the lower face, which resembled a hyperplasia, developed (see Fig. 7-19). This cellulitis cleared after a few days of treatment. After several years of follow-up study, however, all the typical signs of tuberous sclerosis — including adenoma sebaceum over the chin — developed.

*Congenital craniofacial leukoderma* (Fig. 7-20) is commonly distributed in the lower facial segment as well as elsewhere. This condition may be associated with other facial features and neurologic signs.

### Syndromes characterized by mutilated and abnormally positioned lips

The *Lesch-Nyhan syndrome,* which was clearly delineated by Lesch and Nyhan (1964), is characterized by X-linked recessive inheritance, hyperuricemia, choreoathetosis and other static neurologic motor defects, mental retardation (usually severe), and self-mutilation. Boyle and

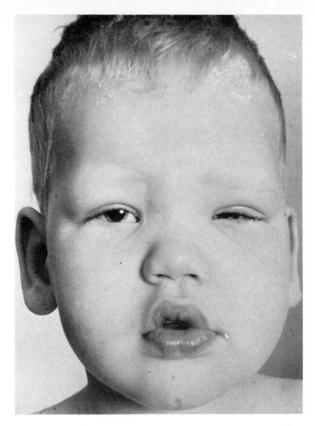

Fig. 7-19. Eighteen-month-old patient with tuberous sclerosis before the development of adenoma sebaceum. There is pronounced edema of the lower face on the left secondary to a cellulitis that developed following a submandibular adenitis.

A

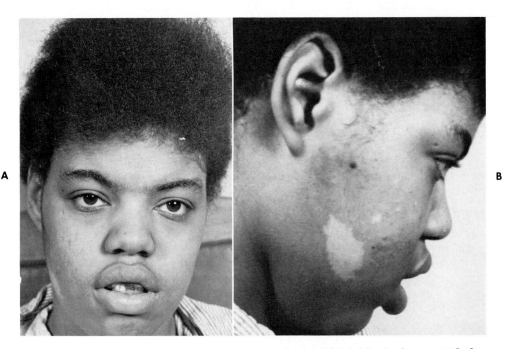

B

Fig. 7-20. Sixteen-year-old girl with congenital craniofacial leukoderma with distribution over the lower face. A, Frontal view showing dull facial expression. Observe patch of leukoderma on the right lateral lower face. Patient is also mildly mentally retarded and has recurrent mixed seizures. The facial hirsutism, thickened lips, and probable gingival hyperplasia are believed to be related to phenytoin administration. B, Right lateral view showing lower facial leukoderma, which was present at birth. Observe protuberant lips.

associates (1970) suggested the presence of a deficiency in the enzyme hypoxanthine-guanine phosphoribosyl (HGP) transferase and conclusively showed that the metabolic defect in the disease was related to an abnormality in purine biosynthesis, as was suggested earlier by Lesch and Nyhan (1964). More recently, McDonald and Kelly (1971) have shown that the disease has more genetic heterogeneity than was previously suspected.

Lesch-Nyhan syndrome has an early onset and may be mistakenly considered to result from birth trauma or hypoxia. Static motor disabilities such as hemiplegia, quadriplegia, diplegia, and choreoathetosis are present early. Progressive symptoms of involuntary movements, restlessness, and self-mutilatory behavior soon develop. The self-mutilatory behavior often includes chewing the lips, banging the head and ears, biting the fingers and toes, and scratching the skin on various parts of the body, including the face.

The facial features of this disease are characteristic but by no means diagnostic. The face may be distorted because of repeated trauma. Evidence of scarring and soft tissue deformity is especially evident around the lips. Calculi and exostosis of the forehead and face may be seen, as well as other old and recent signs of trauma including fresh bruises and abrasions (Fig. 7-21). Choreiform movements of the face, producing frequent grimacing and other peculiar facial expressions, are common.

Several syndromes are very similar to the Lesch-Nyhan syndrome, the diagnosis of which now rests with the typical clinical picture plus the demonstration of the enzyme defect. Disorders easily confused with this syndrome include the syndrome of hyperuricemia, ataxia, and deafness with normal levels of red cell HGP transferase; juvenile gout without neurologic symptoms; severe mental retardation, which may be associated with some self-mutilatory behavior (Fig. 7-22); and child abuse and neglect. Phenylketonuria in the untreated state characteristically is associated with extreme excitability and self-destructive behavior, but seldom to the extent witnessed in the Lesch-Nyhan syndrome.

Schwartz and Jampel (1962) described two siblings with the syndrome that now usually bears their names. In the original description of the *Schwartz-Jampel syndrome*, the siblings had myotonia, blepharophimosis, and joint limitation. Aberfeld and associates (1965), reporting on the same patients, emphasized the uniqueness of the syndrome and described the skeletal manifestations in more detail. Since these reports, several more cases have appeared in the medical literature. Huttenlocher, and associates (1969) suggested the name osteochondromuscular dystrophy.

Affected patients are dwarfed and usually show limitation in motion of the fingers, wrists, spine, hips, or toes. There are joint contractures, kyphoscoliosis or limbar scoliosis, hip dysplasia, pectus carinatum, umbilical and inguinal hernia, and small somatic muscle mass. Small testes

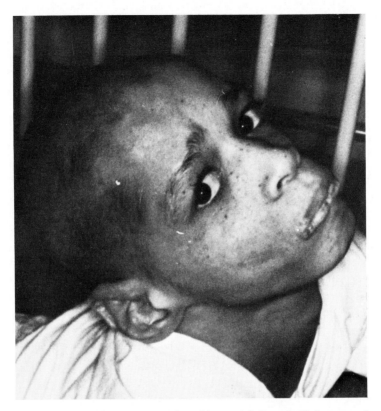

Fig. 7-21. Fifteen-year-old institutionalized boy with Lesch-Nyhan syndrome. Patient is severely retarded and has engaged in severe self-mutilation, as is evident from the mutilated and scarred lips and ears. Patient also has choreoathetosis and quadriparesis. (Courtesy of Dr. Theo Thevaos, Gracewood State Hospital and Training Center and Medical College of Georgia.)

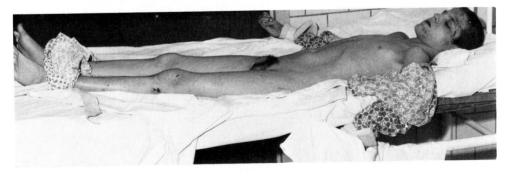

Fig. 7-22. Eighteen-year-old institutionalized male with self-mutilatory syndrome that was proven not to be associated with hyperuricemia. Patient was severely retarded and quadriparetic but did not show choreoathetosis. There is extensive evidence of fresh and old facial and somatic trauma. Patient had to be restrained from damaging himself further. Self-mutilation of the lips appears to occur more often in the Lesch-Nyhan syndrome than in other self-mutilation syndromes.

have been reported in males. Patients are not usually mentally retarded. Seizures may be a feature of the disorder. Many patients have signs and symptoms suggesting a muscular dystrophy or, at least, dysplasia. Muscular weakness, as well as myotonia, has been seen in this disorder.

Patients with the Schwartz-Jampel syndrome have small faces, even in comparison to their small bodies. There reportedly is a saddened, fixed, facial expression that may be an illusion resulting from facial myotonia, blepharophimosis, and oral phimosis, which frequently are present. The lips tend to be puckered, and the mouth is usually small. Although these symptoms are the most pronounced facial features, long eyelashes, increased intercanthal distance, ptosis (occasionally), microcornea and microphthalmia, cataract, severe myopia, short neck, and micrognathia may occur.

Fig. 7-23, A, shows a 3½-year-old patient who is believed to have the Schwartz-Jampel syndrome. The most characteristic facial features consists of the peculiar posture of the lips, which are somewhat puckered. The upper lip seems to be especially puckered, and it is also thin. The nasal philtrum is long and curled inward over the upper incisors, a feature that remains constant as the patient grows older (see Fig. 7-23, C and D). Somatically, there is a strikingly pronounced protuberant abdomen with severe lumbar lordosis, as seen in Fig. 7-23, B. In this lateral view, one can also better appreciate the blepharophimosis of the eyelids and mouth and the mild micrognathia.

A similar syndrome was described by Marden and Walker (1966) in a female infant. This syndrome consists of a fixed facial expression, blepharophimosis, mongoloid slant, esotropia, micrognathia, cleft palate, and low-set ears. This disorder also is associated with large hands and arachnodactyly. One case of the *Marden-Walker syndrome* involved progressive general deterioration. Autopsy showed abnormalities of the vena cava, diffuse dilation of the renal collecting tubules, hydropic degeneration of proximal and distal tubules, and atrophic skeletal muscle.

The *whistling face syndrome* or craniocarpotarsal dysplasia, which was first described in 1938 by Freeman and Sheldon, involves facial abnormalities very similar to those of osteochondromuscular dystrophy. The whistling face syndrome involves no myotonia, although there is reduced motor unit activity of the facial muscles. Muscle histology testing shows sparse and degenerated muscle fibers. Unlike Schwartz-Jampel syndrome, an associated severe dwarfism is not present, and there are usually no severe joint contractures. Affected patients have stiff, immobile, flattened facies, antimongoloid slant, heterotropias, blepharophimosis, mild pseudoptosis, long philtrum, high palate, and lips that protrude as if for whistling. A receding chin and low-set ears also are usually present. Occasionally, one sees ptergyium colli, protruding ears, and an H- or V-shaped groove on the chin. Affected patients usually have normal intelligence.

The *Hallervorden-Spatz disease* is characterized by neurologic

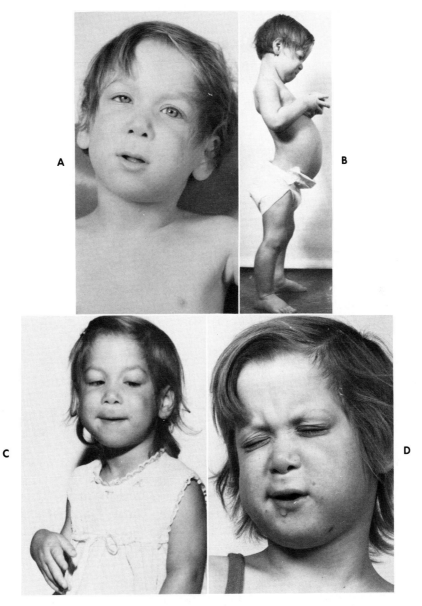

Fig. 7-23. Girl with the Schwartz-Jampel syndrome. A, Frontal facial view at 3½ years of age. Note long philtrum with oral phimosis and small mouth. B, Lateral full-body view at same age showing smallness, extreme lumbar lordosis, and protuberant abdomen, which result from the coexisting myopathy that characterizes this disease. Observe, however, the posture of the mouth and eyes, which may result from myotonia. C, Frontal facial view at 2½ years of age. Note the same abnormal features of the lower face and lips. D, Close-up facial view at 6½ years of age. (See also Fig. 7-25, B.)

deterioration resulting from degeneration of extrapyramidal systems of the brain. The disorder was first described by Hallervorden and Spatz (1922) and has since been related to a possible disturbance in iron metabolism (Szanto and Gallyas, 1966). Hallervorden-Spatz disease involves extensive brownish discoloration in the subthalamic nucleus, lenticular nucleus, and caudate, which is believed to be related to free iron deposits, as well as extensive cerebral cortical neuronal loss. There is a wide range of neurologic symptoms. Clinical symptoms are usually extrapyramidal—including, for example, choreoathetosis, dystonia, and ballismus—although seizures and intellectual impairment also are prominent. Seldom, however, do the mental symptoms dominate. Retinal pigmentary disturbances occur in a high percentage of cases. The disease is inherited as an autosomal recessive trait, although there is a tendency for males to be affected more commonly. The course of the disorder is slow but relentlessly downhill. Death usually occurs in the second decade of life.

Several characteristic facial features are present. There is frequent orofacial dyskinesia, accompanied by constant grimacing and writhing movements of the muscles of facial expression. These movements predominate in the lower face and over a period of years may lead to orofacial contractures (Fig. 7-24). One seldom sees, however, the totally dull facial expression common in other extensive central neurologic degenerative processes. Dystonic postures occur in the neck, leading to torticollis and unusual head positions.

Several other syndromes produce facial distortions similar to those seen in Hallervorden-Spatz disease. These disorders include *perinatal cerebral anoxia, kernicterus, Wilson's hepatolenticular degeneration, dystonia musculorum deformans,* and *Huntington's chorea.* Other so-called extrapyamidal disorders also may rarely be associated with orofacial dyskinesias. Two examples are *Sydenham's chorea,* which, however, is usually a transient phenomenon, and *benign familial chorea,* which more frequently spares the face. In aged persons, *senile orofacial dyskinesias* occur frequently. It is presumed that these dyskinesias result from cerebral arteriosclerotic changes and chronic ischemia of extrapyramidal systems. Drug-induced *tardive dyskinesia* frequently is associated with orofacial involuntary movements.

## Syndromes characterized by microstomia or macrostomia

Seldom does microstomia (excessively small mouth) or macrostomia (excessively large mouth) constitute the major feature of a syndrome. Yet these conditions are found frequently enough in a few conditions to deserve separate note.

**Microstomia syndromes.** In addition to the many other facial features that are more thoroughly discussed in Chapter 6, an unusually small mouth is a characteristic of trisomy 21. This characteristic is of great importance diagnostically, particularly in early life when several more

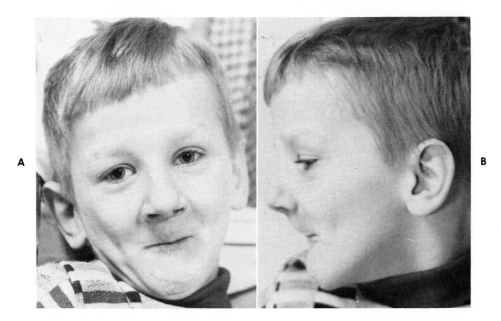

**Fig. 7-24.** Nine-year-old boy with Hallervorden-Spatz disease, which was proven by autopsy also to exist in a similarly affected older brother. **A,** Frontal view showing orofacial dyskinesia and oral posturing as well as pitiful facial expression. Patient is reasonably normal intellectually. **B,** Lateral view showing retraction of the lips.

specific facial features are less obvious. The smallness of the oral cavity gives an illusion of a large tongue (see Fig. 7-25, *A*). A truly small mouth, as seen in trisomy 21, should be contrasted to the apparent microstomia present in the Schwartz-Jampel syndrome, in which the mouth is characterized by phimosis (Fig. 7-25, *B*), and to congenital myotonic dystrophy, in which an apparent microstomia is in fact due to facial diparesis and hypoplasia (Fig. 7-25, *C*).

**Macrostomia syndromes.** Several disorders are characterized by relative macrostomia. These conditions include the *De Lange-Brachmann syndrome*, which has many facial features that are more specific but which characteristically involves a relatively large mouth in comparison to a generally pinched up, hypoplastic face (see Chapter 6), *Williams' syndrome* or the *supravalvular aortic stenosis – elfin facies – idiopathic hypercalcemia syndrome* (see Chapter 6), *Treacher Collins' syndrome, Turner's syndrome,* the *Klippel-Feil anomalad,* and the *Rubinstein-Taybi syndrome* (Chapter 6). Additionally, we have encountered a syndrome, characterized by severe mental retardation, middle facial hypoplasia, epicanthal folds, mild prognathism, and macrostomia, that possibly fits into this category (see Fig. 7-26). Patients with this syndrome have normal chromosomes, so shown by repeated special banding studies. We have named the disorder the *MMM syndrome* (mental re-

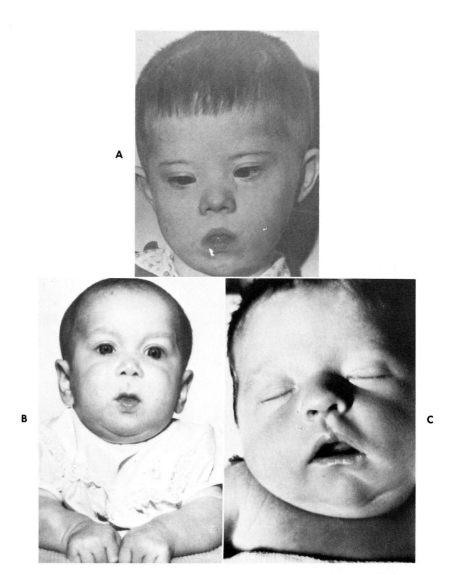

Fig. 7-25. Microstomia or pseudomicrostomia in three patients. **A,** Two-year-old boy with trisomy 21 proven by chromosome study. Note extremely short oral line and shallow oral cavity as well as other facial features of Down's syndrome. **B,** Patient in Fig. 7-23 when three months old. Observe the relative smallness of the mouth because of oral phimosis believed to be related to myotonia of facial musculature. **C,** Three-day-old boy with congenital dystrophia myotonica. Because of the facial diplegia that occurs in this disorder, there is a "tented" upper lip and shortening of the philtrum, resulting in an appearance of relative smallness of the oral line and mouth. (From Swift and others: Am. J. Dis. Child. **129:**734, 1975. Copyright 1975, American Medical Association.)

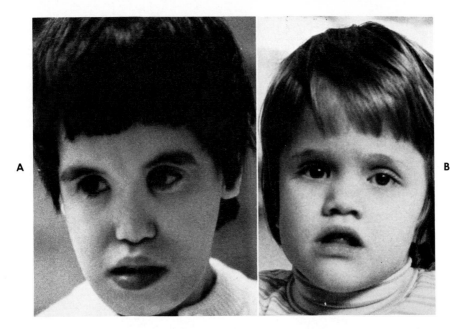

Fig. 7-26. Two severely mentally retarded, institutionalized children with a combination of abnormal facial features consisting of macrostomia, middle facial retraction, and prognathism. A, Eleven-year-old. B, Seven-year-old.

tardation, middle facial hypoplasia, and macrostomia). Another individual we encountered had macrostomia in combination with idiopathic congenital glaucoma and mental retardation (see Fig. 6-31).

## SYNDROMES OF THE PERIPHERAL LOWER FACE
### Syndromes characterized by abnormal chins

Since the chin is merely the most anterior part of the jaw, syndromes of the chin are somewhat difficult to separate from syndromes of the jaw. Several disorders, however, are characterized by isolated chin abnormalities, and they will be briefly discussed here.

Cretinism, the most commonly encountered form of congenital hypothyroidism, will be discussed in a later section of this chapter. Rarely, a physician encounters early-onset forms of hypothyroidism that have not begun in utero. Patients who have such early-onset acquired hypothyroidism show varying symptoms at the onset of the disorder and in later life. One such patient, seen in Fig. 7-27, who was in her sixties when first seen by us, was reportedly normal at birth. In late infancy she suffered from an unclear illness that involved constitutional inflammatory symptoms and that resulted in an inability to be nourished properly, a painful swelling in the region of the thyroid gland, and transient psychomotor standstill. She eventually recovered from the acute illness but thereafter showed poor growth and progressive psychomotor retardation. The

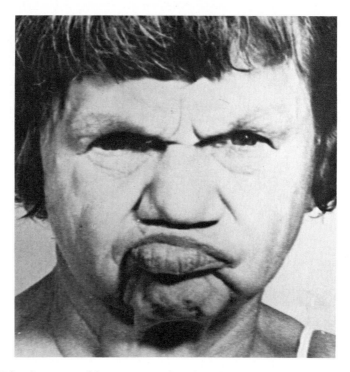

Fig. 7-27. Fifty-five-year-old woman with infantile acquired hypothyroidism with goiter. Note scarring and fibrotic bands extending from the thyroid goiter to the chin. Observe thickened lips and dull, scrawling facial appearance.

swelling persisted and became associated with synechia and subcutaneous fibrous bands that extended to the chin. She lived in a medically disadvantaged community and never sought medical attention until she was institutionalized at a hospital for the chronically mentally retarded many years later. Her abnormalities produced the facial stigmata evident in the photograph. We speculate that this patient suffered from an acute thyroiditis of unknown cause in infancy after a degree of facial development had occurred. This unknown insult produced extensive destruction of the thyroid glands, leaving only enough functioning tissue to be compatible with life and to account for the lack of the other facial stigmata often associated with congenital hypothyroidism.

Triangular chin syndromes. Several disorders are associated with narrow and triangular but normal-sized chins. These conditions include some of the congenital myopathies such as *nemaline myopathy, carnitine myopathy*, and *congenital fiber-type disproportion*. The patient in Fig. 7-28 has a triangular chin in association with a not-yet-fully-classified congenital myopathy. This patient was bright and had no specific neurologic abnormalities. Yet he was born with bilateral talipes equinovarus (Fig. 7-28, *B*) and began to suffer from signs of slowly progressive

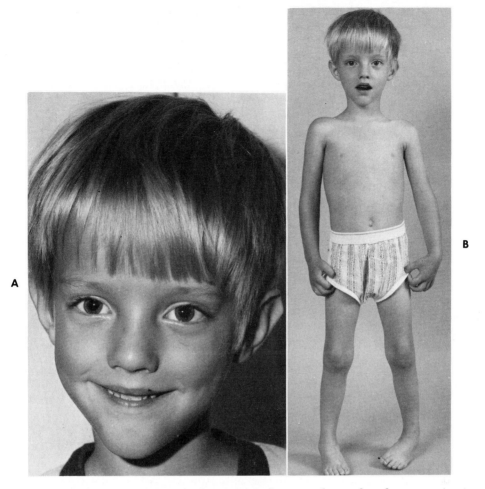

**Fig. 7-28.** Seven-year-old boy with congenital myopathy and arthrogryposis. A, Frontal facial view showing triangularly shaped face with pointed and narrow chin. B, Frontal full-body view. Observe bilateral talipes equinovarus and hip deformity on left and triangularly shaped face. Patient is small but not dwarfed and shows no hypertrophy of limbs, as is seen in Silver dwarfism.

muscular weakness and atrophy approximately 6 months before the photograph was taken. Biopsy showed definite signs of muscular involvement.

The chin is also abnormal in many of the first-branchial-arch syndromes. *The Hallermann-Streiff syndrome* usually is characterized by a pointed, slightly retracted chin in addition to other features of the first-arch syndrome, hypotrichosis, and ocular disturbances. Additionally, the *Silver-Russell syndrome* of dwarfism and other abnormalities may show a pointed or triangular chin that also may be retracted slightly.

Prognathism, or jutting chin, will be discussed in the next section.

## Syndromes characterized by abnormal jaws and cerebral gigantism

Marie in 1886 was the first to describe *acromegaly* and to use the term. The condition later was shown to result from a pituitary tumor. It has since been established that all patients with acromegaly, or pituitary gigantism, do not have neoplastic growths. In patients without such growths, hyperplasia of the functioning pituitary cells responsible for secreting growth hormone produces the signs and symptoms of acromegaly. In these cases, hereditary factors are considered to be important in the development of the condition.

Regardless of cause, excessive amounts of growth hormone in young persons with open epiphyses results in pituitary gigantism. In persons with closed epiphyses, however, acromegaly results. Acromegaly, as the name implies (acro=terminal, extreme; megaly=largeness) consists primarily of enlargement of distal parts of the body, although abnormal growth occurs in a generalized fashion as well. The size of the skull usually increases, and the nose becomes broader and larger than it was before the onset of the condition. The tongue and lips thicken. Particularly obvious, however, is the pronounced growth of the mandible, which occurs both in anterior and horizontal directions. The chin becomes jutting, and the teeth became separated. Fingers and toes enlarge, primarily in thickness rather than in length (Fig. 7-29). Although these abnormalities are characteristic of acromegaly per se, they also occur in pituitary gigantism, but to a lesser degree. In pituitary gigantism the most striking feature is the increased growth of the body in both height and weight. The symptoms of acromegaly and pituitary gigantism also can occur together. Whether such a situation develops seems to depend upon the age of the patient at onset. Various degrees of both syndromes may be seen in both children and adolescents (Kenyon, 1956).

The specific facial features of both pituitary syndromes consist primarily of mandibular hyperplasia, which is associated sometimes with striking prognathism, especially in acromegaly. There is thickening and coarsening of the facial features, especially around the lips and nose, as well as accentuation of the superciliary region and the bony eminences of the eyebrow. The cranioface appears quite large and long. The jaw angles may, however, be normal. The skin over the cranium, as well as over the rest of the body, is quite thick. These features are different from the facial features of the form of cerebral gigantism first described by Sotos and associates (1964). In Sotos' syndrome, there are often other facial stigmata, such as hypertelorism, antimongoloid slant, and large ears. Sotos' syndrome also involves a much duller facial expression that has also been described as silly, or wide-eyed (Fig. 7-30).

**Prognathism syndromes.** The term *cherubism* was used by Jones in 1965 to describe a rather uncommon but very distinctive facial deformity that is first recognized in childhood. The syndrome consists of fullness of the cheeks and bony swelling of the submandibular regions. There may be associated hypertelorism and irregularly placed deciduous teeth.

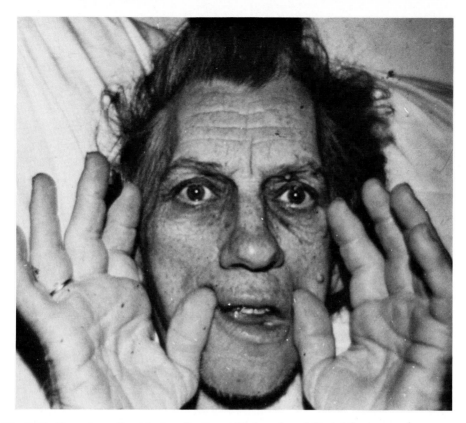

**Fig. 7-29.** Female patient in her forties with hand and facial features of acromegaly. Note superciliary hyperplasia, elongated and coarse facial features, and prognathism. Hands are also enlarged. Patient had a pituitary adenoma.

A rim of sclera may be visible beneath the iris during frontal viewing of the patient. The most commonly associated facial abnormality is prognathism. In cherubism, although the bony changes primarily produce a deformity in the lateral growth lines of the jaw, anterior hyperplasia also occurs (see Fig. 7-31). The angle of the jaw in this condition may be strikingly broad. On occasion there is an impression of midfacial hypoplasia because of the striking mandibular changes. Multilocular bony cystic changes may also affect the ribs, humerus, femur, and carpals, in addition to the mandible or maxilla. The mandibular lesion often regresses somewhat in later life (Jones, 1965).

Several other neurologic syndromes are associated with varying degrees of prognathism. The patient in Fig. 7-32 was mildly mentally retarded and had a mild prognathism. This patient was of normal size, and the results of endocrinologic investigations were normal. He suffered from an unclassified congenital myopathic process characterized by slowly progressive distal wasting and weakness and electric and active myotonia. We identified this previously unrecognized syndrome as *con-*

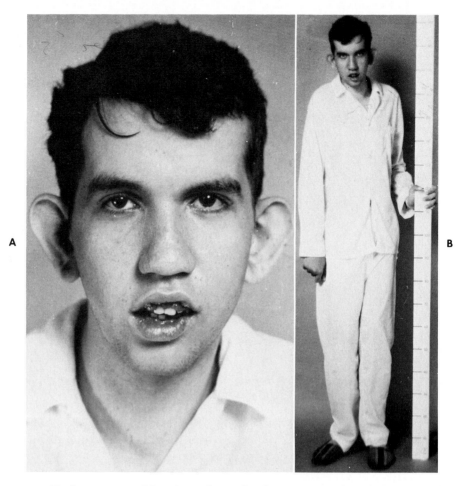

Fig. 7-30. Eighteen-year-old male with cerebral gigantism of Sotos. **A,** Frontal facial view showing elongated facies with mild prognathism, large lips, narrowed angles of the jaw, long nose, mild superciliary hyperplasia, and large protuberant ears. **B,** Frontal full-body view showing height that is excessive (approximately 6 feet 5 inches) when compared to heights of other family members. Patient is mildly mentally retarded and has recurrent seizures and multiple telangiectasia. CT scan showed mild ventricular dilation.

*genital myotonic distal dystrophy with prognathism.* The patient in Fig. 7-33 was discovered at a state hospital for the chronically mentally retarded. He was profoundly disabled intellectually and showed not only pronounced prognathism but also superciliary hyperplasia. His facial features were very coarse, and he was relatively hypopigmented. He had been committed for several years, but even before this time he was considered to be extremely aggressive and difficult to manage. When first examined at 24 years of age, he was quite large but showed no additional stigmata of pituitary dysfunction. A karyotype test once suggested that he had an extra male sex chromosome. Later, however, more sophisticat-

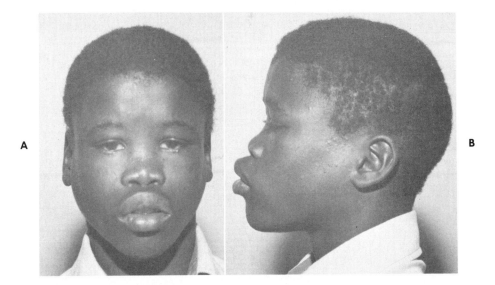

Fig. 7-31. Fourteen-year-old moderately mentally retarded patient with cherubism. A, Frontal view showing excessive hyperplasia of mandibles at angle of the jaw. Also observe prognathism, hypoplastic nasal base, and broad distal nose. B, Lateral view showing mandibular overgrowth and prognathism. Lips are large, and nasal hypoplasia is present.

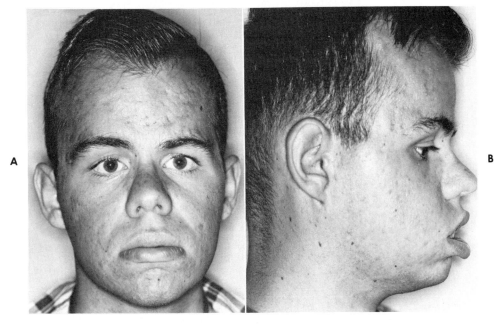

Fig. 7-32. Sixteen-year-old mildly retarded patient with signs of a distally somatically distributed congenital myopathy with myotonia. Patient is small but not dwarfed. A, Frontal facial view showing prognathism. There is an illusion of mild macrostomia. No features of dystrophia myotonica are evident. B, Lateral facial view showing prognathism and enlarged and protuberant lower lip.

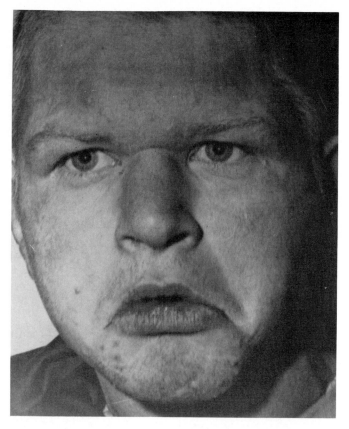

Fig. 7-33. Extremely aggressive 22-year-old institutionalized patient with XYY syndrome. Patient shows prognathism and illusionary macrostomia. Observe coarse facial features with superciliary hyperplasia and extensive facial scarring.

ed studies failed to show any chromosomal anomaly. It is speculated that this patient may have been a mosaic for the *XYY syndrome*, which may be associated with aggressiveness and possibly with facial features similar to his. Such possibly related symptoms of the XYY syndrome have been mentioned, but they are very inconsistently found in persons who are proved to have the syndrome.

**First-branchial-arch syndromes.** The first-branchial-arch syndromes have been discussed in detail in Chapters 3, 4, and 6. Most of these syndromes involve some degree of mandibular hypoplasia and micrognathia. The *Hallermann-Streiff syndrome*, for example, is commonly associated with a triangular chin. The prototype of the first-branchial-arch syndromes, however, is *Treacher Collins' syndrome*, which shows the most pronounced mandibular hypoplasia as well as other features. It has been suggested that Thomson may have described this syndrome in 1846 (Goodman and Gorlin, 1977), but its main features were clearly defined by the great British neurophthalmologist E. Treacher Collins (1900).

Franceschetti and Klein (1949) coined the term mandibulofacial dysostosis for the syndrome.

The main features of the syndrome involve the face, although there have been rare cases in which the syndrome has been associated with congenital heart disease. Mental retardation has been reported only slightly more frequently. There is usually a symmetrical antimongoloid slant caused by hypoplasia of the bony structures of the first branchial arch. Colobomas of the lid have been reported. Ear deformities, usually of the symmetrical type, including absence of the external auditory canal, deformed pinnae, conductive deafness, extra ear tags, and blind fistulas, are frequently encountered. Patients with the syndrome may also have a large nose, narrow nares, and hypoplastic zygomatic arches. There may be an associated high or cleft palate, dental malocclusion, and macrostomia (in about 15% of cases). The most striking feature, however, is a severely hypoplastic mandible with concave undersurface and micrognathia.

## SYNDROMES OF THE ORAL CAVITY

Under ordinary conditions the internal mouth is not visible. In abnormal situations, however, many internal mouth structures can be readily seen, even when the patient is not opening his mouth. Syndromes characterized by abnormalities of the mouth will be discussed in the sections that follow.

### Syndromes characterized by abnormalities of the buccal surface and gums

Gum hypertrophy or *gingival hyperplasia* usually is an iatrogenic condition. Although the commonly used anticonvulsant *phenytoin* characteristically is associated with both clinical and histologic gum changes, other anticonvulsants also may produce minimal gum changes. It is believed that the gingival hyperplasia associated with anticonvulsant medication is caused by an idiosyncratic, low-grade inflammatory reaction. Such changes also seem to characteristic of some of the collagen diseases, namely systemic and discoid *lupus erythematosus* (Meislin and Rothfield, 1968). The tissue changes associated with chronic anticonvulsant administration are not limited to the gingivae. They also involve, to a lesser extent, the lips — especially the inner or buccal surfaces (Fig. 7-34, A). Buccal surface hypertrophy occasionally is even more pronounced than the gum changes (Fig. 7-34, B), especially in the acute period of administration of phenytoin. Since a wide range of neurologic diseases is associated with epileptic seizures, an equally wide range may be associated with lip and gum hypertrophy. Fig. 7-34, A, shows chronic hypertrophy related to long-term phenytoin administration in an institutionalized patient with *tuberous sclerosis.* Observe also the other characteristic facial features of this syndrome. Another buccal surface abnormality, the mucous membrane plaque mentioned in Chapter 4, is not present in

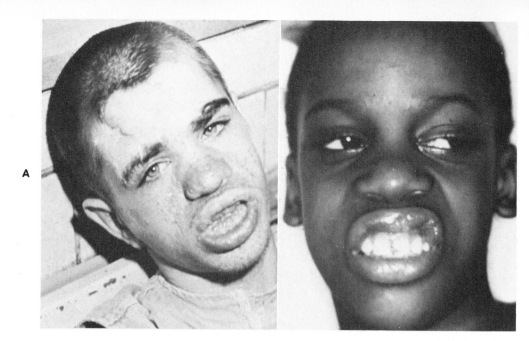

Fig. 7-34. Lower facial abnormalities associated with phenytoin ingestion. A, Patient with tuberous sclerosis undergoing long-term phenytoin administration. Observe marked gingival hyperplasia and hypertrophy of the lips. B, Patient receiving shorter-term phenytoin therapy. This patient shows lip hypertrophy alone. He has subacute sclerosing panencephalitis and has been receiving anticonvulsants for three months. Patient also has an exotropia and demented facial expression.

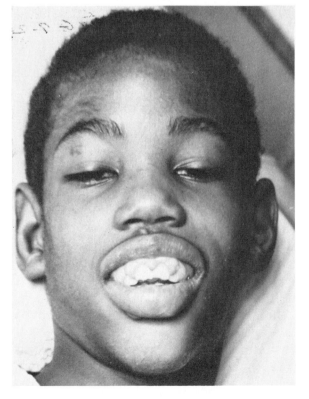

Fig. 7-35. Twelve-year-old boy with Waterman's syndrome of gingival hyperplasia. Patient is mildly demented and has had seizures but is not being given phenytoin.

this patient. Fig. 7-34, *B*, shows the more acute lip and gum changes believed to result from phenytoin administration. The patient in this photograph had refractive myoclonia as a manifestation of *subacute sclerosing panencephalitis (SSPE)*.

There are also several interesting but rare syndromes of idiopathic gingival hyperplasia worthy of comment in this section. Waterman (1969) described a syndrome characterized by gingival fibromatosis, hypertrichosis, epilepsy, and mental retardation that probably should be called *Waterman's syndrome*. Since this initial description, several other cases have been described. In some instances the disease is progressive and is associated with neuropathologic structural changes. In Waterman's syndrome the face is coarse and hirsute, even in infancy before long-term anticonvulsant administration, and neither the gum changes nor the hirsutism seem to be related directly to phenytoin use or dosage. The gingival abnormalities are generalized, and there is little histologic evidence of the chronic inflammation that characterizes phenytoin ingestion and collagen diseases. Seizures and mental retardation as well as other neurologic signs and symptoms are usually present in this slowly progressive disease. The hirsutism sometimes becomes more pronounced during pubescence. The syndrome seems to be inherited as an autosomal dominant trait. A patient with Waterman's syndrome is seen in Fig. 7-35. A slowly progressive neurologic deterioration began in this 11-year-old mentally retarded youngster soon after the onset of seizures at 7 years of age. He was given phenytoin, but the gum hyperplasia was present even before this medication was used. As the seizure disorder progressed, he continued to lose mental and motor skills. He was ataxic and demented and had extensive hirsutism even though phenytoin administration had been stopped years before.

Another rare syndrome characterized by gingival hyperplasia is the *Zimmermann-Laband syndrome* and others, (Laband, 1964). This syndrome is characterized additionally by thick, floppy ears and a bulbous soft nose. There is absence or dysplasia of the nails and/or terminal phalanges and hyperextensibility of the joints. Hepatosplenomegaly may occur. Hypertrichosis and mental retardation occur in a few patients but are not consistent features of the syndrome. Yet another easily distinguished syndrome of hyperplasia of the gums is *Cross' syndrome* (Cross and others, 1967; Witkop, 1971). This is an autosomal recessive disorder characterized by diffuse gum hyperplasia, hypopigmentation, microphthalmia, oligophrenia, athetosis, mental retardation, spasticity, and early death. There may be cloudy corneas, nystagmus, and high-arched palate. There is a reduced number of melanocytes with weakly positive tyrosin reaction of the hair bulbs. *The Murray-Puretić syndrome*, besides showing gum hyperplasia, is characterized by multiple gingival and cutaneous hyaline fibromas. These lesions, which occur in early childhood, are firm, painless, elastic nodules that adhere to the overlying skin of the head and face, causing a coarse facial appearance. There may be associated stunted growth, osseous defects, flexion contractures of the joints appearing early in life, and muscular hypotrophy with reduced subcutaneous tissue. Dysseborrhea and other skin changes may be evident. The disorder is inherited as an autosomal recessive trait (Murray, 1873; Puretic and others, 1962).

Gingival hyperplasia has also been seen in type VII mucopolysacchariodosis and in mucolipidosis I or II cell disease (Leroy and Crocker, 1966).

The histiocytosis syndromes include *eosinophilic granuloma* of bone, the *Hand-Schüller-Christian syndrome*, the *Letterer-Siwe syndrome*, and other *reticuloendothelioses*. These syndromes represent a wide range of clinical patterns in which the underlying common denominator is the histologic development of granulomatous lesions with histiocytic proliferation (Lichtenstein, 1964). From a clinical viewpoint, five basic types of histiocytosis are now identified. The first and most benign type (eosinophilic granuloma) is limited to bone and represents approximately 50% of the cases. A second type (Hand-Schüller-Christian syndrome) also is associated with bone, with minor additional involvement in the nature of anemia and minor skin or mucous membrane eruptions. In addition, there is occasionally pituitary-hypothalamic involvement that produces diabetes insipidus. A third type, which is more fulminating and extensive, is characterized by bone and moderate multiple visceral involvement. This type begins in infancy or early childhood and may be associated with papular skin lesions, seborrhea of the scalp, stomatitis, lymphadenopathy, pulmonary infiltrations, and hepatomegaly. This third type of histiocytosis blends into a fourth type, which shows even more extensive organ involvement and an even more fulminating course. Affected persons are usually infants who have severe hepatosplenomegaly, marked bone marrow suppression, widespread pulmonary infiltration, and generalized debilitating infection. There is even more extensive cutaneous involvement and lymphadenopathy (Fig. 7-36). Some of the signs of the third type and all of the signs of the fourth type correspond to what has been identified as Letterer-Siwe syndrome in the traditional medical literature. A fifth type of histiocytosis corresponds roughly to the formerly used designation of familial reticuloendothelioses, or atypical cases. These cases show, for example, involvement of the central nervous system with cerebrospinal fluid pleocytosis and severe blood abnormalities. This type has a rapid total course with or without skin or lymph node involvement.

From a facial viewpoint alone, the types classically identified as Hand-Schüller-Christian disease and Letterer-Siwe disease can be grouped together. Within the mouth one usually finds gingival hypertrophy with inflammation, necrosis, and retraction, which usually result in loss of teeth. The mucous membranes may show a vesicular inflammation. In addition, there are a variety of skin lesions that, in the acute

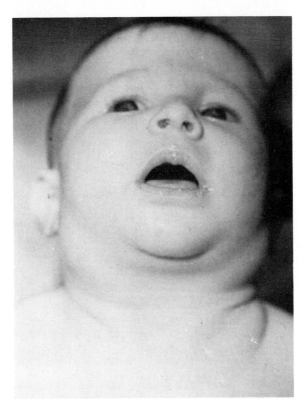

Fig. 7-36. Three-year-old patient with histiocytosis X. Note marked submandibular lymphoadenopathy. Patient was neurologically normal.

phase, may appear as diffuse papular eruptions of vesicular nature or as scaly and/or petechial dermatitis (especially on the forehead and trunk). In the recovery phase or in the chronic phase, the skin over the soma appears moist and denuded.

## Syndromes characterized by abnormal teeth

*Ectodermal dysplasia* was first described by Thurman (1848), but Darwin (1875) pointed out its X-linked recessive nature. The syndrome is suggested in infancy because of unexplained, high body temperatures that develop on hot days especially. Ectodermal dysplasia involves a characteristic clinical triad—hypohidrosis, hypotrichosis, and hypodontia. Dryness of the skin may be severe. The palms and soles are sometimes hyperkeratotic. There is scant axillary and body hair. The mammary glands are often hypoplastic. Mental retardation may occur.

In addition to the classic features of adontia or hypodontia, the facial features are quite characteristic. When teeth are present, they are conical in shape. One typically sees frontal bossing with a wide or square forehead, depressed nasal base, and mild midface hypoplasia (see Fig. 7-

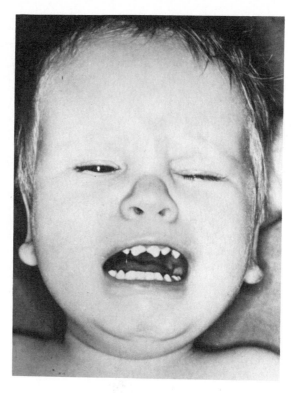

Fig. 7-37. Four-year-old patient with hypohidrotic ectodermal dysplasia. Note hypoplastic teeth and mild hypotrichosis.

37). There may be hyperpigmentation and fine linear wrinkles around the eyes and mouth. The skin is fair. The hair is thin and soft and usually hypopigmented. There are scanty eyebrows and eyelashes. The lips, on the other hand, are relatively fleshy and protruding. There is often decreased formation of tears.

Other teeth abnormality syndromes. There is a wide range of syndromes characterized by abnormal tooth formation. One such syndrome is the congenital form of *dystrophia myotonica*. In this condition malocclusion of the teeth characteristically occurs. Teeth abnormalities are also a feature of many of the first-branchial-arch syndromes, as well as many others discussed in this chapter and other chapters. It should be emphasized that unusually fractured teeth may be the first clue to *child abuse* or to improper dental care, as is characteristic of *child neglect*.

## Syndromes characterized by macroglossia and other tongue abnormalities

Many syndromes are characterized by abnormalities of the tongue. It would be appropriate at this juncture, however, merely to mention some of the more frequently encountered neurologic syndromes associated

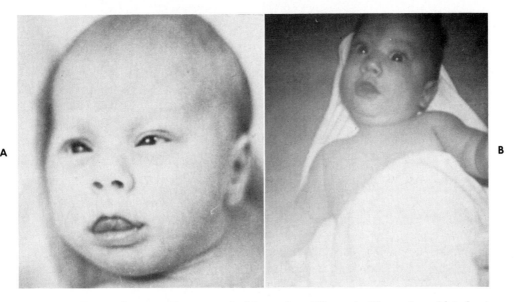

Fig. 7-38. Two infants with congenital hypothyroidism. A, Three-day-old infant with large tongue. Observe dull facial expression. This baby also has mild mongoloid slant and esotropia. B, 3-month-old infant showing macroglossia. Notice thickened skin and retraction of eyelids.

with hallmark abnormalities of the tongue. Some of these conditions have been mentioned in previous chapters.

It is extremely important that *cretinism*, also called agoitrous cretinism, athyreotic cretinism, and nongoitrous hypothyroidism, be recognized early in life before the development of unresolvable mental retardation and dwarfism. Through careful facial viewing, a physician may detect one of the early signs of abnormality. The tongue is characteristically large even at birth and often protrudes from the mouth. In addition, there is a large head, as well as puffiness of the face, pallor, low hairline, mild hypertelorism, narrow palpebral fissures, thickening of the eyelids, flat nasal base, hoarse cry, open mouth, short neck, hypotonia, and hyporeactivity. Later, delayed dentition, psychomotor and growth retardation, obvious characteristic dwarfing, abnormal myotatic reflexes, yellow skin color, prominent abdomen, and (sometimes) muscular hypertrophy develop (see Figs. 7-38 to 7-40).

In early infancy, *trisomy 21* may be confused with other syndromes associated with macroglossia—especially cretinism—because of the hypotonia and hyporeactivity. The macroglossia in Down's syndrome, however, is not a true largeness of the tongue. It is rather a relative largeness that results from a relatively small oral cavity. In later life, however, when the differential diagnosis is not nearly as important, the tongue in mongolism is deeply furrowed and truly large.

The *mucopolysaccharidoses* and several of the mucolipidoses (such

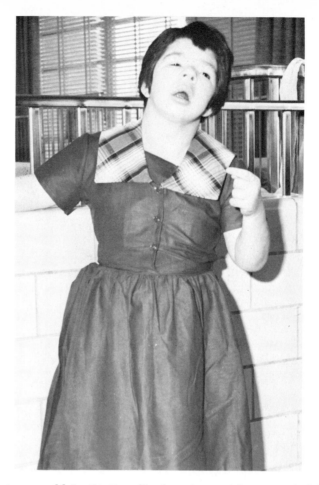

**Fig. 7-39.** Thirty-year-old institutionalized patient with congenital hypothyroidism. This patient, who has not been treated, was severely retarded and dwarfed when her condition was discovered in adulthood. Note coarse facial features with large tongue. Hair is coarse, and skin appears thick.

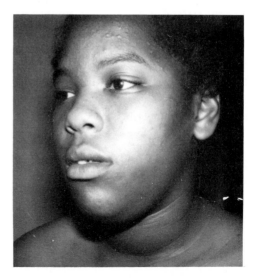

**Fig. 7-40.** Thirteen-year-old mildly mentally retarded patient with acquired goiter. Note that neck is enlarged in region of thyroid gland.

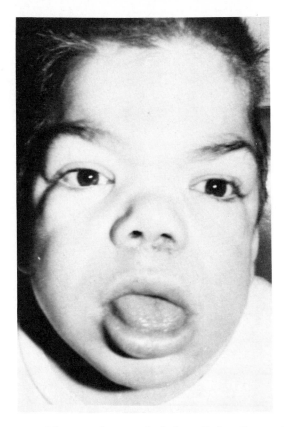

Fig. 7-41. Sixteen-year-old severely retarded, dwarfed patient with Hurler's syndrome (MPS IH). Patient is institutionalized and has multiple-system involvement. Note characteristic coarse facial features as well as macroglossia. Lips are also quite large.

as I cell disease) are also associated with abnormally large tongues (Fig. 7-41). The other stigmata of the mucopolysaccharidoses enable one to distinguish these diseases from other disorders associated with macroglossia.

The *Melkersson-Rosenthal* syndrome is characterized by a large furrowed tongue (see Fig. 7-42).

*Sturge-Weber disease* may be associated with macroglossia in rare situations.

The *Beckwith-Wiedemann syndrome* is also characterized by macroglossia. In addition, this syndrome is associated with high birth weight, mild to moderate mental retardation, large habitus later in life (affected persons usually fall at the ninetieth percentile and thus are not true giants), omphalocele, umbilical hernia, neonatal polycythemia, and abdominal and cardiac organopathy. Patients may have cryptorchidism, clitoromegaly, hemihypertrophy, microcephaly, exophthalmos, nevus flammeus, prognathism, dental malocclusion, ruddy complexion, linear fissures on ear lobes, abnormal ears (punched-out depressions of posteri-

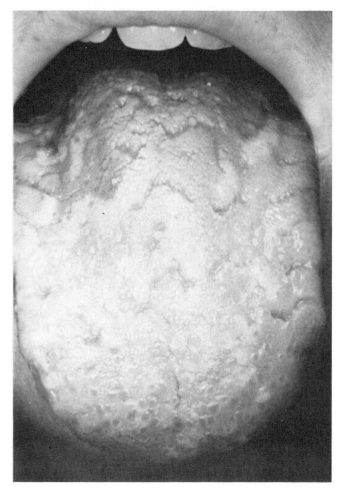

Fig. 7-42. Close-up view of tongue of person with macroglossia and lingua plicata. This patient, who is also shown in Fig. 7-4, has Melkersson-Rosenthal syndrome. (Courtesy of Dr. Thomas Swift, Medical College of Georgia.)

or pinnae), and midface retraction. A diagnosis of Beckwith-Wiedemann syndrome is suggested at birth if one finds macroglossia, omphalocele, and hypotonia in a baby with a high birth weight. Hypoglycemia, hypocalcemia, and polycythemia are common neonatal problems. (see Fig. 7-43.)

*Werdnig-Hoffmann disease* is a wide-ranged neurologic deterioration of the anterior horn neurons of the spinal cord and brainstem. The disease begins in infancy and in most instances results in death (about 75% of affected persons die in early childhood; about 25% survive but with limited neurologic function). The disease is one of the many so-called floppy-baby syndromes that are characterized by severe generalized hypotonia of the muscles, hyporeflexia, and paresis in infancy. One of

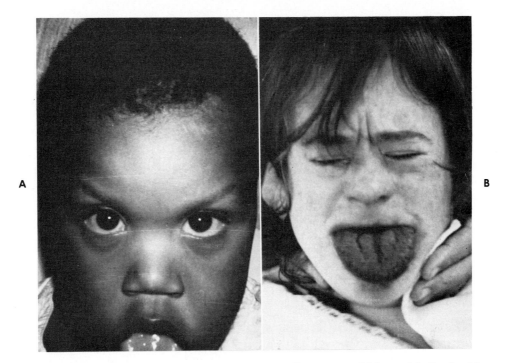

Fig. 7-43. Two patients with macroglossia. A, Three-year-old boy with Beckwith-Wiedemann syndrome. Unfortunately, the tip of the tongue is not visible in this photograph. B, Eight-year-old girl with true macroglossia and trisomy 21. The macroglossia described in Down's syndrome usually is an illusion resulting from the smallness of the oral cavity. (A, Courtesy of Dr. Patricia Hartlage, Medical College of Georgia.)

the characteristic and most helpful bedside signs that can be used to distinguish this disease from a wide variety of other disorders associated with muscular hypotonia concerns the tongue. In Werdnig-Hoffmann disease the motor neurons of the hypoglossal cranial nerve deteriorate, a feature uncharacteristic of all the other floppy-baby syndromes. Thus one usually sees severe atrophy and often fasciculations (Fig. 7-44), which may take the form of diffuse writhing movements within the muscle mass of the tongue. These movements result from denervation of the neurons of the hypoglossal nucleus in the medulla oblongata.

A rare but interesting syndrome of children, which is often associated with abnormal tongue posture, has been called the *happy puppet syndrome* (Angleman, 1965). Affected children usually have had life-long neurologic problems, including severe hypotonia at birth and often quadriparesis. Other neurologic deficits have also been described in the infantile and childhood periods. These children are almost always severely microcephalic and severely to profoundly mentally retarded. Seizures, usually of a myoclonic type, are present. Ataxia develops in late infancy or childhood and is usually associated with a peculiar titu-

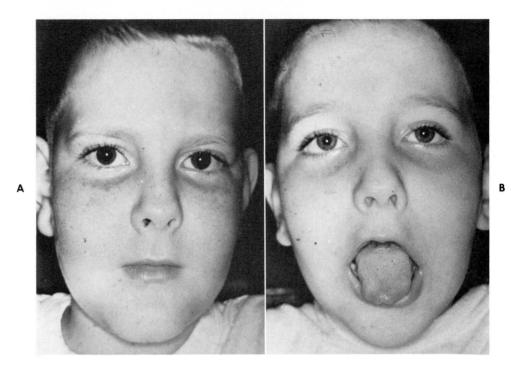

Fig. 7-44. Fourteen-year-old boy with a chronic form of Werdnig-Hoffman progressive spinal muscular atrophy. A, Full facial view at rest showing no abnormalities. B, Full facial view after tongue protrusion. Observe atrophic tongue especially on the right lateral border. Constant wormian movements representing fasciculations were seen both at rest and on protrusion of the tongue.

bation of the head and trunk when the child is sitting or standing. This titubation results from mild myoclonia. Most abnormal movement disappears at rest and during sleep. A patient usually has a happy, unconcerned expression quite unlike that seen in patients with disorders causing similar intellectual and motor impairment, who tend to be dull and apathetic. The combination of happy expression and titubation account for the syndrome's name. An additional peculiar characteristic of this syndrome is the tendency toward paroxysms of unexplained laughter. A few children have a tendency to protrude their tongues during the paroxysms and at other times as well. The tongues are usually long and thin and, when protruded, tend to curl upward on the sides (see Fig. 8-40).

## SYNDROMES OF THE NECK
### Syndromes characterized by abnormal head posture

*Dystonia musculorum deformans* is characterized by progressive dystonia and distortions of the body. It is now recognized that there are two hereditary forms of this disease, an autosomal dominant type and an autosomal recessive type. Other syndromes that closely resemble dys-

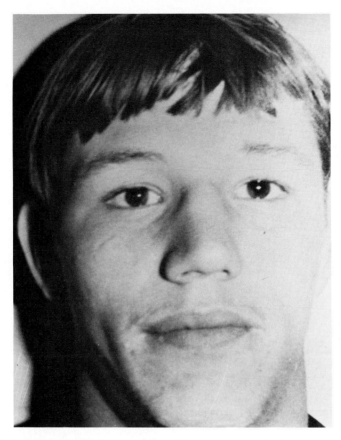

Fig. 7-45. Relatively normal appearing 18-year-old with dystonia musculorum deformans. Observe mild torsion of face and head to the right and broad and highly muscular neck.

tonia musculorum deformans clinically are now placed under the category "symptomatic dystonias" (Zeman and Dyken, 1967). These conditions include dystonia following or associated with perinatal cerebral hypoxia or trauma, carbon monoxide poisoning, Wilson's hepatolenticular degeneration, Hallervorden-Spatz disease, and others (Swaiman and Wright, 1975).

Dystonia musculorum deformans begins in childhood or early adulthood, usually between 5 and 15 years of age. The onset is usually insidious, with intermittent posturing or slow tonic or dystonic movements of the foot, neck, or arm (Zeman and Dyken, 1967). Thereafter, there is usually steady progression and involvement of other parts of the body. Over a period of years, the dystonic movements and postures become severe enough to cause severe incapacity. Grotesque distortions of the body may be seen, with marked somatic pretzel-like deformities. In the symptomatic dystonias, the onset is usually earlier, the progression is less pronounced and stereotyped. No form of the disease, however, is totally static, even those forms that follow brain damage.

The face is usually not a primary site of involvement in the dystonias, although athetotic writhing of facial muscles occasionally is seen because of associated orofacial dyskinesias (Fig. 7-45). The major effect on the face in dystonia musculorum deformans is a secondary one related to the posture of the head resulting from sustained contraction of the muscles of the neck. Dystonia can be differentiated from other involuntary movements by its tendency to involve proximal musculature more commonly than distal musculature. The neck typically is involved in dystonia musculorum deformans at some time in the disease progression. The neck involvement takes the form of torticollis or retrotorticollis

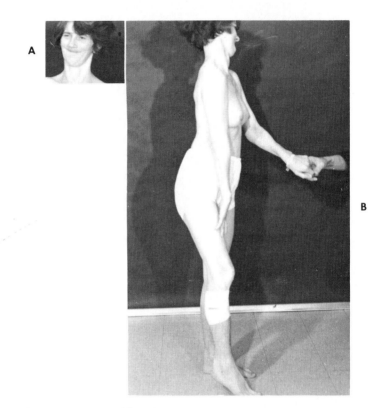

Fig. 7-46. Forty-two-year-old patient with dystonia musculorum deformans. Patient was hospitalized at a hospital for the chronically mentally retarded. Although she had normal intelligence, she did poorly on numerous psychometric tests because of her motor and speech disabilities. A, Frontal view showing facial abnormalities. Note lower facial deformity secondary to dystonic movements and postures of muscles of neck and face. Grimacing and torted mouth posture were characteristic. Observe torticollis to the right. B, Lateral body view. Patient had difficulty standing without aid. Abnormal "torted" movement and posture of the right lower extremity and dromedary position of pelvis and back were characteristic. Bilateral cryogenic thalamotomies had been performed several months before these photographs were taken. Prior to that time, this patient was nonambulatory and had even more severe twisting deformities of body and extremities.

(Fig. 7-46) primarily, although antecollis is also seen rarely (Fig. 7-47). Dystonia may be defined as an abnormal fluctuation in the tone of a muscle. This fluctuation alternates from hypertonia (excessive tone) to hypotonia (deficient tone), with hypertonia predominanting. Dystonia usually takes the form of an excessive tension in the muscle, causing forced, sustained movement of the parts of the body affected by the predominant action of the muscle involved. Excessive muscular activity, however, occurs in both antagonistic and synergistic muscles during a dystonic movement or posture. The extent of the movement and the ultimate posture seem to depend on the amount of force exhibited by the affected muscles. It is common in advanced cases of dystonia musculorum deformans to see a "strained" facial expression and muscle tension in unaffected muscle groups in an effort to counteract the primary muscle action. In torticollis, it is common to see a great deal of hypertrophy of

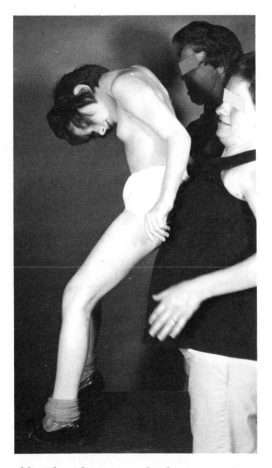

**Fig. 7-47.** Ten-year-old girl with severe, slowly progressive antecollis resulting from dystonia musculorum deformans. She had flucuating hypotonic-hypertonic flexions in muscles of neck. Patient also showed somatic dystonia and could not walk or stand without aid. Symptoms improved following thalamotomies.

the neck muscles, which become similar to the muscles of a well-trained athlete.

The facial grimacing in dystonia musculorum deformans is not as extensive as the grimacing one might see in some of the other similar involuntary movement disorders. (Refer to the discussion of Hallervorden-Spatz disease on p. 320.) Wilson's disease can be distinguished from true dystonia musculorum deformans by the characteristic "wilsonian risus" of this type of symptomatic dystonia. The "strained expression" and tilted face and head with anterior neck muscular hypertrophy, on the other hand, characterized dystonia musculorum deformans.

Haar and Dyken (1977) have described an autosomal dominant condition characterized by congenital hemiplegia. In affected patients, hypoplasia and athetosis developed on the same side in early childhood. This syndrome was believed to represent a static encephalopathy rather than a degenerative process per se. The patient in Fig. 7-48 showed the facial

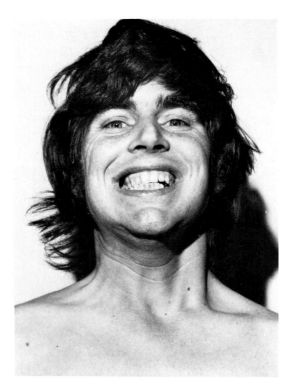

Fig. 7-48. Twenty-one-year-old male with hereditary hemiplegia, hemihypoplasia, and hemiathetosis. Photograph was taken after patient was asked to actively show teeth and to tense platysma muscles. Observe lack of platysma contraction on the left and asymmetrically bulging sternocleidomastoid muscle on the same side. The patient is hemiplegic on the left and has a mild unilateral facial paresis on that side. Note that the left shoulder is held slightly lower than the right and that the contours of the trapezius muscles are different from each other because of long-standing wasting of facial nerve–innervated musculature (that is, the platysma). (From Haar, F., and Dyken, P.: Neurology 27:849, 1977.)

characteristics of this syndrome when he was asked to forcibly show his teeth and contract his neck muscles. One sees a relative paresis of the affected platysma, allowing the sternocleidomastoid to stand out. The affected sternocleidomastoid muscle is hypoplastic in comparison to the normal one. There is mild facial paresis on the left side.

## Syndromes characterized by dolichostenocollis

It has been our impression, in our dealing with many children who have mental retardation and a host of other neurologic disorders, that there is an association between these disorders and dolichostenocollis, which literally means "long, thin neck." Since we see many patients with neuromuscular diseases in which the muscles of the face, neck, and shoulder girdle are wasted, it is possible that the appearance of a long, thin neck is only an illusion. On the other hand, many patients have been seen with various cytogenic and developmental disorders in which "dysmorphism" is characteristic. We believe that dolichostenocollis is an important feature in helping to characterize these diverse neurologic disorders.

**Neuromuscular disorders.** It is well known that many of the muscular dystrophies are characterized by long and thin necks. One of the most common muscular dystrophies in which this phenomenon is seen is myotonic dystrophy or *dystrophia myotonica* (see pp. 301). It has been stated that patients with myotonic dystrophy typically have long and slender necks that resemble the okapi, a forest mammal, of the Congo region in Africa that is related to the giraffe but smaller. The appearance, of course, is caused by the loss of muscle bulk, primarily in the sternocleidomastoid muscles. (See Fig. 7-49.) The illusion of dolichostenocollis is heightened by the characteristic thin facies and the loss of muscular bulk in the surrounding shoulder girdle areas. For the same reasons, patients with *facioscapulohumeral muscular dystrophy* also give the illusion of having long and thin necks. Other myopathies—usually of benign, congenital chronic, or "dysplastic" types (the term "dysplastic" is used because of the frequent occurrence of congenital physical defects and associated dysplastic or dysmorphic abnormalities in structures and tissues not directly related to the muscle), such as *nemaline myopathy*—often are associated with dolichostenocollis.

**Cytogenic disorders.** A host of primary chromosome defects, especially those involving the X chromosome, are characterized by a long neck. The *XXY or Klinefelter's syndrome* is usually associated with a long neck (this condition is the opposite of Turner's syndrome, or monosomy X, with its characteristic short, broad neck). A patient with Klinefelter's syndrome is seen in Fig. 7-50. This person has other abnormalities as well, including an abnormal head tilt caused by weakness and some wasting of the lateral neck muscles on one side. Patients with the other extra-X syndromes also tend to have dolichostenocollis in addition to other clinical features. In addition to their occurrence in sex chromosome abnormalities, long necks are predominant in several rarer au-

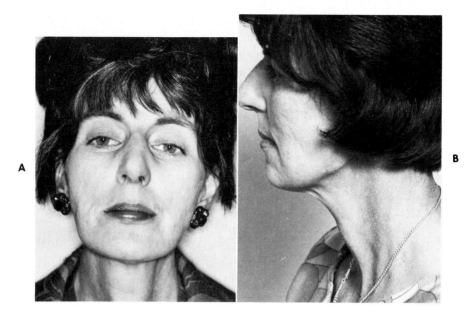

Fig. 7-49. Forty-year-old woman with adult-onset dystrophia myotonica. A, Frontal view showing facial stigmata of adult-onset disease. Observe thin neck resulting from bilateral atrophy of sternocleidomastoid muscles. B, Lateral view showing "okapi" type neck also resulting from bilateral wasting of sternocleidomastoids.

tosomal chromosome disorders such as *trisomy 8 syndrome*, the *supernumerary isochrome 18 syndrome* (+18 pi syndrome), *de Grouchy's syndrome* (18 q− syndrome), and the *cat's-eye syndrome* (22 trisomy and 22 q+ syndrome).

**Nonchromosomal dysplastic syndromes.** In some syndromes associated with dolichostenocollis the basic defect is not known but a developmental or dysgenic process is probably active. An example of this type of long-neck syndrome would be *Marfan's syndrome*. In Marfan's syndrome the basic defect is believed to be one of faulty collagen and elastic tissue, resulting in diffuse somatic abnormalities characterized by arachnodactyly, dolichostenomelia, vascular aneurysms, lens changes, and tall, thin habitus. *Cleidocranial dysplasia* may involve a seemingly long neck due to drooping of the shoulders, which is related to the total or partial absence of the clavicles. The rare *multiple mucosal neuroma syndrome*, a neurocristopathy (cristo=crest), is characterized by dolichostenocollis, associated with asthenic body build and muscular wasting. The *osteodysplasty of Melnick and Needles* (Melnick and Needles, 1966) is characterized by a high forehead, exophthalmos, full cheeks, micrognathia, and large ears. This rare syndrome, which also includes many skeletal and bony defects in the radius, tibia, clavicle, scapulae, pelvis, and hips, is characterized by dolichostenocollis. In addition, a long, thin neck may be associated with *Sotos' syndrome of cerebral gigantism. The N syndrome*, a rare malformation disorder associated with

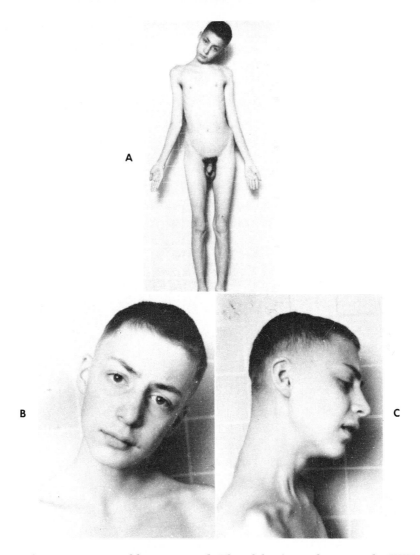

Fig. 7-50. Seventeen-year-old patient with Klinefelter's syndrome or the XXY syndrome. A, Frontal body view showing typical habitus and posture. Observe feminine appearance, dolichostenomelia with increased carrying angle of upper extremities, and tall and thin habitus. Patient has normal secondary sex characteristics. Patient also has myopathy of uncertain type. Head is tipped to one side because of localized weakness of trapezius muscle on the left. B, Frontal facial view showing tilt of head to left and no facial distortion like that often seen in disturbances involving the primary torters of the head. Patient also is slightly microcephalic. C, Right lateral facial view showing dolichostenocollis.

multiple congenital anomalies and mental retardation, also involves a long, thin neck (Hess and others, 1974).

One of us (PRD) has studied long-necked individuals in state mental institutions. Of 3000 patients whose cases were reviewed, five were found to have mental retardation of varying degrees and intelligence quotients ranging from 30 to as high as 70. Each of these patients had an

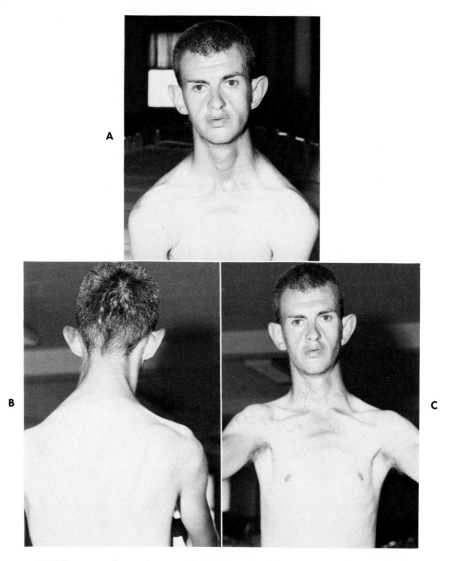

Fig. 7-51. Mildly to moderately retarded 21-year-old patient with giraffism not related to neuromuscular disease or chromosome defect. A, Frontal facial view showing extremely long neck with normal-appearing nuchal musculature. Note the somewhat dull facial expression. B, Posterior view of the dolichostenocollis. C, Frontal view showing dolichostenocollis when shoulders are abducted and arms elevated. Although no neuromuscular disorder was demonstrated by extensive electromyographic study and muscle biopsy with full histochemical analysis, the protruding ears, which are evident in all views, might suggest a neuromuscular problem.

excessively long and thin neck (see Fig. 7-51). Complete histories of these patients were taken, and morphologic and neurologic examinations were performed. Each underwent chromosomal analysis, although not all analyses were done with the newer banding techniques. No chromosomal abnormalities were uncovered. Neurologic symptomatology was variable, although all affected individuals showed generalized asthenia or frail body habitus. No definite evidence of a myopathic process was uncovered. Roentgenograms of the cervical vertebrae were normal in four of the persons, except that the cervical vertebrae were all unusually long and interbody or disc spaces were also generous. In one person, a normally formed extra cervical vertebrae was discovered. The condition of these five patients was named *giraffism,* although this term is recognized as not conforming to the rules of naming new syndromes as expressed by the First International Workshop on Genetic Disorders organized by the National Institute of Health in 1975 (Goodman and Gorlin, 1977). It was established at this meeting that syndrome names that may have an unpleasant connotation to an affected person or his family should be avoided.

## Syndromes characterized by brachycollis and pterygium colli

A malformation first described by Klippel and Feil (1912) is characterized clinically by short neck caused by abnormal fusion or formation of vertebrae, especially in the high cervical region. X-ray film may show a wide variety of cervical vertebral fusions and other anomalies. Several types of the malformation may be differentiated through roentgenographic study (Jarcho and Levin, 1938).

The most striking feature of the *Klippel-Feil anomalad,* of course, is the shortened neck with low posterior hairline (Fig. 7-52). There may be many other associated clinical features. There is usually painless limitation of head movements. One may see flaring of trapezius muscles extending from the mastoid region to the shoulders. This phenomenon gives an initial impression of pterygium colli, but there is seldom an associated cord of subcutaneous tissue associated such as that seen in true pterygium colli. Upward displacement of the scapulae from birth, a condition called Sprengel's deformity, is frequently associated with the Klippel-Feil anomalad. There may be cervicothoracic scoliosis. A variety of neurologic abnormalities may be associated, including mirror movements and/or bimanual synkinesis. The synkinesis is believed to result from an abnormal decussation of the pyramidal tract in the medulla, which in turn is perhaps related to a bony fusion defect. Cranial nerve palsies are common, as are hemiplegia, quadriplegia, and sensory defects. Occasionally, the Klippel-Feil deformity is associated with a variety of cerebellar dysfunctions such as ataxia, dysmetria, and nystagmus. These latter symptoms are believed to be related to pressure on the cerebellum from impaction of neural and meningeal tissue in the foramen magnum.

Mental retardation is not always a feature of this abnormality, but it is frequently present. When present, its severity is believed to be proportional to the severity of other associated cerebral anomalies. In addition, recurrent seizures are seen much more frequently than in the general population.

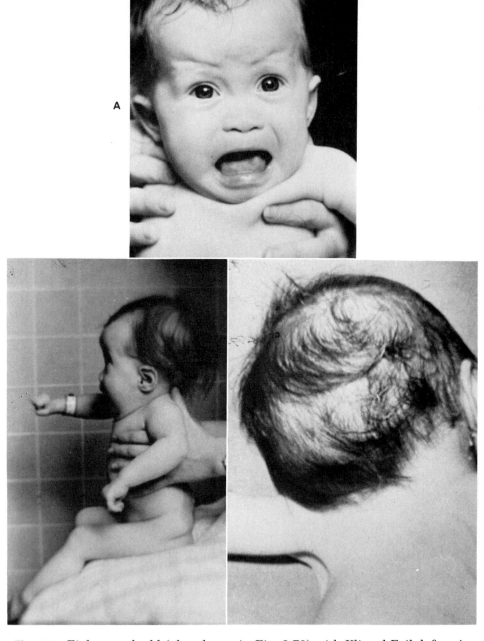

Fig. 7-52. Eight-month-old (also shown in Fig. 6-72) with Klippel-Feil deformity. A, Frontal view showing brachycollis, nasal base hypoplasia, and mild hypotelorism. Observe burying of chin on chest as a result of shortened neck. B, Lateral facial view showing extreme brachycollis and shortening of neck. Other facial features of Klippel-Feil deformity are present as well. C, Posterior view showing asymmetrical osseous deformity of neck.

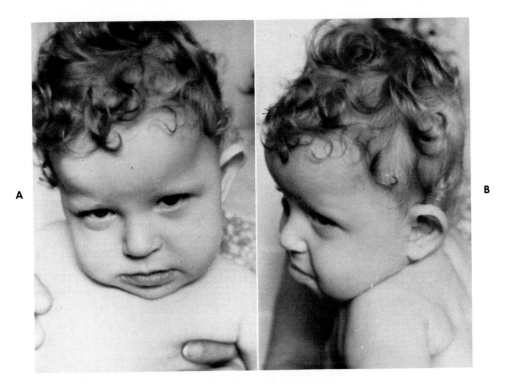

Fig. 7-53. Fifteen-month-old child from a family of patients with hereditary spastic paraplegia. **A,** Frontal view showing shortened neck. Observe burying of chin in chest and positioning of eyeballs. **B,** Lateral view showing shortened neck and secondary facial features related to this defect. Patient also has the Klippel-Feil anomaly.

Technically, the face is not the major site of involvement in cases of the Klippel-Feil anomalad. Still, the face displays typical abnormal features. The head appears to be placed directly on the thorax, both from front and side views (Fig. 7-53). The face is distorted and often asymmetrical. There may be heterotropia and/or nystagmus. Affected patients may have a high-arched or cleft lip and palate and bifid uvula. The mouth is often widened. (See Fig. 7-54, A.)

Turner (1938) described the classic features of the syndrome that bears his name. Several females he examined had short stature, cubitus valgus, pterygium colli or webbed neck, and many signs of sexual infantilism. It was later shown that the disorder is caused by a missing X chromosome. It is now known that there are two types of *Turner's syndrome.* The most common type is caused by a monosomy of the X chromosome. In persons with the second type, there is a full complement of 46 chromosomes, but there is a deletion of one of the short arms of one of the X chromosomes. The cause of the chromosomal defect is unknown, the condition does not appear to be inherited. There is no evidence that maternal age is a factor, as in trisomy 21. The X chromosome

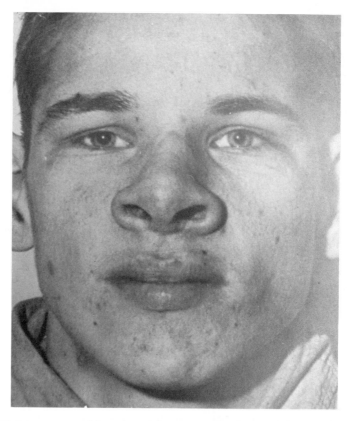

**Fig. 7-54.** Eighteen-year-old male with extremely short neck resulting from the Klippel-Feil deformity. Patient is also mildly mentally retarded and shows classic mirror movements, which sometimes are associated with anomalies at the occipital-cervical junction presumably because of faulty decussation of the pyramidal tract. Observe the brachycollis and the secondary facial features.

in most cases is of maternal origin. The condition is believed to cause about 5% of all spontaneous abortions. Fully 95% of persons with monosomy X form die in utero. Turner's syndrome is said to represent 1 in 2500 female live births.

In both types of the chromosomal disorder, one finds a long list of abnormalities. Besides the primary clinical features of the syndrome, one may find a shield-like chest, wide-spaced nipples, coarctation of the aorta, multiple pigmented nevi, hypoplastic toenails, keloid formation, and renal anomalies. The affected infant often has lymphedema of the hands and feet, which disappears by the second year. Intestinal telangiectasia is sometimes found. The redundant skin of the neck and the characteristic lymphedema at birth allow for early diagnosis, even at birth. Performing a buccal smear is an easy way to confirm the diagnosis. If Turner's syndrome is present, a chromatin-negative pattern will be shown. Pubescent or older patients have elevated gonadotropin levels and depressed 17-ketosteroid levels. Osteoporosis is sometimes observed,

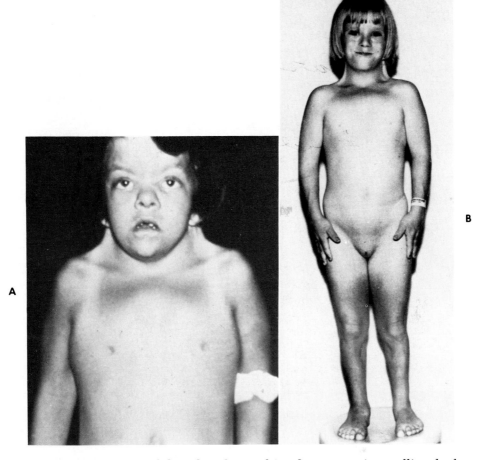

**Fig. 7-55.** Two patients with broad necks resulting from pterygium colli and related to Turner's syndrome or the XO syndrome. A, Fourteen-year-old mildly retarded patient (also shown in Fig. 6-73). Note pronounced pterygium colli and brachycollis. Observe secondary facial stigmata, including mild hypertelorism, downturned mouth, and antimongoloid slanting. Patient also shows typical chest appearance of Turner's syndrome, poorly developed secondary sexual characteristics, and dwarfism. B, Thirteen-year-old girl with Turner's syndrome (also shown in Fig. 6-52). Observe pterygium colli and other somatic and facial features of the syndrome. (B, Courtesy of Dr. Charles Linder, Medical College of Georgia.)

especially of the hands and feet. Study of dermatoglyphic patterns will show greater than average total finger ridge counts. This finding is the opposite of that in individuals with extra X-chromosome material.

The face has characteristic features. In general, it is broad, sometimes being described as heart-shaped (see Fig. 7-55). This shape is due primarily to the pterygium colli. Associated with the webbing is a low hairline on the neck. There may be evidence of premature aging. Various ocular abnormalities may be present, including ptosis, cataract, heterotropia, epicanthal folds, and blue sclera. Color blindness, interestingly, occurs in a high percentage of patients (about 7%). Also related to the

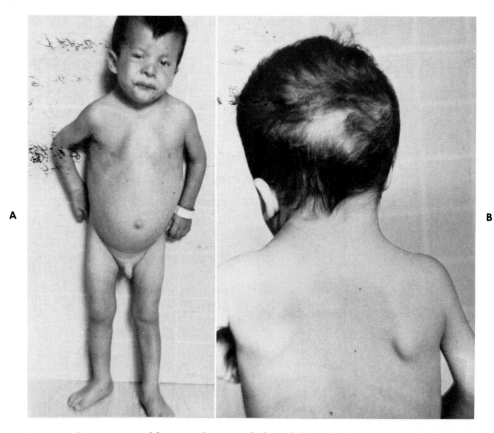

Fig. 7-56. Seven-year-old severely retarded and dwarfed patient with Noonan's syndrome. A, Frontal view showing brachycollis resulting from mild pterygium colli. Observe secondary facial characteristics and ocular hypertelorism. B, Posterior view showing pterygium colli and low posterior hairline. The results of chromosome studies were normal for this patient, who was institutionalized.

pterygium colli are depressed corners of the mouth and high-arched palate. Dental malocclusion occurs frequently. The ears are prominent and often low-set (Horowitz and others, 1976). Micrognathia occurs frequently (Engel and Forbes, 1965; Ferguson-Smith, 1965).

Several patients, both male and female, with a phenotypic resemblance to patients with Turner's syndrome, were reported by Noonan and Ehmke in 1963. These patients, who had normal chromosomes, for a time were said to have "pseudo-Turner's syndrome." The term "male Turner's syndrome" was also used. Such persons are now considered to have a similar, but separate, disorder called *Noonan's syndrome*. In this condition the pterygium colli is not as striking; hypertelorism and more severe degrees of mental retardation predominate. While patients with Turner's syndrome tend to have coarctation of the aorta, those with Noonan's syndrome more commonly have valvular pulmonary stenosis (see Fig. 7-56) Noonan and Ehmke, 1963).

# CHAPTER EIGHT

# Syndromes of the total face

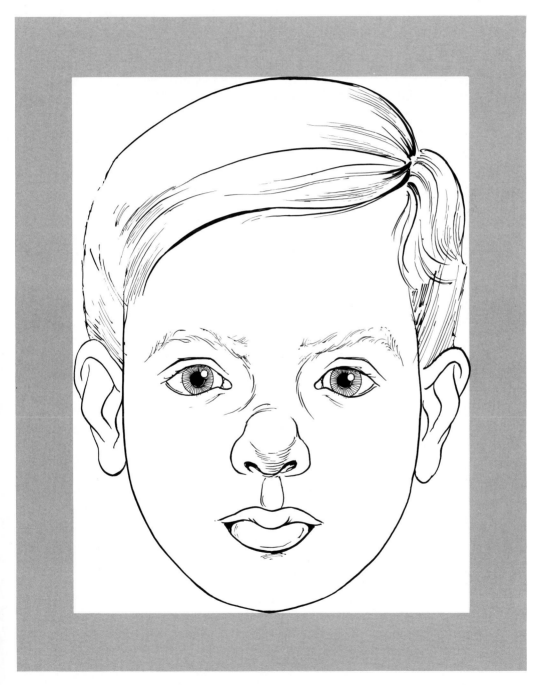

An attempt has been made in previous chapters to classify abnormal facial features by anatomic division. Such a classification is difficult, as witnessed by the fact that many syndromes involve more than one segment. Various major disorders with multisegmental involvement have already been discussed in this book. In addition, the diseases discussed thus far generally involve true, easy-to-define anatomic abnormalities. Yet there are many facial abnormalities that are subtle and that cannot be clearly delineated scientifically or structurally. These more subjective abnormalities may be characterized, for example, by a disturbance in a patient's "expression" rather than simple heterotropia, a bulge in the neck, frontal bossing, or a combination of several multiple-segment abnormalities. These are the vaguest, and in some regards the most interesting, of all of the abnormalities of the face. This final chapter, therefore, not only will reemphasize the important syndromes that involve more than one segment but also will discuss the syndromes that are characterized by abnormalities in general facial expression.

## SYNDROMES OF MULTISEGMENTAL INVOLVEMENT
### Syndromes characterized by abnormalities in total facial contour and size

**Dolichostenofacial syndromes.** The dolichostenofacial syndromes are characterized by an excessively long and narrow face. ("Dolicho" is the stem word meaning "long," and "steno" is the stem word meaning "narrow.") Excessive length and narrowness usually go together, but occasionally each occurs alone. Examples might be *de Lange's syndrome*, which is characterized by short yet extremely narrow facies, and *Zellweger's syndrome*, which typically involves a long yet reasonably wide face. Dolichofacies or dolichostenofacies very often, but not always, is associated with dolichocephaly.

Since *Marfan's syndrome*, which has been discussed briefly in Chapter 6 and Chapter 7, was first described in 1896, many investigators have added additional features, including ectopia lentis and cardiovascular abnormalities. The disease is transmitted as an autosomal dominant trait (Marfan, 1896; McKusick, 1972).

Affected patients characteristically have arachnodactyly, dolichostenomelia, sparse subcutaneous fat, kyphoscoliosis, pes planus, pectus excavatum et carinatum, hyperextensibility of the joints, hernias, muscular hypoplasia and hypotonia, dilation and/or dissection of the aorta, aortic regurgitation, loose mitral valve and mitral regurgitation, and numerous other connective tissue defects. From a neurologic viewpoint, such patients are susceptible to multiple cerebral aneurysms. Genu recurvatum is often present.

Besides dolichostenofacies, facial features include dolichocephaly, high-arched palate, mandibular prognathism, ectopia lentis, iridodonesis, and blue sclera. Severe myopia may be a frequently encountered feature. (See Fig. 8-1.)

Rarely are all the defects, which are basically of mesenchymal origin,

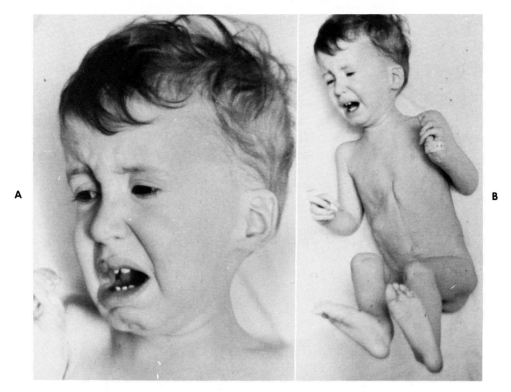

Fig. 8-1. Nine-month-old boy with Marfan's syndrome. **A,** Oblique facial view. Observe dolichstenoofacies, low-set and "jug" ears, long concave nose, high-arched palate, and irritability. **B,** Full-body view. Note long thin soma, dolichostenomelia, long and narrow feet, and arachnodactyly. Patient is of normal psychomotor development and did not have subluxation of the lenses or other ocular findings. (See also Fig. 6-13.)

present together. Because of the major clinical habitus, abnormalities are usually suggested at birth. Slit-lamp examination may reveal the subluxation of the lens, often in an upward and temporal direction, in about 70% of cases. Measurements are helpful: the lower body segment is longer than the upper segment (that is, the distance from pubis to sole is greater than that from pubis to vertex), the arm span is greater than the height, and the longest digit is usually more than twice the length of the longest metacarpal. Marfan's syndrome is one of the best examples of dolichostenofacies as well. The body and extremities are also elongated and narrow or thin. As mentioned before, arachnodactyly, dolichostenomelia, narrow chest with a variety of deformities, and narrow and high-arched hard palates are characteristic dysplastic features of the disease.

In Marfan's syndrome, abnormal collagen contributes to abnormal elastin formation. This biochemical defect accounts for other features seen in the syndrome, namely aortic and cerebral aneurysms.

The closely related *syndrome of congenital contractural arachno-*

*dactyly,* which was probably the correct category for the condition of one of the original patients of Marfan, also is characterized by dolichosteno- facies (Lowry and Eurichon, 1972). Affected patients have ocular prob- lems but usually have miosis rather than frankly dislocated lenses. They have characteristically deformed, "crumpled" auricles. They are tall and have little subcutaneous fat. Other features include arachnodactyly, severe contractures involving the fingers, toes, and other joints, kypho- scoliosis, and chest deformities. The contractures are present at birth. Cardiovascular disease and dislocated optic lenses are not usually present in this syndrome, which is inherited as an autosomal dominant trait. It is highly likely that this syndrome is a variant of Marfan's syn- drome rather than a separate disorder. Reported cases of osteogenesis imperfecta combined with Marfanian features (Epstein and others, 1966) also are probably variants of Marfan's syndrome, as are the dis- orders of patients who have marfanian features and dystrophia myo- tonica (Dyken, 1966).

*Homocystinuria* was initially described by Gerritsen and associates

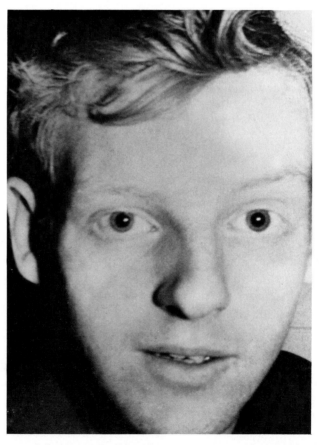

Fig. 8-2. Patient with homocystinuria. This patient was hypopigmented and mild- ly mentally retarded. Observe the mild dolichofacies. He had poor vision, but sub- luxated lenses were not identified as the cause.

(1962) and by Carson and Neill (1962). The enzymatic defect in this disorder, a deficiency or an absence of cystathionine synthetase, was discovered in 1964 (Goodman and Gorlin, 1977, p. 288). The enzyme deficiency produces the characteristic homocystinuria and methionemia. The syndrome is characterized clinically by ectopia lentis (dislocated lens). It is believed that the dislocated lenses are usually displaced downward, as opposed to the situation in Marfan's syndrome, in which there is upward displacment. Myopia, martanian habitus, mental retardation (rare in Marfan's syndrome), hypopigmented and fine hair, erythematous flush in the malar region, irregularly aligned teeth, dolichocephaly, arterial or venous thrombosis, recurrent thrombophlebitis, childhood cerebrovascular accidents, livedo reticularis (mottled skin changes), nervousness, osteoporosis with pathologic fractures, and recurrent epileptogenic seizures are often features of this syndrome. The most striking marfanian feature is dolichostenofacies, although it is usually not as severe as in Marfan's syndrome. (See Figs. 8-2 and 8-3.)

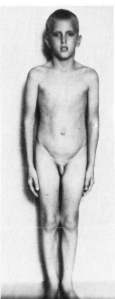

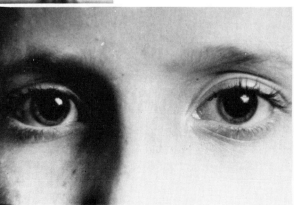

Fig. 8-3. Nine-year-old boy with homocystinuria. A, Full-body view showing no major abnormalities. Patient is hypopigmented and shows borderline mental retardation. B, Close-up view of eyes. The pupils were artificially dilated in an attempt to make the patient's subluxated lenses visible. The lens edges, however, are not appreciated in this photograph.

*Zellweger's syndrome,* or the cerebrohepatorenal syndrome, is characterized by severe neonatal and infantile symptoms. The major signs are severe muscular hypotonia, severe psychomotor retardation, seizures, hepatosplenomegaly, cryptorchidism and hypospadias, congenital heart disease, flexion contractures of the fingers and knees, ulnar deviation of digits, talipes (clubfoot) albuminuria, hyperbilirubinemia, hypoglycemia, high serum iron and iron-binding capacity, and renal cysts. From a facial viewpoint, one sees some features reminiscent of trisomy 21, including brachycephaly, flattened occiput, Brushfield spots, epicanthal folds, mongoloid slant, and low-set ears. The face is long and rectangular but not necessarily narrow. The forehead is broad and flat, the jaws are broad, and the cheeks are puffy. (See Fig. 8-4). There is often ocular hypertelorism, and sometimes there are puffy eyelids, glaucoma, corneal clouding, cataracts, retinopathy, micrognathia, and high-arched and narrow palate. Roentgenograms of the ribs, acetabula, and patellae may show calcified stippling. The mortality rate is very high. Most infants die within the first year of life. Postmortem examination reveals a variety of malformations of the brain, renal cysts, heavy iron deposition in liver, kidney, and bone marrow, and diffuse interstitial fibrosis of the liver. This syndrome is inherited as an autosomal recessive trait. It has been speculated that a defect in energy metabolism resulting from a structural disturbance in mitochondria produces the abnormalities in iron metabolism (Bowen and others, 1964; Dauks and others, 1975; Gilcheist and others, 1975).

*Klinefelter's syndrome,* which is associated with an extra complement of X-chromosome material (that is, XXY), has been discussed elsewhere (see Chapter 7). Although the habitus is more strikingly abnormal than the face in affected patients, there is a tendency toward dolichostenofacies (Becker and others, 1966).

The *N syndrome* of Hess and associates (1974) is characterized by a long and narrow facies as well as dolichocephaly and other features, the most common of which are scalloped upper eyelids and sunken orbits. This disorder is a rare entity that to this juncture has been reported only in two brothers.

The *supernumerary isochrome 18 syndrome,* or +18 pi syndrome, is characterized by a mildly elongated and narrow facies as well as many other facial and somatic abnormalities (Condron and others, 1974).

**Brachyfacial and fat facial syndromes.** The brachyfacial and fat facial syndromes involve excessively wide, broad, round, or flattened facies. The midfacial line, which extends from the vertex point to the mental point, also may be abnormally short.

*Albright's hereditary osteodystrophy* is now the recommended name for the disorders previously called pseudohypoparathyroidism and pseudo-pseudohypoparathyroidism (Albright and others, 1942; Albright and others, 1952). There are, however, slight variations between the two conditions. Pseudohypoparathyroidism involves abnormalities in cal-

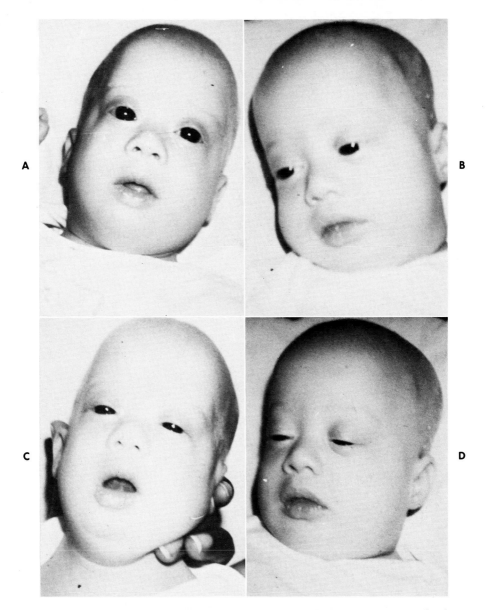

Fig. 8-4. Seven-month-old twin female infants with Zellweger's cerebrohepatorenal syndrome. A, More mildly affected twin. Note dolichofacies. Face is long and rectangular rather than narrow. Observe mild mongoloid slant and other features reminiscent of trisomy 21. B, More severely affected twin. Observe similar facial stigmata. C, First twin several weeks later. D, Second twin several weeks later.

cium and phosphorus blood levels, while pseudo-pseudohypoparathyroidism does not. The two conditions produce similar phenotypes. Females are affected twice as often as males. Affected patients are short, sometimes are obese, and usually have only mild mental retardation. They have osseous disturbances, short nails, subcutaneous and ectopic bone formation, tetany, convulsions, short teeth, excessive dental caries, lenticular opacities, and enamel hypoplasia. The most characteristic feature, however, is a "rounded" facies (Fig 8-5, *A*) that is sometimes accompanied by ptosis. Milder forms involve less pronounced facial and somatic changes (Fig. 8-6). Especially unique, both clinically and roent-

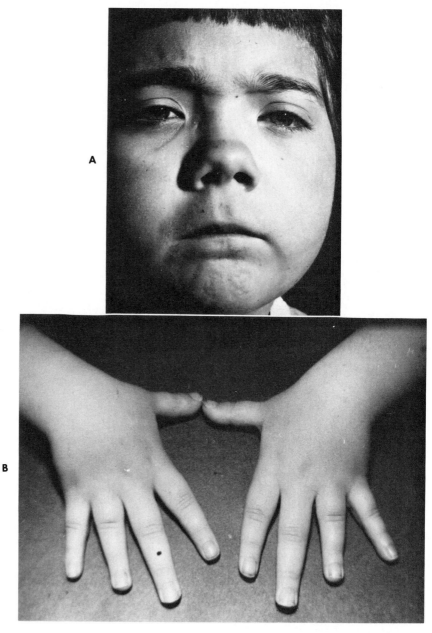

Fig. 8-5. Fifteen-year-old female with Albright's hereditary osteodystrophy (pseudopseudohypoparathyroidism). **A**, Coarse and round facies. **B**, Bilateral hypoplasia of fourth intercarpal bones producing shortening of fourth digits.

genographically, are shortened metacarpal and metatarsal bones of the fourth and fifth digits (Fig. 8-5, *B*). X-ray film also may show soft tissue calcifications and short digits in general. There may be electrocardiographic abnormalities. Infants with this syndrome may develop laryngospasm caused by hypocalcemia.

The basic defect in osteodystrophy is believed to be a deficiency of parathormone-sensitive adenylcyclase in bone and kidney. Therefore, one observes normal secretion of parathormone, but its function at the end organ is deficient.

*Turner's syndrome* must be distinguished from Albright's disease, for it, too, is characterized by brachyfacial contour and occurs more often in females. The distinction is usually easy because Turner's syndrome is associated with pterygium colli and gonadal dysgenesis.

*Prader-Willi syndrome* is characterized less by brachyfacies than by a fat and chubby facies. Nevertheless, the face tends to be more brachyfacial than dolichofacial (see Fig. 8-7). In addition, the forehead is prominent, and microcephaly and bitemporal narrowing tend to be present. This syndrome is also characterized by obesity, hypogonadism, and mental retardation. In the neonatal period severe hypotonia is characteristically present (Prader and others, 1956).

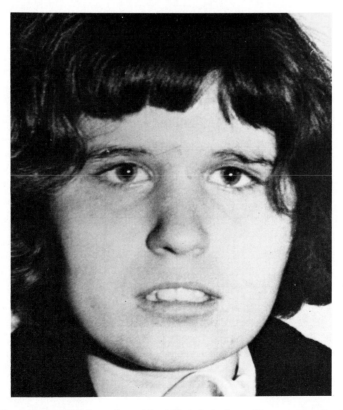

Fig. 8-6. Fifteen-year-old female with Albright's hereditary osteodystrophy. Patient is mildly mentally retarded. Observe round facies.

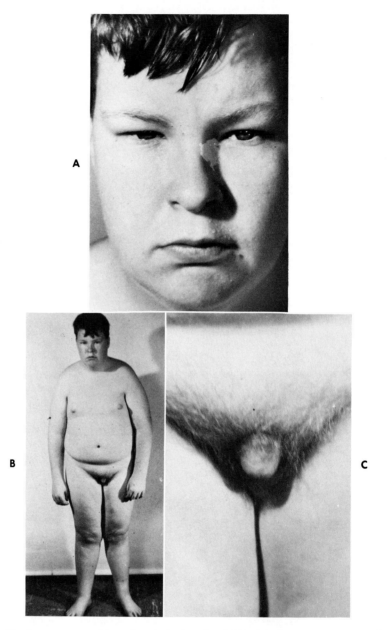

**Fig. 8-7.** Eighteen-year-old male with Prader-Willi syndrome. **A,** Frontal facial view showing fat, rounded facies. Observe dull expression and mild pseudomongoloid slanting related to facial obesity. **B,** Frontal body view showing extreme somatic obesity, small penis and testes, pes planus, and folds of skin on lower abdomen. **C,** Close-up view of genitalia showing female hair distribution and small penis and scrotum.

In the neonatal and infantile periods, hypotonia is by far the most remarkable feature of the disorder. This feature is associated with poor sucking, crying, and swallowing abilities and sometimes with hypothermia. Later, psychomotor retardation becomes more evident. Then, hypogonadism is recognized, with small penile size being most prominent, and obesity develops. There is usually a ravenous appetite with strikingly pathologic polyphagia. As the obesity worsens, it becomes clearer that the penis, hands, and feet are small compared to other body parts. There is progressive atrophy of muscle mass and thickening of skin. The testes may be small and the scrotum atrophic; but these structures are less severely affected than the penis. Cryptorchidism may be present. Females have small labia majora and minora. Adults have sparse axillary and pubic hair, irregular or absent menses, and sparse beard and often have high voices. Occasionally, there is mesobrachyphalangy of the fifth finger, clinodactyly, and/or a simian crease.

The facial features are also distinctive. The face is fat, with the cheeks and the underside of the chin being most prominent. There is a prominent forehead but relative microcephaly, especially in later life. Heterotropias are common. The palpebral fissues are said to be almond shaped, a feature observed early in life even before severe obesity ensues. The palate is high and narrow. The mouth is often held open. There is a triangularly shaped upper lip, but seldom is a full "tented" upper lip—as seen in facial diplegia—present. Micrognathia and dental caries are common, the latter often resulting from defective enamel. Microdontia may be present.

It has been postulated that the Prader-Willi syndrome results from an as-yet-undiscovered hypothalamic defect. In later life especially, the obesity becomes so great that the pickwickian syndrome of hypersomnambulism may develop because of chronic respiratory insufficiency. The clinical characteristics follow a rather stereotypic course from the neonatal period to adult life. An affected newborn is usually a male, although affected females have been reported (Cohen and Gorlin, 1969). The newborn is usually moderately ill and has fairly severe degrees of hypotonia and unresponsiveness. The hypotonia is self-limited and seldom lasts past the second year of life. Obesity is uncommon at birth. In fact, the baby is often underweight. An excessive appetite sometimes develops soon after birth, but weight gain is dramatic regardless of daily caloric intake. The attainment of motor and mental milestones is delayed, sometimes dramatically. In males particularly, hypogonadism is obvious later in childhood. It usually takes the form of smallness of the phallus rather than testicular atrophy. In early and middle childhood hypomentia and obesity become more evident, and by puberty hypogonadism is obvious in both males and females. Mental functioning seldom exceeds the trainable-mentally-retarded level, and more profound levels of mental retardation are common. A variety of studies has noted a disorder of the diencephalon in patients with Prader-Willi syndrome, although no distinct, always-characteristic patterns of dysfunction are seen. Some physicians have preferred to call this syndrome the 4 H syndrome (hypotonia, hypomentia, hyperobesity, and hypogonadism) (Dunn, 1968).

*Fröhlich's syndrome* does not represent a specific disease entity. It was first described in 1901 by Fröhlich, who examined an obese male child with hypogonadism. Later, it was determined that this patient suffered from a suprasellar craniopharyngioma. Hypogonadism is a difficult-to-evaluate finding in persons with obesity. There is, of course, some tendency for optical illusion in severely obese prepubescent male children. Rather than small genitalia, the abnormality in such children may be the excessive folds of fat in the prepubic regions. This fat tends to cover the phallus and testes. It is proper to use Fröhlich's syndrome as a preliminary diagnosis in a fat, hypogonadal youngster, especially if other acute symptoms suggest a central nervous system mass in the suprasellar region. These masses are usually craniopharyngiomas. It is possible that the syndrome also can be produced by diseases other than neoplasms. The round, fat, or chubby face is seldom as severe as that encountered in the Prader-Willi syndrome (Gomez and others, 1975, p. 673).

The *Laurence-Moon-Biedl syndrome* in its complete form is characterized by obesity, polydactyly, retinitis pigmentosa, mental retardation, and hypogonadism (Bisland, 1951). Facial features are not specific for this syndrome, but a chubby, fat, or wide face is usually present.

*Cushing's syndrome,* which is the name given to a characteristic pattern of obesity in association with hypertension, is the result of sustained high levels of serum hydrocortisone. Hypercortisonism may be intrinisic because of adrenal cortical or pituitary hyperfunction, or it may be iatrogenic as a result of corticoid therapy. The condition was first described by the American neurosurgeon Harvey Cushing (1932). Cushing attributed the symptoms to a basophilic adenoma of the pituitary gland. It was later assumed that adrenocorticotropin generated the hypercorticism. It is now believed that the syndrome almost always results from the iatrogenic effects of heavy use of corticoids, from adrenal hyperplasia, or from adrenal functioning tumors. The exogenous form of this disorder may be referred to as the *"Cushingoid" syndrome.* In Cushing's syndrome, there is the characteristic somatic form of obesity with "buffalo hump," but there is relatively little fat on the limbs. Other stigmata include stunted growth, plethoric skin, oily and erupted skin, purple cutaneous stria, hypertrichosis, listlessness, apathy, and mental dullness. Affected persons have a characteristic accumulation of fat on the cheeks and chin. The cheeks tend to be reddened, and acne may develop even in young children. Hypertrichosis of the face may occur. The 6-year-old youngster in Fig. 8-8 suffered from dermatomyositis and required large doses of alternate-day corticosteroids to allow continued remissions of his severe muscular symptoms. He had been receiving

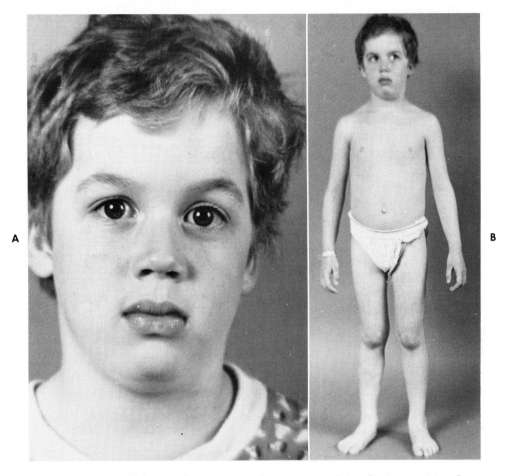

**Fig. 8-8.** Six-year-old boy with recurrent dermatomyositis who is receiving large doses of glucocorticoids. **A,** Facial view showing facial obesity and edema secondary to hypercorticoidism (Cushingoid facies). Observe mild erythema over malar region, which is possibly related to the dermatomyositis. **B,** Full-body view showing abdominal distribution of obesity, mild anterior tilt to the pelvis, and pes planus. Musculature is actually quite deficient in bulk.

steroids for well over a year when the photograph was taken. Fig 8-8, *A* shows the rounded, edematous appearance to the face and the particular puffiness of the cheeks. In addition, there is a plethoric appearance to the malar region. The facial expression, however, is alert and inquisitive. Fig. 8-8, *B* shows some of the somatic stigmata of both the corticosteroid effect and the muscular problem. The patient shows a mildly protuberant abdomen because of paraspinal and pelvic muscle weakness. The youngster's natural facial and somatic habitus was asthenic.

The *cri-du-chat syndrome* (cat's-cry or 5 p− syndrome) is characterized by hypertelorism (see Figs. 6-53 and 6-54). In addition, affected patients have a round, broad facies that is particularly evident in infancy.

There are other unique facial and somatic abnormalities in this syndrome, which has been discussed in Chapter 6 (Lejeune, 1963).

The *fetal face syndrome* involves a characteristic broad, flattened face that resembles that of a fetus of 8 weeks' gestation (see Chapter 1). Persons with this syndrome have relative hypertelorism, a disproportionately large cranium, frontal bossing, S-shaped lower lids, a short and upturned nose, a triangularly shaped mouth with downturned corners, short stature, mesomelic brachymelia, stubby hands, vertebral abnormalities, rib defects, and hypoplastic genitalia (Robinson, 1969).

**Coarse facial syndromes.** Both the syndromes that will be discussed in this section have been described in greater detail elsewhere in this book. *De Lange's syndrome,* or the *Brachmann-De Lange syndrome,* has been discussed in Chapter 6. This very distinctive syndrome is easily recognized because of many facial and somatic abnormalities. The "pinched" quality of the face, which is particularly evident in the middle face, accounts in part for the midline eyebrow so characteristic of this syndrome. The midline eyebrow is, however, only one of the facial features whose presence leads to the diagnosis of the syndrome. The face in De Lange's syndrome is small, even when the microcephaly and the dwarfed body, which are also typical of this syndrome, are taken into account. Usually there is a short yet narrow face. The second most distinctive facial feature is a coarseness. A third distinctive feature is excessive facial hair.

The *mucopolysaccharidoses* are a group of diseases characterized by an abnormal excretion of mucopolysaccharides in the urine and by abnormal deposits of glycolipids in various tissues of the body, including the brain. The first of the mucopolysaccharide syndromes was described by Hunter (1917). Hurler (1919) described a more severe variation, and Sanfilippo (1963) described yet another variation. McKusick (1972) was able to classify the mucopolysaccharidoses into six main types. Since this classification, many new variations have been discovered (McKusick, 1975). For the purpose of this chapter, however, only three of the mucopolysaccharide syndromes will be emphasized. Each is reasonably common, involves abnormal facial features, and has neurologic implications.

*Hunter's syndrome* (MPS IIA and IIB) is characterized by a sex-linked type of inheritance. Affected males often are born with abnormal facial stigmata that are more striking than the macrocephaly that is also present. The facial features are coarse and somewhat grotesque, but the stigmata are not as extensive as in *Hurler's syndrome* (MPS IH, IS, IH/S), which is a more severe, autosomal dominant condition. Superciliary hyperplasia, extensive eyebrow formation, hirsutism, thickened skin (often with patches that resemble on orange peel), and large ears (especially the earlobes) are prominent facial features, in addition to a rather severe macrocephaly that usually results from a true megalencephaly (see Fig. 8-9). Rarely, hydrocephalus has also been reported in both Hunter's and Hurler's syndromes. The megalencephaly results

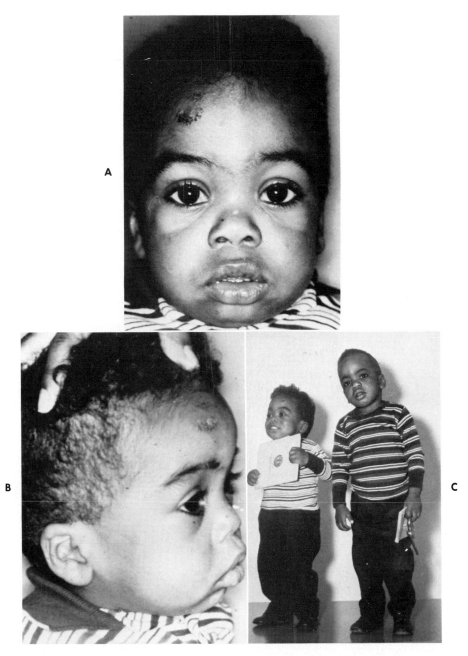

Fig. 8-9. Brothers with Hunter's syndrome (MPS IIA). **A,** Frontal facial view of 2½-year-old with milder stigmata of this disorder. Observe coarse features, including thick lips, midline brow, superciliary hyperplasia, broad nose, and large lobules. **B,** Lateral facial view of same patient. **C,** Better appreciation of disorder is obtained by comparing face of younger brother to that of older brother who is also shown in Fig. 6-92, *A.* Both brothers have somatic as well as facial stigmata of the syndrome.

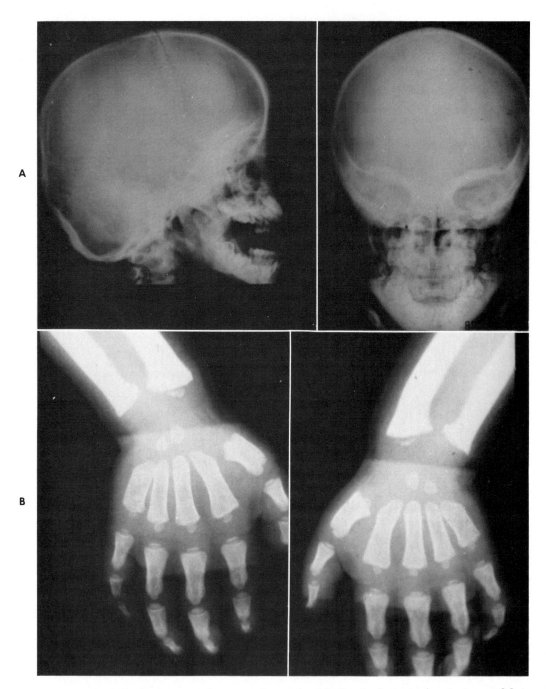

Fig. 8-10. Hurler's type of mucopolysaccharidosis. A, Anterior/posterior and lateral skull roentgenograms showing hyperostosis of roofs of orbits and base of skull and J-shaped sellae. B, Hand roentgenograms showing ulnar deviation, abnormal tilt of terminal ends of both radius and ulna so that they face each other, and hyperostosis.

from deposits of glycolipids in neurons and glia. Such deposits also accumulate in interstitial sites and, to a lesser degree, in intracranial nonneural tissue.

Hunter's and Hurler's syndromes are quire similar clinically even though they may be separate biochemically and genetically. The extent of the clinical features differs, however, in the two diseases. Hunter's syndrome seldom is associated with corneal opacity, whereas Hurler's syndrome is. The syndromes are different in systemic manifestations as well. Hurler's disease usually is characterized by more extensive cardiac involvement and more somatic bony deformity (Fig. 8-10). These features decrease the life expectancy of persons affected with Hurler's syndrome. Mild variations of Hunter's syndrome (MPS IIB) may not be associated at all with mental retardation, but retardation of mild to moderate degree usually is present. Profound mental retardation is usually seen in Hurler's disease.

*Sanfilippo's syndrome* represents another disease in this complex of separate diseases with common characteristics. This disorder, which is one of the more recently described diseases in this group, is characterized by an almost totally neurologic presentation. Although affected infants might appear reasonably normal for several years, subtle facial and somatic stigmata suggesting the mucopolysaccharidoses are evident early in life. In late infancy or early childhood, developmental standstill becomes evident and tends to develop into frank deterioration as time continues. The general neurologic functioning of affected individuals may decline over several years, and they finally die, usually in the second or third decade of life. The facial appearance, therefore, changes in Sanfilippo's disease (see Fig. 8-11). Neurologic deterioration and facial change also may occur, to a lesser degree, in the other variations of the mucopolysaccharidoses.

The entire group of *mucopolysaccharidoses*, as well as the *mucolipidoses, fucosidosis,* and *mannosidosis,* are characterized by coarse facial features, with Hurler's, Hunter's, and Sanfilippo's varieties involving the most severe coarseness (see Fig. 8-12). These facial abnormalities include—in addition to the features already discussed in Chapters 6 and 7 under sections on hypertelorism—defects of the ears, the lips, and the mouth and tongue, as well as a considerable number of features that cross facial segments, such as facial hirsutism. The cranioface is large in comparison to the cranioface of De Lange's syndrome. One may observe a superciliary hyperplasia with predominant eyebrows that sometimes meet in the midline, thickened facial skin, and a general largeness of facial features to the point of grotesqueness in the more severe forms of mucopolysaccharidosis. The craniofacial deformity is contributed to by excessive ossification of the superciliary bony structures and the base of the skull (Fig. 8-10, *A*). This ossification is similar to the processes that occur in the hands (Fig. 8-10, *B*). *Sanfilippo's syndrome* shows prominent neurologic symptoms with severe deteriorating mental retardation

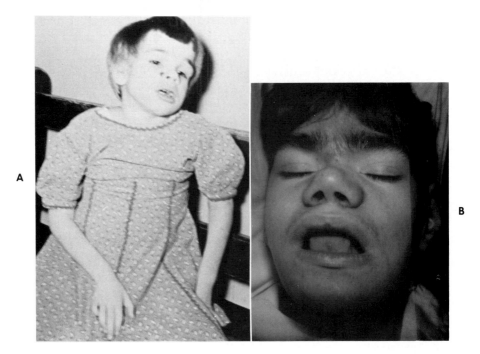

Fig. 8-11. Two patients with Sanfilippo's type of mucopolysaccharidosis (MPS III). A, Twelve-year-old patient with coarse facial features. Observe ulnar deviation of hands and atrophy of radial surface. Ear lobules are not as large as in MPS IIA. B, Eighteen-year-old with extreme facial coarseness similar to that of previous patient.

but without as severe facial segmental abnormalities. Coarse facial features without prominent facial abnormalities in a severely retarded, neurologically deteriorating child or young adult is an especially important diagnostic clue to the mucopolysaccharidoses, with the exceptions pointed out in Fig. 8-12, A and B.

Similarly, mild facial features may be the only clue to the diagnosis on clinical grounds of the probably related diseases now usually designated the mucolipidoses. At least three and possibly five or more of these disorders are now identified. These diseases, plus the disorders called fucosidosis and mannosidosis, another group of diseases now called the sialase deficiencies, and the types of generalized gangliosidoses characterized by GM$_1$ ganglioside accumulation, all show mildly coarse facial appearances that vaguely resemble the more severe facial coarseness seen in the classic mucopolysaccharidoses (Swaiman and Wright, 1975, p. 359).

### Syndromes characterized by facial emaciation and aging

Several neurologic syndromes are characterized by craniofacial changes that suggest malnutrition and/or aging. Yet the affected pa-

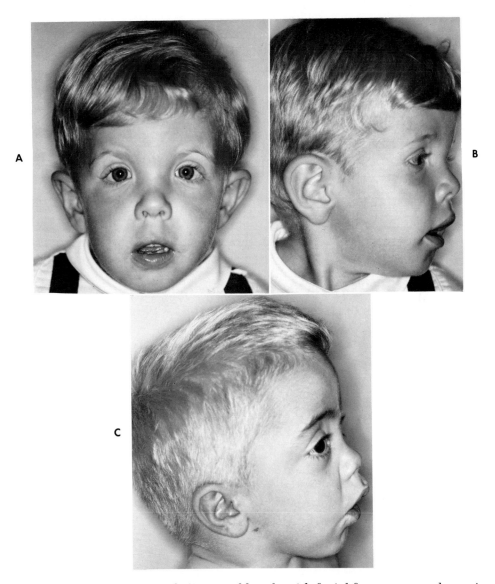

Fig. 8-12. A, Frontal view of 2½-year-old male with facial features vaguely reminiscent of the mucopolysaccharidoses. This patient showed transient excretion of
urinary mucopolysaccharides. It was later determined, however, that no abnormal mucopolysaccharides had been excreted in the urine. This youngster was
considered to have pseudomucopolysaccharidosis, which is a variation of normal. Observe the slightly coarse facial features including mildly broad nose,
mildly thick lips, slightly large ear lobules, and mild superciliary hyperplasia. B,
Lateral view of same patient. C, Lateral view of patient in Fig. 5-40, who has
proved MPS IIB. Note the characteristic facial appearance of even the milder
forms of mucopolysaccharidosis.

tients may be quite young and taking the usual nutritional requirements for their ages and cultures. It is convenient to break these syndromes down into (1) those in which the features of emaciation predominate and (2) those in which the features of premature aging predominate.

**Facial emaciation syndromes.** A relatively common disorder in pediatric neurologic practice is the so-called *diencephalic syndrome* (Russell, 1951). This syndrome is inexactly named, for it usually results from an infiltrating glioma of the anterior hypoalamus that originates in the optic nerve. The association of this syndrome with neurofibromatosis in infancy is common. Affected infants or young children with lesions at this anatomic site may have disturbances in nutrition, vision, and emotional reactions but have few other neurologic signs of an expanding mass lesion. The lack of specific neurologic deficits, which characterize other brain tumors, results from this lesion's histologic character and its location in the the hypothalamus. Affected infants show, on occasion, profound generalized emaciation, sometimes following a brief growth spurt, despite normal or ravenous appetite and adequate or even extraordinary caloric intake (Fig. 8-13). Yet such an infant tends to remain seemingly cheerful, if not euphoric. Hyperactivity can occur. Abnormal eye movements, such as nystagmus or simple jittery eye, are seen, along with occasional poor vision. The diagnosis may be suggested purely on the basis of the characteristic facial appearance. The facies shows features of emaciation combined with a relatively cheerful and unconcerned expression (Addy and Hudson, 1972). (See Fig. 8-13). Both isotope brain scan and contrast and air encephalography show a neoplastic mass originating in the optic nerve and extending into the anterior hypothalamus.

*Cockayne's syndrome* is now believed to be a sudanophilic leukodystrophy. This latest view is based upon findings of patchy demyelination in the central nervous system of affected individuals. Cockayne's syndrome was first described in 1936 (Cockayne, 1936). Severe neurologic symptoms and signs are present. Affected children usually have severe mental retardation, ataxia, intention tremor, peripheral neuropathy, optic atrophy, primary retinal degeneration, nystagmus, and sensorineural deafness. Such individuals have short stature with poor muscular development, disproportionately long limbs with large feet and hands, kyphoscoliosis, increased anterior-posterior diameter of the chest, flexion contractures, cryptorchidism, and photosensitive skin. Facial features include microcephaly, slender noses, cataracts, prominent ears, carious teeth, and narrow palate. The most striking facial feature, however, is an emaciated, senile, and "pinched" appearance resulting from loss of facial subcutaneous tissue, sunken eyes, and sparse hair. Sometimes the hair shows premature graying. The symptoms of neurologic degeneration begin in the first to second year of life. Death usually occurs in late childhood to early adulthood. There is an autosomal recessive inheritance with predilection for males (Moosa and Dubowitz, 1970; Paddison and others, 1963).

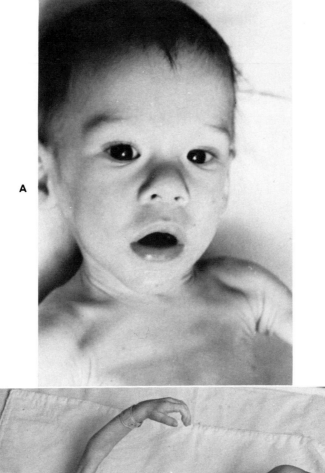

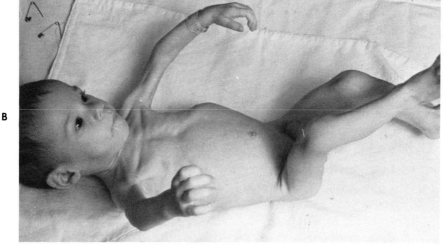

Fig. 8-13. Six-month-old male with the diencephalic syndrome caused by a posteriorly infiltrating optic glioma. A, Facial view showing unconcerned expression and wasting of subcutaneous tissue. Observe subcutaneous atrophy around shoulders and upper trunk as well. B, Full-body view showing extensive emaciation, which was present in spite of high caloric intake.

*Continued.*

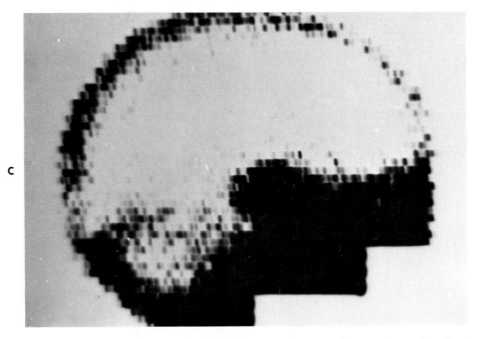

Fig. 8-13, cont'd. C, Lateral cranial isotope scan showing abnormal uptake of technetium in a neoplasm of the anterior hypothalamus.

We studied a possible variant of Cockayne's syndrome. The youngster in Fig. 8-14 was 7 years old when first examined for gradually progressive loss of intellectual functioning. He was not dwarfed and was considered to be reasonably normal intellectually and in all other ways until he was about 3 years old. Associated with intellectual decline was gradual generalized wasting of the musculature and subcutaneous tissue but without specific paresis or selectivity to skeletal muscle. This wasting bore no relationship to caloric intake. He slowly became more uncoordinated but had no specific neurologic abnormalities suggesting either proprioceptive, cerebellar, or peripheral nerve dysfunction. The reflexes were slightly depressed throughout. Vision and hearing were intact. He had a dull facial expression, facial emaciation, a small nose with anteverted nostrils, large ears, normal cranial hair, and slight facial hirsutism. Somatic hirsutism was also observed. Extensive endocrinologic studies were performed, and the results were normal. Air and contrast encephalography (Fig. 8-14, C) showed a slightly dilated anterior projection of the third ventricle but no other abnormalities and certainly no evidence of a mass lesion. The patient's condition was followed for 1½ years, during which time he continued to slowly lose mental abilities. When we last saw him, he still had no specific neurologic abnormalities but had continued to lose weight for unexplained reasons. He was judged to be at a low-trainable level of mental deficiency, which was

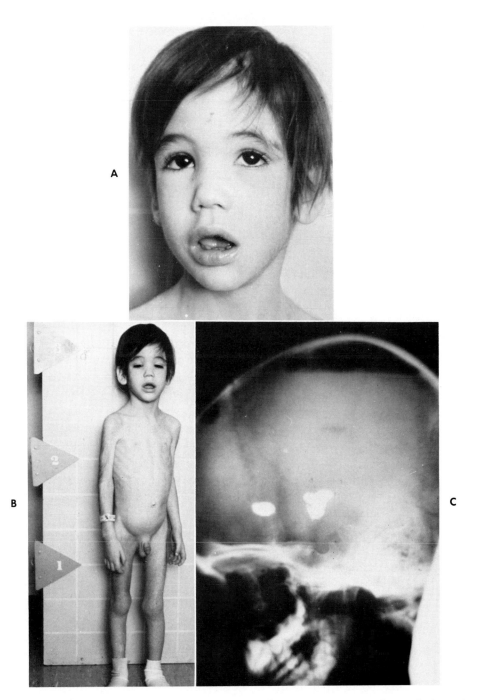

Fig. 8-14. Eight-year-old patient with a dementia-emaciation syndrome believed to be similar to Cockayne's syndrome. A, Facial view showing dull expression, subcutaneous atrophy, and hirsutism. B, Full-body view showing marked, generalized subcutaneous atrophy. C, Encephalography with opaque dye instilled into ventricles. Air has been artificially injected inadvertently into subdural space. Observe contrast material outlining the anterior third ventricle, which is slightly dilated, and the inferior frontal horn, which is of normal size.

considerably lower than when he was first seen. His condition was considered to be a variant of Cockayne's syndrome.

*Donohue's syndrome* or leprechaunism waa first described in 1948 (Donohue, 1948). The syndrome was originally described in a child with an elfin-like face, hirsutism, and multiple endocrine abnormalities, Later, the resemblance to the classic Irish leprechaun was alluded to because of the early development of aging characteristics overlying the elfin-like face. Affected infants show mental and motor retardation, low birth weight, and some signs of sexual precocity. Occasional cryptorchidism may occur, however. One sees severe muscle and subcutaneous wasting with redundant folds of skin, particularly about the distal extremities. Progressive marasmus occurs, showing itself in the face as well as over the entire body. Microcephaly is common. The face is more grotesque than elfin-like. There is hypertelorism with prominent eyes. The ears are low-set and large. The nose is broad at the tip with flaring nostrils and flattened nasal base. The mouth is wide and the lips are thick. The appearance of emaciation, however, is the most outstanding of all the facial abnormalities. There are similarities between Donohue's syndrome and congenital lipodystrophy. Persons with leprechaunism have low fasting blood sugar levels, prolonged responses to insulin, and sometimes hyperinsulinemia. Electron microscopic studies of the liver have shown a large number of intracellular microfilaments in pericanalicular areas (Donohue and Uchida, 1954). The basic defect in Donohue's syndrome may be abnormal adipose tissue.

*Congenital lipodystrophy*, or Lawrence-Berardinelli syndrome, is characterized by a congenital absence of all subcutaneous fat. The absence of facial fat produces a characteristic gaunt, emaciated appearance. There may be similarities to the clinical features of Donohue's syndrome, as well as to those of Cockayne's syndrome (Berardinelli, 1954; Senior and Gellis, 1964).

The *N syndrome* has been discussed in the section on abnormally dolichofacial contours on p. 364. Persons with this rare syndrome have a somewhat emaciated appearance with sunken eyes and thin facies (Hess and others, 1974).

**Facial aging syndromes.** There is a host of uncommon syndromes characterized by facial features suggesting premature aging. These disorders are sometimes difficult to separate from the group of syndromes discussed in the preceding section on emaciation. The best example is the *Hutchinson-Gilford syndrome* or progeria. Jonathan Hutchinson (1886) first described the syndrome in an article entitled "Congenital Absence of Hair and Mammary Glands." Eleven years later, Gilford presented a second case and coined the term progeria, which comes from the Greek word meaning "prematurely old" (Goodman and Gorlin, 1977). The classic features of this syndrome are usually present in the first year of life and include cachectic dwarfism with stooped posture, atrophic inelastic skin, absence of subcutaneous fat, atrophic and furrowed

nails, redundant and wrinkled skin (over the hands especially), protuberant abdomen, poorly developed muscles, joint enlargement with
some limitation of movement, other orthopedic deformities, and poor
sexual development at puberty. The cranioface may be disproportionate
with a relatively large cranium and a small facies. The eyes are prominent. The nose is narrow and may be beak-like, and the palate is narrow.
The most striking feature, however, is the aged, senile facial appearance
with thin skin and paper-thin wrinkles. The hair is sparse and prematurely gray. Loss of eyebrows and eyelashes is common in later life.
Premature arteriosclerosis is present regularly, and death usually occurs
in the second decade of life, with coronary heart disease found frequently
to be the cause. Although mental retardation is not usually present, this
disease is considered of importance to the pediatric neurologist because
of the rare presence of typical neurologic complications of the aged, including stroke, hypertensive cerebral changes, and so on.

The patient in Fig. 8-15 has a facial and somatic aging syndrome, yet

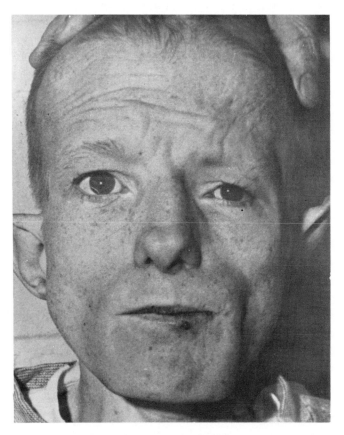

**Fig. 8-15.** Eighteen-year-old severely dwarfed patient with severe mental retardation and signs of excessive aging. This patient had many features suggesting
that he suffered from a form of progeria.

it is difficult to classify this condition as any one of the full syndromes listed before. This patient, who looked at least 40 years old, was 16½ years of age when he was first seen. At that time, he had been in a state hospital for the mentally retarded for at least 5 years. His mental level was judged to be in the range of profound mental retardation, which was approximately what it was when he was first hospitalized. The first records note that, even at 10 or 11 years of age, he appeared to be prematurely old. He was considered small but not dwarfed, with his height being slightly more than 5 feet. Facial emaciation was quite extensive, but more striking were the extensive, fine wrinkles of the skin and the flecks of what appeared to be senile keratosis over the face and arms especially. The nose was long but not necessarily beak-like. The ears were deformed. Cranial and body hair were sparse. The results of neurologic examination were unremarkable, except for some mild hyperreflexia. Further personal historical information prior to his hospitalization had not been obtained, and a full family pedigree could not be developed. At the time of a short follow-up examination, it was reported that the patient had had intermittent episodes of hypertension. He is considered to have a variant of the Hutchinson-Gilford syndrome.

In 1902 Gilford described another rare disorder, which was characterized by mild features of premature aging and dwarfism with normal body proportions (Gilford, 1902). These conditions have now come to be called *pituitary dwarfism.* There are three types now distinguished. *Type I* or primordial dwarfism is due to isolated growth hormone deficiency. *Type II* or Laron's type involves an excessive level of growth hormone, and *Type III* or panhypopituitarism, which is of autosomal recessive inheritance, is similar to nongenetically controlled panhypopituitarism (Goodman and Gorlin, 1977). In type III pituitary dwarfism, all anterior pituitary hormones are deficient. Persons with pituitary dwarfism, type I, have smooth skin, but as aging ensues premature and excessive facial wrinkling occurs (Laron, 1974; Rimoin and others, 1966).

The *Rothmund-Thomson syndrome* is characterized by short stature, poikiloderma atrophicans, cataract, multiple bony abnormalities, and saddle-shaped nose. The cutaneous lesions closely resemble other dermatologic syndromes. The facies can be easily distinguished from that of progeria (Kirkham and Werner, 1975).

*Werner's syndrome* is characterized by balding and premature graying of cranial hair. There is a scleroderma-like facial skin change resulting in an appearance of premature aging. Affected individuals have a beaked nose, juvenile cataract, retinitis pigmentosa, macular degeneration, short stature, mild mental retardation, sexual immaturity, subcutaneous calcification, osteoporosis, premature arteriosclerosis, and mild neurologic defects (Epstein and others, 1966).

*Montreal-type dwarfism* was described by Fitch and associates (1970) as a form of bird-headed dwarfism with features of premature senility. Affected patients appear to have facial and somatic features similar to those found in Seckle's bird-headed dwarfism but in addition show premature aging features, including adult male baldness patterns.

*Gerodermia osteodysplastica hereditaria, or the wrinkly skin syndrome,* is a rare syndrome that has thus far been seen only in the members of one Swiss family. The condition involves short stature, various osseous abnormalities, and a variety of other dysmorphic features, including muscular hypotonia and paresis resembling those found in some of the benign congenital myopathies. Affected patients have characteristic facial features that, besides signs of premature aging, include large sagging cheeks, microcornea, myopia, keratoconus, micrognathia, and dental anomalies (Gazit and others, 1973).

*Turner's syndrome* has been discussed in more detail elsewhere (see Chapters 6 and 7). In addition to more pronounced facial abnormalities, the facial features of premature aging are reported to be associated with this syndrome.

The *Potter facies,* which is seen in neonatal infants, is characterized by redundant and wrinkled skin, giving an aged facial appearance. In addition, one may see hypertelorism, a prominent fold at the inner canthus extending below the eye, a flattened nasal tip, micrognathia, and low-set, posteriorly rotated, large ears with deficient cartilage. (See Fig. 6-66.) This face also has an appearance that suggests emaciation. The Potter facies, when associated with bilateral renal agensis or dysgenosis, has been referred to as *Potter's syndrome* by some authors (Cain and others, 1974).

## Syndromes characterized by diffuse cutaneous pigmentary lesions

Discussed in this section are prototypes of disorders characterized by diffuse changes in skin pigmentation, including syndromes both of hypopigmentation and of hyperpigmentation.

**Diffuse hypopigmentation syndromes.** *Oculocutaneous albinism* has been known for many years and was originally differentiated in modern medical terms in blacks and American Indians. As early as 1904, the enzymatic defect causing this condition was known (Goodman and Gorlin, 1977). It has now been shown that two biochemically and genetically distinct forms of oculocutaneous albinism exist. These are the tyrosinase-positive and the tyrosinase-negative types. Albinism means "condition of whiteness." As a sign or symptom it may be seen in many disorders (1) as a universal defect (such as in the oculocutaneous forms), (2) as a partial defect (such as in albinism associated with a white lock of forehead hair, as seen in Waardenburg's syndrome), or (3) as a diffuse but localized phenomenon (as in ocular albinism, which does not have cutaneous stigmata). Both types of oculocutaneous albinism, as well as ocular albinism, may be associated with poor vision and photophobia (due to retinal hypopigmentation). There is, additionally, a wide range of other ocular defects in albinism, including heterotropia, nystagmus (often of an ocular or pendular type), refractive errors, coloboma of the iris, congenital pupillary membranes, partial aniridia, and capsular cataract. The exposed skin in oculocutaneous albinism is often erythematous, wrinkled, or folded—especially on the face, neck, and hands. The tyrosinase-negative type is characterized by milk-white hair, pink to reddish skin color, and light gray to blue irises with no pigment flecks and a prominent red reflex. Very rarely, affected persons also have freckles and pigmented nevi. The tyrosinase-positive type is more common in blacks and dark-complexioned persons. The hair becomes yellow, golden, red, or brown with age. The irides are blue to brown and have flecks of pigment especially on the pupillary border. The red reflex is usually absent. Freckles and pigmented nevi are common. Deaf-mutism, polydactyly, mental retardation, and epilepsy are seen in a high percentage of patients with both types of albinism. Affected persons typically "squint" in an effort to shelter the eyes from light. The disorder often involves a dull facial expression that is related to associated mental slowness.

*Phenylketonuria* is associated with diffuse hypopigmentation of skin and other tissue due to the relative deficiency of tyrosine and the competitive inhibition of tyrosine by hyperphenylalanine. This metabolic defect results from a deficiency in phenylalanine hydroxylase, which causes phenylalnine to be catabolized to tyrosine, which is essential for melanin metabolism. Patients with phenylketonuria are seldom as severely hypopigmented as patients with albinism, yet the hypopigmentation may be severe. In blacks especially, phyenylketonuria may be confused with the tyrosinase-positive form of albinism. (See Fig. 8-16.) In classic untreated phenylketonuria, there usually is profound mental retardation. In a few atypical cases, no mental deficiency is observed (Crome, 1962; Jervis, 1937).

*Cross' syndrome* is a very rare disorder, first described in 1967, that is characterized by gingival fibromatosis, microphthalmia, oligophrenia, athetosis, spasticity, and moderately severe hypopigmentation of the skin over the face and body. Signs and symptoms occur in infancy. The severe neurologic handicap and the near-blindness that characterize this condition allow for easy differentiation from similar syndromes. Hair bulb tests show a reduced number of melanocytes, and tests for levels of tyrosinase have weakly positive results (Cross and McKusick, 1967). (See Chapters 6 and 7.)

The *Tuomaala-Haapanen syndrome* is characterized by brachymetapody (abnormal shortness of metacarpal or metatarsal bones), anodontia, hypotrichosis, and albinoid traits. The skin of the face and soma is albinoid. There may be esotropia, double rows of eyelashes, myopia, hypoplastic tarsus, ocular nystagmus, and hypoplastic mandibles. There is hypotrichosis of the head, face, and body and severe shortening of all digits except the thumbs and halluces. There is shortened stature (Tuomaala and Haapanen, 1968).

**Diffuse hyperpigmentation syndromes.** Many syndromes are characterized not by hypopigmentation, as in albinism, but by diffuse hyperpigmentation. The types of hyperpigmentation that are related to medical

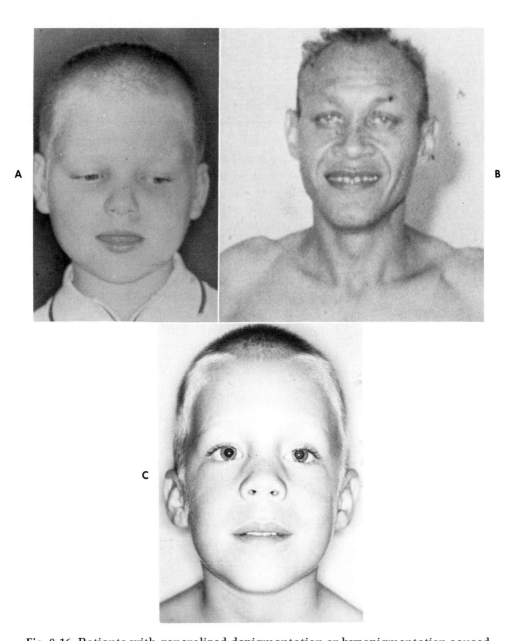

Fig. 8-16. Patients with generalized depigmentation or hypopigmentation caused by disturbances in phenylalanine metabolism. A, Five-year-old twin brother of patient in Fig. 5-52, A. Observe dull facies and generalized hypopigmentation. Patient had clinically and biochemically typical phenylketonuria. B, Thirty-five–year–old black patient considered to have oculocutaneous (tyrosinase-positive) albinism until urinary studies showed excessive quantities of phenylacetic and phenylpyruvic acid and hyperphenylalaninemia was demonstrated. Patient was moderately mentally retarded but showed biochemically typical phenylketonuria. C, Eight-year-old normal child with phenylketonuria that was atypical in that he had all the biochemical stigmata of PKU but no clinical stigmata except for universal hypopigmentation. He was never treated for PKU during the period in which his case was followed. It was later reported that another physician had placed him on a phenylalanine-restricted diet and that, after 8 years on this diet, the patient continued to be normal mentally, behaviorally, and neurologically. Two siblings had similar clinical pictures.

syndromes are varied. Included are (1) a bronzed type such as that associated with *Addison's disease* (Fig. 8-17); (2) a slate-gray type, as is characteristic of *hemochromatosis;* and (3) a diffuse bluish-gray type, as is typical of chronic silver ingestion (argentosis). The bronzed type of hyperpigmentation is the only type related specifically to neurologic diseases (which will be discussed later in this chapter). The entire concept of the *leukodystrophies* has been a subject of interest to neurologists for some time, but it is a subject whose nosology is still quite confused. Leukodystrophy refers to a classification and not a disease. The term is used to refer to a group of specific diseases, all of which are characterized by a deterioration of central nervous system white matter. The reasons for this loss of myelin are unknown, but most of the diseases in this group are presumed to result from genetic defects. The use of the term leukodystrophy therefore infers the exclusion of diseases of sporadic demyelination, such as those due to infections or to autoimmune reactions, as is presumed to be the basis of multiple sclerosis (Swaiman and Wright, 1975, p. 117). Some investigators do not adhere to these strict definitions, unfortunately. The great Schilder himself described what he considered to be three separate diseases (Schilder, 1912; 1913; 1924), only two of which are now thought to be examples of leukodystrophy

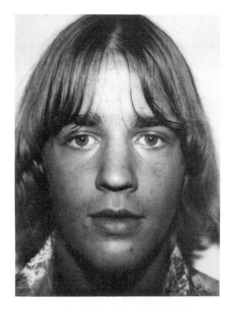

Fig. 8-17. Seventeen-year-old patient with laboratory findings of Addison's disease. This patient had long-term behavioral symptoms and showed nonspecific neurologic signs but displayed no definite symptoms of neurologic deterioration. Note alert facial expression and diffuse bronzing type of hyperpigmentation. He was believed to have a forme fruste of adrenoleukodystrophy, since a brother had the more classical form of that disease.

(Poser and Van Bogaert, 1958). These diseases, now believed to be examples of adrenoleukodystrophy, metachromatic leukodystrophy, and subacute sclerosing panencephalitis, respectively, are even now often erroneously called "Schilder's disease," as if they were variations of the same disease process. They are not. Since the original descriptions and subsequent reports of "Schilder's disease," it has been shown that *subacute sclerosing panencephalitis* is in fact caused by a measles-like virus and the host's reaction to it and therefore is not technically a leukodystrophy. It is now accepted that *metachromatic leukodystrophy* is an autosomal recessive inherited disease that results from an absence of, or a deficiency in, arylsulfatase. This condition is a prototype, therefore, of the leukodystrophies. The initial case of Schilder—which he called encephalitis periaxialis diffusa (Schilder, 1912), although there was little resemblance to usual encephalitis—on clinical grounds seemed to involve sporadically occurring instances of rapidly declining neurologic function in a male juvenile in whom an autopsy showed extensive demyelination of the white matter. Although one cannot be certain from studying Schilder's original report, studies of similar patients have shown that in most instances the disease has a sex-linked type of recessive inheritance. In these cases there is a high incidence of associated adrenal insufficiency. Some patients have a bronzing type of cutaneous hyperpigmentation. Others have a history of prominent gastrointestinal symptoms resulting from presumed adrenal crises. Some patients have few clinical indications of adrenal insufficiency, but postmortem examinations show mild to extensive abnormalities in the adrenal cortex. These pathologic signs are not directly related to the effects of the neurologic debilitation and seem to be primary to the adrenals. The clinical neurologic course of this sex-linked leukodystrophy, now preferably called *adrenoleukodystrophy (ALD)*, is variable as well (Schaumberg and others, 1972). Once it was believed to be an invariably rapidly deteriorating disease, with death usually occurring within months to years. A few reports of death occurring within a matter of days are documented. More recently, chronic forms of ALD have been described (Estrada and others, 1979), as well as late-onset types consisting of mild neurologic symptoms. These types are identified as adrenomyeloneuropathy (AMN). Cases of ALD and AMN appear to occur in the same families and possibly represent effects of modifying alleles. The patient viewed in Fig. 8-17 is 17 years old and has typical addisonian bronzing, behavioral changes, mild neurologic symptoms, and evidence of mild glucocorticosteroid insufficiency. (He has a brother with more severe neurologic symptoms and signs.) The 14-year-old patient in Fig. 8-18, on the other hand, had rapidly deteriorating neurologic functions that are more typical of patients with adrenoleukodystrophy. He died shortly after this photograph was taken after an illness that lasted only 2½ years. He had a diffuse bronzing of hyperpigmentation, was severely demented, and showed decorticate posturing and blindness.

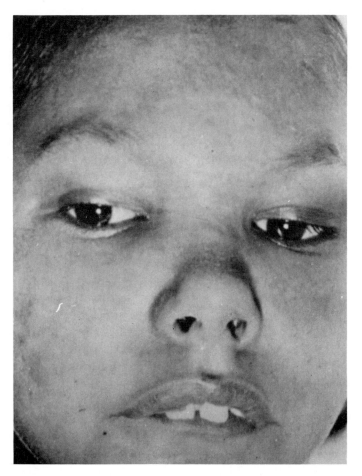

**Fig. 8-18.** Fourteen-year-old patient with typical adrenoleukodystrophy with bronzing of addisonian type. Observe dull facial expression. Patient died soon after this photograph was taken, after an illness of approximately 2½ years.

A similar type of addisonian bronzing has been reported in a patient with GM₂ gangliosidosis (Dyken and Zeman, 1964). This syndrome was also associated with a severe degree of blood eosinophilia (up to 18,000 total eosinophil count) and other cutaneous abnormalities (flat hemangioma on the hypothenar eminence and extensive "mongol" spots). The patient and his entire family were examined in detail. A younger brother also developed Tay-Sachs disease and also ultimately underwent full systemic and neuropathologic studies, which reportedly showed no major systemic abnormalities but revealed the typical central nervous system pathology of GM₂ gangliosidosis. Several members of this family —including the father and several of his siblings, a niece, the mother, and an uncle—also has granular muscular degeneration of varying degrees (see Fig. 8-19) (Dyken and Zeman, 1964).

**Diffuse skin blemish syndromes.** Several other syndromes are charac-

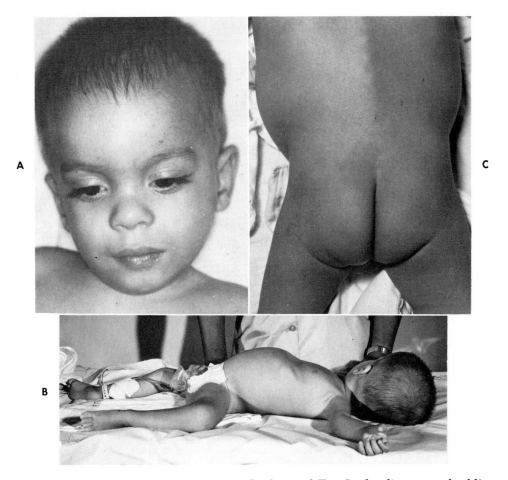

Fig. 8-19. Eighteen-month-old male with classical Tay-Sachs disease and addisonian type of hyperpigmentation. A, Facial view showing dull expression, hyperpigmentation, mild macrocephaly, and mildly coarse facial features. B, Fullbody view showing diffuse bronzing and debilitated condition. The macrocephaly can be better appreciated in this view. C, Posterior trunk view showing bronzing and "mongoloid" spots of the lumbar area, a nonspecific cutaneous finding. (From Dyken, P., and Zeman, W. J.: Neurol. Neurosurg. Psychiatry 27:29, 1964.)

terized by skin blemishes that are not differentiated by area of anatomic involvement. One form of *neurofibromatosis* (von Recklinghausen's disease, which has been mentioned in previous chapters) tends to be associated with hyperplasia of the soft tissues of the face (see Fig. 6-5). More commonly occurring in cases of neurofibromatosis, however, are neurofibromas diffusely scattered over the face and body (see Fig. 8-20). These lesions are not usually associated with symptoms of a neurologic nature, unless they are related to segmental neuropathies and radiculopathy or associated defects such as brain tumor, systemic neoplasm, simple mental retardation, or epilepsy.

*Cowden's syndrome* was first differentiated by Lloyd and Dennis

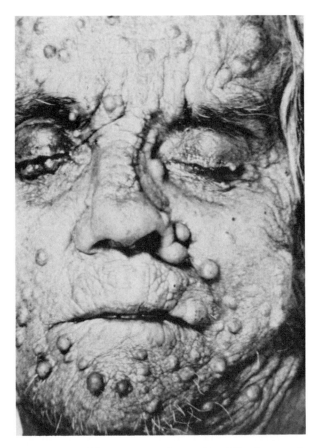

Fig. 8-20. Fifty-four–year–old woman with von Recklinghausen's neurofibroma-tosis. Note multiple neurofibromas of the face. Patient had no neurologic signs believed to be related to this neurocutaneous disorder. She presented with a cere-brovascular accident believed to be associated with arteriosclerosis. (From Dyken and others: Pediatr. Basics 6:10, 1972.)

(1963). Goodman and Gorlin (1977) claim that sixteen cases have been reported in persons ranging in age from 8 to 64 years. Autosomal domi-nant inheritance with variable expressivity occurs. Mild mental retarda-tion occurs in about 50% of cases. Hypertrichosis of the face and body is seen at birth, associated with generalized hyperkeratotic papillomatosis of the lips, gingivae, and ears and the oral, pharyngeal, and nasal mu-cosa. One sees flesh-colored papules about the face, an adenoid facies, and high-arched palate. Fibroadenomas tend to occur in the breasts and may become malignant. Thyroid disorders may be associated with this syndrome. One finds menstrual irregularities, cystic changes in the ova-ry, fibroid uterine tumors, hamartomatous polyps throughout the gas-trointestinal tract, scoliosis, and cysts of the bone. The most pronounced and characteristic features of this syndrome are facial fibromatosis — especially of the gums and nares — and hirsutism. Recurrent seizures and severe retardation have also been noted in one institutionalized patient with this syndrome. This cutaneous syndrome has many similarities to tuberous sclerosis (see Chapter 7 especially).

*Sjögren-Larsson syndrome,* which was first described in 1957, consists of congenital ichthyosis, spastic paralysis, and mental retardation. The disease is progressive, and most patients die before the third decade (Gilbert and others, 1968; Sjögren and Larsson, 1957). There is usually moderate hyperkeratosis, as well as scaling of the face and scalp, sparse cranial hair, enamel defects, increased separation of the teeth, insensitivity to oral pain, and dysarthria. Retinal degeneration and a flat nose, and ocular hypertelorism sometimes are seen. The disease seems to have a proclivity for Scandinavians. The most striking and distinctive facial feature is the hyperkeratosis, which is evenly distributed over the entire face. This feature is usually combined with the dull facial expression of the profoundly mentally deficient.

The *Ehlers-Danlos syndrome* may produce vaguely characteristic facial appearances due to marked hyperextensibility of the skin. Particularly in older persons with the syndrome, one sees excessive scarring, redundant skin folds around the eyes, and easy bruisability, which may result in facial skin changes. Angioid streaks are found in the retina. There are now seven known types of Ehler-Danlos syndrome. There is a susceptibility to cerebral aneurysms and early cerebrovascular accidents in affected patients (Beighton, 1970; McKusick, 1972).

*Cutis laxa* or generalized elastolysis (Goltz and others, 1965) is a syndrome very much like Ehler-Danlos syndrome. This disorder involves fragmented and granular elastic fibers of the skin, as shown by biopsy. There usually are no neurologic complications.

*Darier's syndrome,* or pseudoxanthoma elasticum (PXE), was described in 1896. This syndrome is associated with yellowish skin that becomes lax, redundant, and relatively inelastic and that produces a face characterized by exaggeration of the nasolabial folds and skin creases. Vision is decreased as a result of the presence of macular pigmentary mottling and angioid streaks. Somatic skin often becomes thickened and coarsely grooved, especially around the neck. Hypertension, gastrointestinal hemorrhage, and psychiatric disorders are seen in some cases. Other neurologic symptoms may be associated, including dementia and cerebral atrophy as demonstrated by CT scan (McKusick, 1972).

The *DeSanctis-Cacchione syndrome,* a type of xeroderma pigmentosum, is characterized by mental retardation, dwarfism, microcephaly, choreoathetosis, cerebellar ataxia, sexual immaturity, sensorineural deafness, retarded bone age, and the other cutaneous features of xeroderma pigmentosa. The skin abnormality consists of freckle-like lesions in exposed areas, especially on the face, beginning in the first year of life. There is photosensitivity of the skin as well as photophobia. The lesion usually starts with erythema, which is followed by vesicles and finally by scarring. There is progressive atrophy of the tissue around the nose, mouth, and eyes, with spots of hyperpigmentation and hypopigmentation and some keratosis. Malignancy occurs often. The disorder is an autosomal recessive trait (Reed and others, 1969).

The multiple lentigines or *Leopard syndrome* consists of the following classic clinical features, whose first letters spell the word "leopard" (Goodman and Gorlin, 1977; Gorlin and others, 1969):

L, lentigines (multiple)
E, electrocardiographic abnormalities
O, ocular hypertelorism
P, pulmonary stenosis
A, abnormalities of genitalia
R, retardation of growth
D, deafness (sensorineural)

Moynahan, however, has pointed out only three major signs – generalized lentigines, genital hypoplasia, and childish behavior (Moynahan, 1962). The lentigines are dark brown and flat and between 1 and 5 mm in diameter. They are seen especially around the face and neck (sparing the mucosal surface) and are diffusely distributed. A variety of other neurologic symptoms may be associated with the syndrome, including ptosis. There may be muscular hypoplasia, paresis, and weakness. Scapular winging is common. There may be a variety of dysplastic features including mild pterygium colli, epicanthal folds, low-set ears, pectus carinatum or excavatum, and hyperflexibility of the metacarpophalangeal joints. The disorder produces distinct electromyographic abnormalities that suggest a diffuse neuromyopathy. The lentigines, which are usually abundant by the time the patient is 4 or 5 years old, remain the most striking and diagnostic feature of the disorder, although some patients have all the findings except the lentigines. The pulmonary stenosis may be valvular, infundibular, or supravalvular. In addition, pulmonary valvular dysplasia, hypertrophic cardiomyopathy, atrial septal defect, and muscular subaortic stenosis have been observed in the syndrome. Since pulmonary stenosis is prominent, this syndrome must be distinguished from Noonan's syndrome. The disease is an autosomal dominant trait with high penetrance and variable expression (Sevanez and others, 1976). Perhaps related is the syndrome of *central facial lentiginosis*, which is associated with mental retardation (usually of mild degree) and with brachycephalic contour of the cranium. (See Fig. 8-21.)

The *Urbach-Wiethe syndrome*, also called lipoid proteinosis and hyalinosis cutis et mucosae, is characterized facially by relatively large, yellowish white, waxy nodules diffusely spread over the face. Pustules and bullous lesions may also develop. The oral tissues may also be infiltrated by yellow-white plaques. The lips may have a cobblestone appearance, and the tongue becomes thick and loses its papillae. Hyperkeratotic lesions occur on the knees, elbows, and fingers. Progressive hoarseness and seizures make this rare syndrome an important one to be recog-

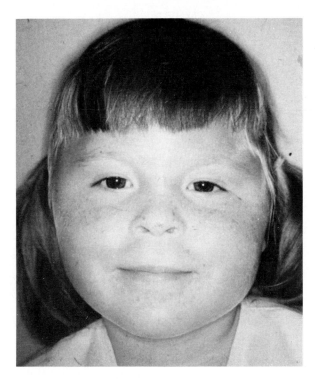

**Fig. 8-21.** Pleasant-appearing 8-year-old with extensive facial lentiginosis. Patient is mildly mentally retarded and also showed brachycephaly. (See also Fig. 5-14, *A.*)

nized by the pediatric neurologist. Bilateral intracranial calcification is noted suprasellarly in the hippocampus, caudate nucleus, globus pallidus, amygdaloid, falx cerebri, and/or temporal lobes — usually in the early juvenile period. It has been speculated that this autosomal recessive disorder is due to a disturbance in glycoprotein metabolism (Newton and others, 1971; Urbach and Wiethe, 1929).

*Parry-Romberg disease,* or hemifacial atrophy, is closely related if not identical to *coup de sabre* (see p. 276), which has also been called linear facial scleroderma (Fig. 8-22). Parry-Romberg disease is a degenerative disorder that tends to involve skin, subcutaneous tissues, bones, and underlying organs and tissues in an atrophic fashion. The progressive atrophy may remit spontaneously. It is believed that the disorder may represent an autoimmune reaction to a variety of noxious stimuli and that it could be related to the collagen diseases.

Several syndromes of which skin blemishes are a part have already been discussed in detail in previous chapters. Besides tuberous sclerosis, these disorders include *Sturge-Weber syndrome,* the *half-and-half syndrome,* and *leprosy* (Fig. 8-23).

**Other disorders with generalized cutaneous and/or subcutaneous involvement.** Several disorders characterized by extensive, generalized

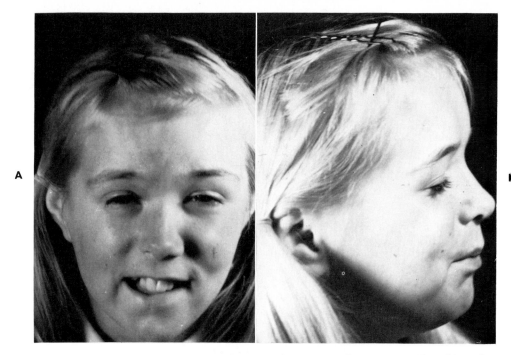

Fig. 8-22. Thirteen-year-old girl with hemifacial atrophy or Parry-Romberg disease. A, Frontal view showing extensive atrophy of the entire right side of the face. Atrophic areas are slightly hyperpigmented. B, Right lateral view showing atrophic side of face. (Courtesy of Dr. Raymond Chun, University of Wisconsin.)

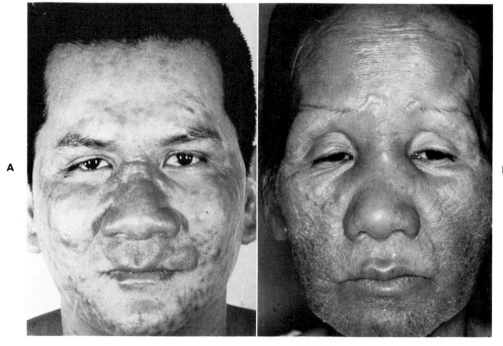

Fig. 8-23. A, Patient with lepromatous leprosy and diffuse facial infiltration by *Myocobacterium leprae* especially involving cooler areas of skin (earlobes, nose, upper lip, and other facial prominences). B, Patient with lepromatous leprosy. Partial alopecia of eyebrows and lids is present. Mild weakness of lower face is apparent. (A, Courtesy of United States Public Health Service Hospital, Carville, Louisiana, and Dr. Thomas Swift, Medical College of Georgia.)

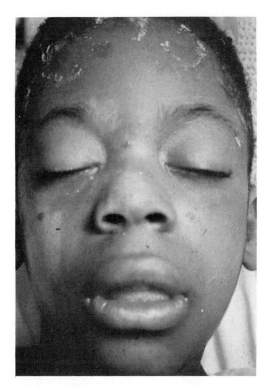

Fig. 8-24. Appearance of patient with tuberous sclerosis before typical adenoma sebaceum develops. This patient also has a large patch of facial leukoderma. Patient is severely hyperactive and mentally deficient. He had fallen asleep just before the photograph was taken.

cutaneous and/or subcutaneous involvement have been discussed in previous chapters but should be mentioned again. These include tuberous sclerosis with leukoderma and adenoma sebaceum (Fig. 8-24), the Klippel-Trénaunay syndrome with cavernous hemangioma (Fig. 8-25), the Riley-Smith syndrome with mixed hemangioma (Fig. 8-26), and the Sturge-Weber syndrome with craniofacial nevus flammeus (Figs. 8-27 and 8-28). All these conditions have characteristic features that extensively involve the cutaneous and subcutaneous tissues of the entire cranioface.

## SYNDROMES OF ABNORMAL FACIAL EXPRESSION

The final section of this chapter — and, in fact, of the entire book — is appropriately reserved for the diseases characterized by abnormal changes in facial expression. These abnormalities can sometimes be explained on the basis of known anatomic facts. In most instances, however, one has great difficulty in explaining why a given expression is abnormal. The difficulty results not from a lack of eloquence on the part of the examiner but rather from the mysteries of facial viewing itself —

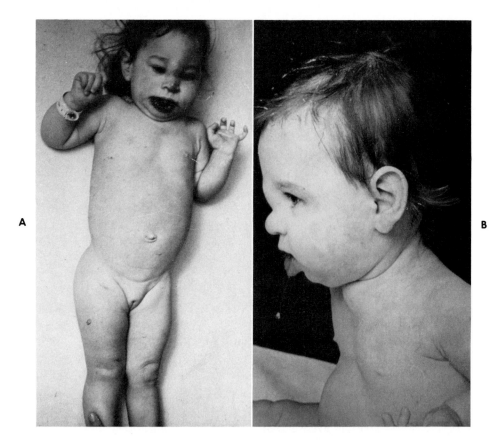

**Fig. 8-25.** Patient of 14 months with the Klippel-Trénaunay syndrome. **A,** Frontal full-body view showing cavernous hemangioma of the left side of the entire face that extends to the midline and stops. Observe the hypertrophy of the opposite lower extremity resulting from the hemangioma and subcutaneous and osseous hypertrophy. **B,** Lateral facial view.

mysteries that continue to intrigue those of us who are interested in facial diagnosis. When I (PRD) was a house officer, one of my respected professors once made a diagnosis of a brain tumor in a patient who, on a logical basis, could not have had a brain tumor. Not only was the patient's history inconsistent with the presence of such a lesion but the clinical and laboratory examinations did not support it. A total novice in facial viewing, for medical purposes at any rate, and a rash young man, I asked the respected professor what on earth made him think that the patient had a brain tumor when all the evidence spoke against it. The kindly gentleman answered, "Because he *looked* like he had a brain tumor." To my amazement, the patient turned out to have a brain tumor. A subtle dullness of facial expression, a mild intermittent heterotropia, combined with great experience and medical judgment—these were the ingredients of the professor's diagnosis. They turned out to be far more important than formal neurologic examinations and endless laboratory

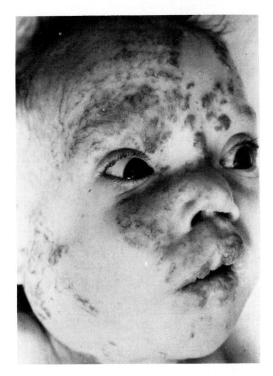

**Fig. 8-26.** Three-month-old male with mixed type of hemangioma extending predominantly over the right side of the face and involving upper, middle, and lower segments. The hemangioma consists of a deep cavernous component, which accounts for the enlargement of subcutaneous tissue and the "bag of worms" character of the lesion, and a more superficial, dermal component, which accounts for the spotty appearance. The latter component represents the nevus vasculosus type of hemangioma—a type of capillary hemangioma sometimes called a "strawberry" or "button" nevus. Extensive laboratory investigation, including angiography and brain scan, showed that the mixed facial hemangioma in this particular patient was associated with no neurologic deficits.

tests. Such subtle aspects of abnormal facial viewing are the concerns of this final section.

## Syndromes characterized by facial immobility

Neurologic, myoneurojunctional, muscular, cutaneous, subcutaneous, and osseous lesions may produce an immobility of facial expression. Syndromes characterized by this feature are *Moebius' syndrome*, as a prototype of the neurogenic lesion; *myasthenia gravis*, as the prototype of a myoneural junctional lesion; *dystrophia myotonica*, as the prototype of a muscular lesion; *scleroderma*, as a prototype of a cutaneous lesion; *facial lipodystrophy*, as a prototype of a subcutaneous lesion; and the *whistling face syndrome*, as an example of an osseous lesion. Each of these disorders, as well as many others, has been discussed in previous chapters. In many of these syndromes the facial expression is

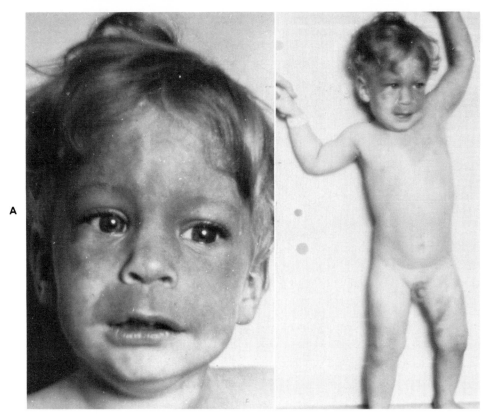

Fig. 8-27. Boy of 2½ years with Sturge-Weber syndrome. A, Facial view showing extensive bilateral nevus flammeus type of capillary hemangioma that involves both sides of the face fairly equally. No buphthalmos is present. B, Full-body view showing involvement of most of the left upper extremity and spotty involvement of other body parts. Patient appears surprisingly normal, showing only mild psychomotor delay and mild motor signs and symptoms.

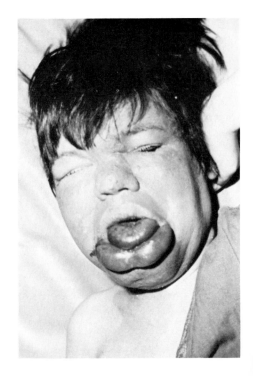

Fig. 8-28. Patient with severe bilateral craniofacial nevus flammeus with secondary trauma to lip and tongue. (This patient is also shown in Fig. 7-14, B.) (From Dyken and others: Pediatr. Basics 6:10, 1972.)

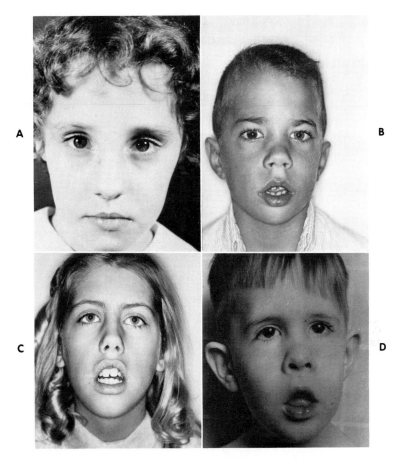

Fig. 8-29. Series of photographs of patients with congenital and adult types of dystrophia myotonica. The photographs are arranged so that the patient with the lowest intelligence quotient (A) appears first and the one with the highest (J) appears last. A, Eight-year-old; IQ=42. B, Seven-year-old; IQ=50. C, Ten-year-old; IQ=59. D, Five-year-old; IQ=66.

*Continued.*

fixed and unchanging after normal environmental stimuli. Dullness of expression is usually, but not always, present in these syndromes. The dull facial expression associated with facial immobility may give the false impression of mental deficiency.

**Facial diparesis syndromes.** Dystrophia myotonica is a good example of a disorder that gives a false impression of mental deficiency, although in some cases this disease is also associated with true mental deficiency. A large number of patients with dystrophia myotonica have been tested with formal psychometric procedures by unbiased psychologists. It has been found that many have intelligence quotients within the range of normal. The montage of facial photographs in Fig. 8-29 shows a group of patients of different ages who had unbiased tests to measure their intelligence. The patients in these photographs had proved dystrophia myoton-

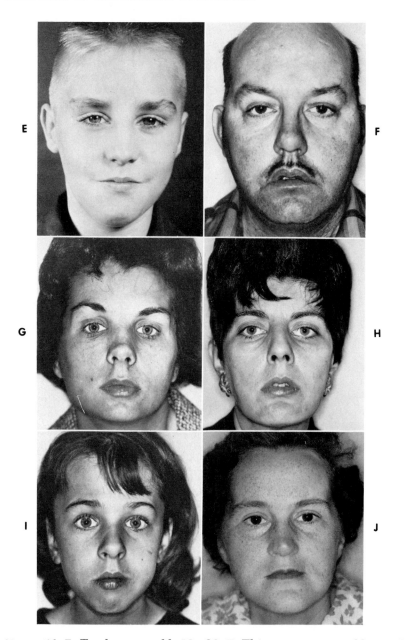

Fig. 8-29, cont'd. E, Twelve-year-old; IQ=80. F, Thirty-two–year–old; IQ=88. G, Twenty-eight–year–old; IQ=96. H, Twenty-nine–year–old; IQ=105. I, Twelve-year–old; IQ=115. J, Thirty-six–year–old; IQ=122.

ica of varying ages of onset. Their conditions ranged from mild to fairly severe forms. Many of the patients appear to be intelligent, but all patients have at least mild forms of facial immobility. When intelligence quotients were compared to facial expressions, it was obvious that dullness of facial expression tended to correlate more with facial immobility rather than with low intelligence. The montage is arranged so that the patient with the lowest intelligence quotient, a child with trainable mental retardation, is shown first (Fig. 8-29, *A*). The intelligence quotients of those that follow are progressively higher. The IQ of the final patient (Fig. 8-24, *J*) is in the high range of normal.

Similar facial immobility is encountered in many other syndromes associated with facial diparesis, including *nemaline myopathy, facioscapulohumeral muscular dystrophy,* and *Moebius' syndrome* and its many variants, such as the *hypoglossia-hypodactylia syndrome,* the *oromandibular-limb hypogenesis syndrome, Hanhart's syndrome,* and the *ankyloglossum superius syndrome.*

**Other immobile face syndromes.** Several rare syndromes characterized by immobile facies are not associated with facial weakness per se. Examples are the *whistling face syndrome,* which involves a typically stiff, immobile, and flattened facies and chin. The lips are held in a position resembling that used for whistling. (This syndrome has been discussed in Chapter 7.) Perhaps related is the *Marden-Walker syndrome,* which is characterized by a fixed facial expression, mildly opened mouth, and micrognathia. The *Schwartz-Jampel syndrome* also involves a somewhat fixed facial expression that is believed to be secondary to fairly constant facial myotonia. (See Figs. 7-23 and 7-25, *B*).

## Syndromes characterized by dementia or mental retardation

Included in this section are some of the diseases and syndromes associated with mental deficiency, static mental dysfunction, frank dementia, or progressive mental dysfunction. It is not our objective to be comprehensive. We will merely discuss some of the important facial features of prototype syndromes. It should be emphasized that a glimpse of a face or even a detailed facial study should not be used in lieu of detailed neurologic testing in cases involving dementia or in lieu of detailed psychometric and neurologic testing in cases involving mental deficiency. (See Figs. 8-30 and 8-31.)

**Mental retardation syndromes.** Simple mental deficiency involves, a sizable segment of our population and can be of varying magnitudes, ranging from profound to borderline mental retardation. At the far end of a bell-shaped curve of mental capacity (in the third percentile and below) are found those individuals with severe and profound types of mental retardation. Many of these persons have a variety of neurologic signs and symptoms besides severe mental deficiency. A large variety of associated facial abnormalities is recognizable. Although simple viewing of the face is no substitute for complete neurologic and psychometric assessment, a dull facial expression may be a clue to the existence of mental deficiency. The degree of dullness of facial expression in some instances seems to be directly related to the severity of the mental deficiency. What constitutes a dull facial expression? This is a difficult question to answer completely, but a dullness of the eyes, a flattening, of the face, and a lack of alertness, accompanied sometimes by an open mouth,

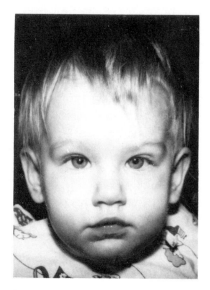

Fig. 8-30. Seven-month-old infant with psychomotor retardation and myoclonic ataxia–plus syndrome. Patient has a mild esotropia on the left. Facial expression is dull and expressionless, but facial musculature is normal.

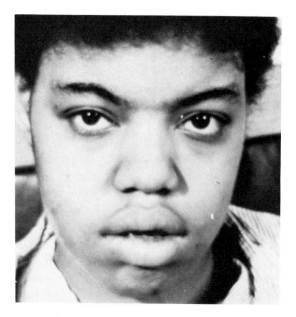

Fig. 8-31. Fifteen-year-old juvenile with mild mental deficiency. Patient has congenital craniofacial leukoderma with birthmark on lower face and recurrent seizures. Note the dull facial expression, which was thought to be unrelated to the dosage of anticonvulsants she was receiving at the time of this photograph.

drooling, and drooping eyelids, are some of the more obvious features contributing to this appearance. It is important to distinguish this dull facial expression from the immobility seen in many of the neuromuscular diseases described earlier, such as *dystrophia myotonica.* A dull facial appearance may result from a mental defect as well as from a flattened "extrapyramidal" facies. These distinctions are not always easily made. The 7-month-old infant in Fig. 8-30 has a disorder discussed in previous chapters as *myoclonic ataxia–plus.* She is delayed in the attainment of psychomotor milestones, possibly because of motor disability. She also is profoundly delayed in social, adaptive, and language areas of development, and she has a typically constant, dull facial expression. This facial expression is not accounted for by deficits in facial mobility. It is speculated that the child is mentally deficient, although she is too young at this stage for an examiner to be certain. She also has mild esotropia, which is seemingly worsened by the normal relative dystopia canthorum frequently seen in children of her age.

The patients in Fig. 8-32 have been seen in illustrations in previous chapters. The patient in Fig. 8-32, *A,* has *von Recklinghausen's disease*

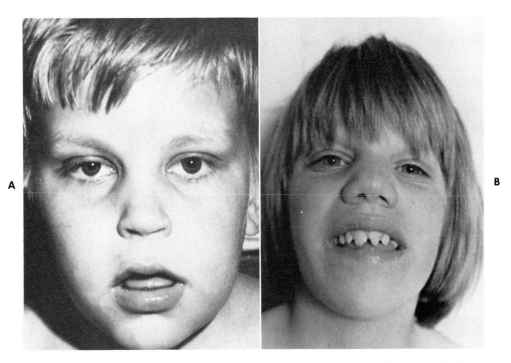

Fig. 8-32. Two patients with von Recklinghausen's disease. **A,** Patient with fairly severe mental deficiency who had a midbrain glioma when this photograph was taken. Observe mild proptosis of the right eye and dull, vacant facial expression. **B,** Patient with fairly severe mental deficiency showing silly yet dull facial expression common to mentally deficient patients. Patient also had seizures and dwarfism.

and a glioma extending into the mesencephalon. He has always been moderately mentally retarded. He has a dull facial expression that is related to his mental deficiency as much as it is to his other problems. Observe the open mouth, the slightly protruding tongue with barely controlled saliva, and the vacant eyes, in addition to a very slight asymmetry to the eyeballs caused by mild proptosis. (See also Fig. 6-4, *A*.) The patient in Fig. 8-32, *B*, also is trainably mentally retarded and has seizures. Observe the dull eyes, blank facies, and slightly open mouth. This patient also has *von Recklinghausen's disease* but shows no evidence of a brain tumor. There is a mild asymmetry to the eyes. She has an animated facial expression, yet the eyes are dull, the mouth is opened slightly, and the tongue is slightly projected forward in the mouth. She appears to be drooling. She is dwarfed and moderately mentally retarded.

The patient in Fig. 8-33, who was 37 years old when the photograph was taken, was hospitalized at an institution for the mentally retarded. She was severely retarded and was examined as part of a family study for another disease that this patient did not have. Observe the facial characteristics of this degree of mental deficiency.

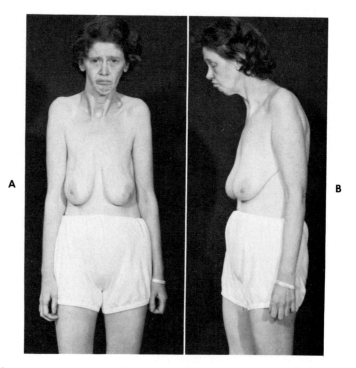

**Fig. 8-33.** Thirty-seven–year–old woman with severe mental deficiency who was discovered at an institution for the chronically mentally retarded. Patient shows a vacant expression with a somewhat saddened and flattened facial appearance. **A**, Frontal view. **B**, Lateral view.

**Dementia syndromes.** The dull facial features of mentally retarded persons differ only in degree from the facial expressions seen in some of the neural degenerations and dementias. *Subacute sclerosing panencephalitis (SSPE)* has been mentioned earlier in this chapter in relationship to the leukodystrophies. It is not known whether this disease is caused by the measles (rubeolla) virus or one like it or by as-yet-unclear reactions of the body to this virus. It is reasoned that, when harbored in the central nervous system, the organism acts as a "slow" virus in a manner similar to those of several other slow viruses associated with disorders such as *Jakob-Creutzfelt disease* and *kuru* (Horta-Barbasa, 1970). Several clinical forms of SSPE are known to exist, including an acute fulminating form (about 10% of cases) and a slowly progressive chronic form (also about 10% of cases). Only about 80% of cases, therefore, follow a subacute, downhill course, and a sizable number of these apparently spontaneously remit. The classic form of the disease shows not only signs of dementia but also rapidly progressive neurologic signs such as myoclonus, ataxia, incoordination, spasticity, dyspraxia, cortical blindness, dysphasia, dysgnosia, other involuntary movements and postures, and seizures. Affected patients frequently also have choreoretinitis. Several stages of clinical involvement have been delinated by Jabbour (1975)—stage I (behavioral, mentation defects), stage II (convulsive, motor signs), stage III (coma, opisthotonus), and stage IV (autism, vegetative). Myoclonus is the most commonly encountered type of involuntary movement. It begins in stage II and extends into stage IV. When well developed in stage III, the myoclonus is regularly repetitive, occurring as frequently as 8 to 15 times per minute. The myoclonus is of the "massive" variety—meaning that many muscle groups are involved at one time, causing a fairly stereotyped repetitive pattern (Jabbour, 1969). Massive myoclonus may not be symmetrical, however (see Fig. 8-34, *B*). In SSPE one may find a typical electroencephalographic pattern (especially in stage III, when massive myoclonus predominates). Additionally, serum and cerebrospinal fluid show pronounced elevation in levels of measles titers and IgG. Other than the signs of dementia, the facial features are nonspecific. Figs. 8-34 and 8-35 show four patients with proved SSPE. The patient seen in Fig. 8-34, *A*, was one of the first in whom the measles virus was cultured from the brain. Shortly thereafter, he was one of the few SSPE patients to experience a remission that seemed to be related to the administration of a variety of treatments aimed at improving immune responses. He received hyperimmunization with killed-measles-virus vaccine and packed leukocyte transfusion. Soon afterward, the neural deterioration ceased. When the photograph was taken, he was cortically blind and demented. This photograph shows the dull and demented facial expression that is nonspecific but characteristic for this disease. The patient in Fig. 8-35, *A* and *B*, who had stage III SSPE, went into a remission and dramatically improved in neurologic functioning after a different viral infection. He is currently

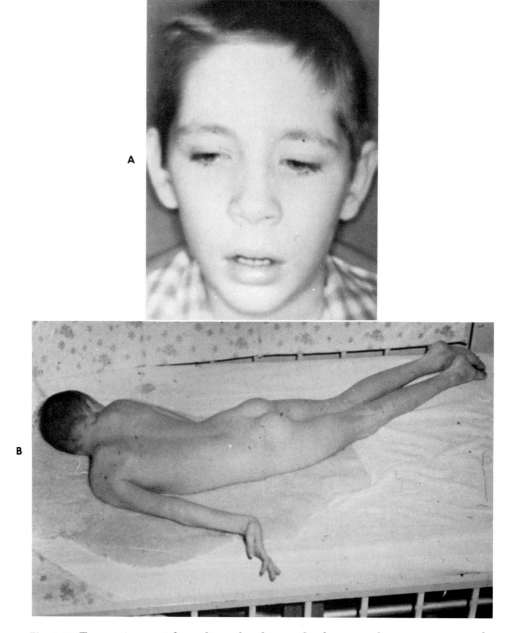

Fig. 8-34. Two patients with moderately advanced subacute sclerosing panencephalitis. A, Twelve-year-old patient with dull, demented expression that can be
contrasted to those of patients with more static encephalopathies seen in Figs. 8-
26 to 8-28. B, Another twelve-year-old patient, who was at a stage III level of involvement with the disease. Photograph shows one of the repetitive massive
myoclonic spasms. Observe somatic contortions typical of this disease.

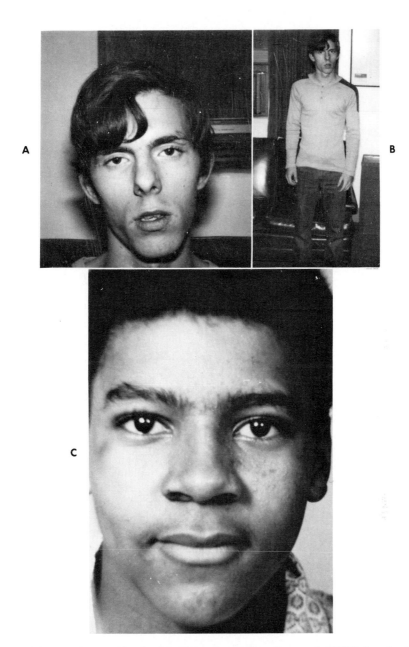

Fig. 8-35. Two patients who had had moderately advanced SSPE that had gone into remission. A, Facial view of 18-year-old who, 2 years before the time of the photograph, was totally bedridden and having repetitive massive myoclonic jerks several times per minute. During hospitalization in this condition he suffered from a nonspecific viral illness and then began to slowly recover to the point that speech returned, myoclonia disappeared, and he began to walk. Now he shows mild to moderate mental residual effects but is able to carry out most motor activities. Observe dull facial expression. B, Full-body view. Ambulation is normal. C, Patient of 15 years with proved SSPE. He also experienced a remission that was possibly brought about by use of an antiviral agent. Observe the residual dull facial expression.

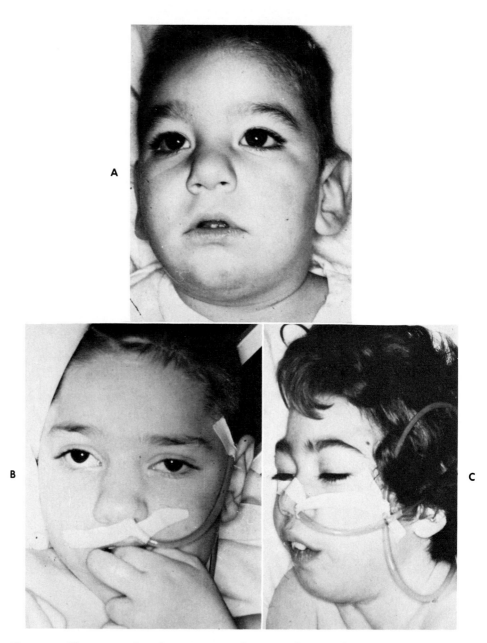

**Fig. 8-36.** Three unrelated patients with acute forms of neuronal ceroid-lipo-fuscinosis (Bielschowsky-Jansky type). A, Two-year-old patient early in course of disease. Note dull facial expression. B, Five-year-old patient with very advanced disease. Note demented, oblivious expression. Also observe exotropia and naso-gastric tube. There was preservation of some purposeful movements of upper extremities. C, Six-year-old patient with terminal disease. Note severely dement-ed facial expression and obliviousness to environment. (See also Fig. 6-64, A.)

being treated with antiviral agents while in remission. Although he has a lowered IQ, his facial expression is reasonably alert. The patient in Fig. 8-35, *C*, who had proved SSPE, was treated with an antiviral agent. Although the downhill progression had slowed somewhat before the treatment, the treatment seemed to bring improvement. It is presumed that the antiviral agents that have been proved to be effective in this disease work through improving cellular immunity. This patient has remained stable while still being treated with the antiviral agent and anticonvulsants.

The neuronal ceroid-lipofuscinoses (NCL) (Zeman and Dyken, 1969) are a group of syndromes previously called the amaurotic familial idiocies. There are seven major clinical subdivisions of this group of diseases—acute infantile, acute late infantile, acute adult, chronic juvenile, chronic adult, transitional, and atypical forms (Dyken and Trefz, 1979). The acute types are characterized by acute course and clinical dynamics, sometimes with fulminating symptoms of myoclonus, refractory seizures, and rapidly progressing dementia and motor signs. The acute infantile, acute late infantile, and acute adult types have also been called the Santavuori-Haltia or Finnish, Bielschowsky-Jansky, and Zeman-Dyken types, respectively (see Fig. 8-36). The acute types have been also identified as the *Bielschowsky-Jansky syndrome* (Fig. 8-36). The chronic types have a slower course and usually a later onset. The most common chronic type, the juvenile, shows predominant dementia and blindness. This type also has been called the Spielmeyer-Sjögren type (Fig. 8-37). The transitional form of NCL may involve features of both the acute and the chronic forms, whereas the atypical forms are quite variable.

*Tay-Sachs disease*, or $GM_2$ gangliosidosis, has been discussed in detail in Chapter 5. This disorder is a good example of an infantile disease producing dementia, as are *metachromatic leukodystrophy* (Chapter 5), *Krabbe's disease* (Chapter 6), *Alper's disease, Alexander's disease, Canavan's disease, Pelizaeus-Merzbacher disease,* and some of the other, even more rare, infantile and juvenile dementias. *Opticocochleodentatic (OCD) degeneration* (Muller and Zeman, 1965) is characterized by progressive facial dementia and debilitation over a period of years. (See Fig. 8-38.)

*Adrenoleukodystrophy* (ALD) also involves facial features that suggest dementia. There is a somewhat characteristic "wide-eyed stare" without unpleasant facial expression, as in the patient in Fig. 8-39. This patient had an unusual, slowly progressive form of ALD characterized by slow dementia, autistic behavior, and mild neurologic signs over a 12 year period. The patient in Fig. 8-40 had a form of the disease with a more typical, rapidly downhill course that led to death within 2 years of the onset. This patient's three brothers, all of whom also died of the disease, had almost identical clinical pictures.

Compare the facial expressions of four patients with adrenoleuko-

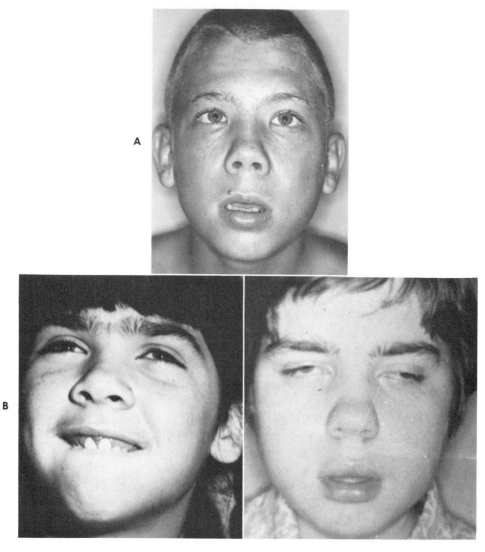

Fig. 8-37. Three unrelated patients with the chronic forms of neuronal ceroid-li-pofuscinosis (Spielmeyer-Sjögren type). **A,** Fifteen-year-old male who had had the disease for 8 years but who showed only mild mental deficiency and blindness. Observe mildly dull facial expression. **B,** Thirteen-year-old female with moderately advanced disease. She had had 3 years of progressive dementia and blindness. Observe dull and silly facial expression and right exotropia. Gingival hyperplasia and hirsutism are caused by phenytoin ingestion. (See also Fig. 6-63, *A.*) **C,** Eighteen-year-old female who had experienced 10 years of slow-ly progressive dementia and blindness. Observe demented facial appearance and exotropia. Some facial features are caused by phenytoin ingestion. (See also Fig. 6-63, *B.*)

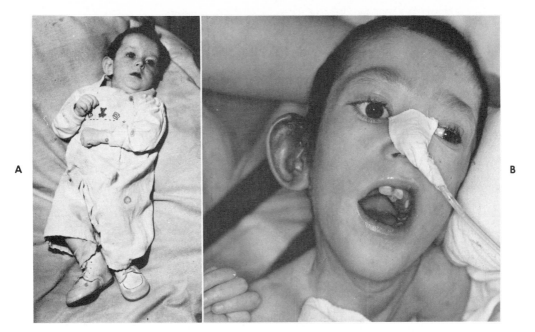

**Fig. 8-38.** Patient with opticocochleodentatic (OCD) degeneration. (This patient is the brother of the patient in Fig. 5-48 and 6-65.) **A,** Full-body view at 8 months of age after beginning of pyramidal tract signs. Observe reasonably alert but dull facial appearance without heterotropia. Patient shows bilateral decorticate posturing and cortical thumbs. **B,** Facial view of same patient at 14 years of age, soon before death. Observe diffuse facial emaciation and necrotic ear on right caused by faulty posturing of this totally vegetative patient. Patient has mild left exotropia. Observe cortical thumb on left. Severe microcephaly is obvious.

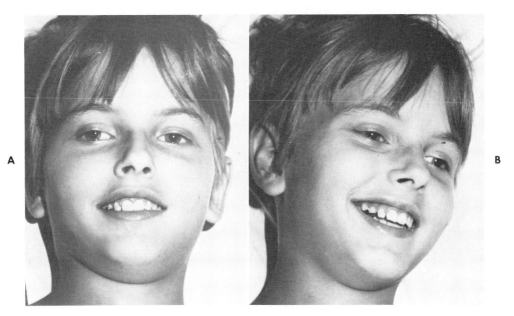

**Fig. 8-39.** Fifteen-year-old male with a history of approximately 12 years of gradually failing mental and neurologic functions. He was at first considered to have Addison's disease, but adrenoleukodystrophy was the proper diagnosis. (This patient is the younger brother of the patient in Fig. 8-17.) **A,** Frontal view showing bronzed hyperpigmentation and silly, unconcerned facial expression. **B,** Oblique view.

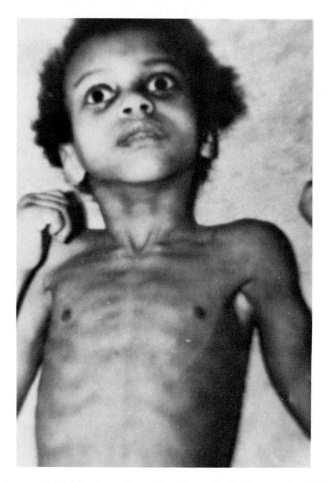

**Fig. 8-40.** Eight-year-old black male with adrenoleukodystrophy. Note the startled, wide-eyed facial expression typical of the advanced stages of this disease. Patient also has a mild right exotropia and decorticate posturing. Muscular wasting is present. Patient had disease course of about 1½ years and died several months after this photograph was taken.

dystrophy at various stages of the disease process. Fig. 8-17 shows a patient before major neurologic illness; Fig. 8-39 shows early dementia and autism; Fig. 8-40 shows a patient with advanced disease; Fig. 8-18 shows the terminal appearance. Affected whites are deeply bronzed. Blacks, if their skin pigmentation is changed at all, may be pale in comparison to other family members.

## Syndromes characterized by peculiar facial expressions

Not all degenerative diseases of the central nervous system are characterized by dementia. In some diseases that are closely related to those

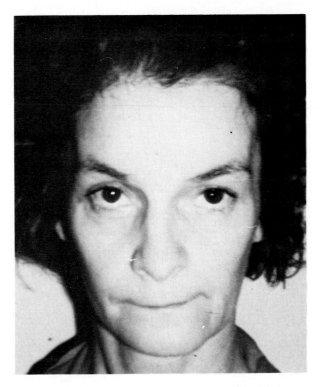

Fig. 8-41. Thirty-eight–year–old woman with Huntington's chorea. Note demented, somewhat grimacing, and pitiful facial expression. There are illusions of
mild ptosis and thin lips because of chorea of the facial muscles and voluntary
"cover-up" movements. (Courtesy of Dr. Patricia Hartlage, Medical College of
Georgia.)

mentioned in the previous section, peculiarities of expression predominate.

**Extrapyramidal facies.** The facial appearance in the dementias can be
contrasted to that found in central nervous system degenerations not
characterized by striking dementia. For example, in *Parkinson's disease*, there is a characteristic global facial appearance that is believed to
be due to the destruction of "extrapyramidal" systems. In parkinsonism,
the substantia nigra is often severely affected. Those with the extrapyramidal type of "masked" facial expression have bright and animated
eyes and other stigmata that distinguish their appearance from that of
persons with the dementia prototyped by Huntington's chorea.

*Huntington's chorea*, especially the so-called rigid form, involves a
fairly characteristic "demented" facial appearance. The face is usually
expressionless. One sees gaunt features that possibly result from long-
term nutritional problems and limitation of the ability to open the mouth
fully. These facial features are not as striking in the hyperkinetic forms
of the disease. In these forms, there is much more grimacing and constant facial movement during wakefulness. Yet, underlying these features is the impression of mental dullness. (See Fig. 8-41.)

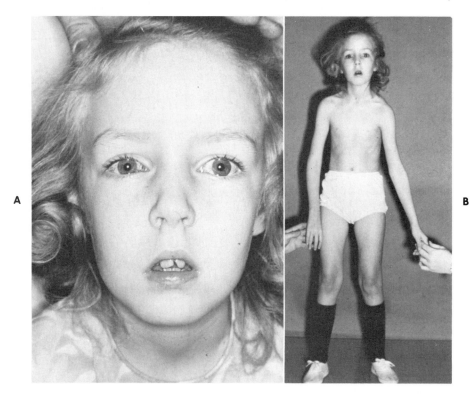

Fig. 8-42. Moderately advanced 9-year-old girl with ataxia-telangiectasia. (This patient is also seen in Fig. 6-34, *A*.) A, Facial view showing bilateral conjunctival telangiectasia. Observe flat, expressionless parkinsonian-like facies characteristic of advanced disease and probably resulting from involvement of extrapyramidal system. B, Full-body view. Patient can barely stand with help. Observe wide-based stance. (From Dyken and others: Pediatr. Basics 6:10, 1972.)

In children, a distinction can also be made between the typical facial appearance characteristic of juveniles with the various forms of dementia and the appearance of those with *ataxia-telangiectasia* (a more pronounced extrapyramidal type of degeneration). In the former there is a flattened, dull facial expression, often with mild bilateral pseudoptosis, whereas in the latter there is a mask-like, wide-eyed, staring facial expression. (See Fig. 8-42, which shows this wide-eyed, vacant stare that is similar to the masked facies of parkinsonism.) Figs. 8-43 and 8-44 show patients with mild telangiectasia. The wide-open, mask-like facies that characterizes ataxia-telangiectasia and, to a lesser extent, Parkinson's disease, may result from disturbances in the substantia nigra and the striatonigral motor system. Such an explanation might also account for the wide-open facial appearance seen in some patients with adrenoleukodystrophy and, to some extent, in the happy puppet

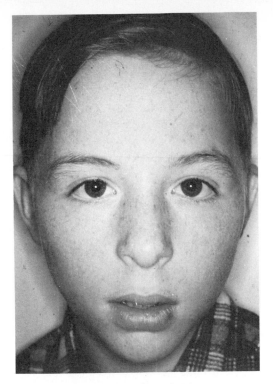

**Fig. 8-43.** Sixteen-year-old patient with mild ataxia. Telangiectasia of lateral conjunctiva is barely detectable. Note expressionless face. Patient had late-developing telangiectasia but early ataxia, frequent sinopulmonary infections, and absence of IgA. Patient also had severe immobility of eyeballs, and family history showed that a sister also was affected with the disease.

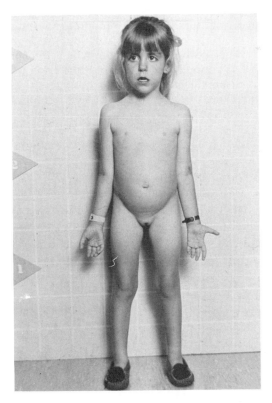

**Fig. 8-44.** Five-year-old girl also shown in Fig. 6-34, *B*. Note flat, expressionless, parkinsonian facial expression and wide-based stance. Telangiectasia is present but mild at this early stage.

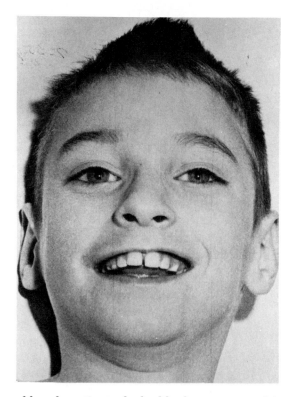

Fig. 8-45. Six-year-old male patient who had had severe, repetitive mixed seizures since early infancy. Many of the earlier seizures were classified as infantile massive myoclonic spasms. The more recent seizures were of a simpler, myoclonic drop or akinetic type. Patient was severely mentally retarded and had microcephaly and severe motor disability (quadriparesis, nonepileptogenic myoclonia, and ataxia). Note the consistently silly and smiling facial expression. This patient often would protrude his tongue. When propped up to sit, he would experience a peculiar titubation of the head and body related to inconstant myoclonia. Patient resembled a small, happy puppet, and he was considered to have Anglemann's happy puppet syndrome (see Chapter 7).

syndrome. (See Fig. 8-45 and Chapter 7.) Persons with multiple sclerosis may have a similar facial appearance. Fig. 8-46, A, shows a lady with internuclearis ophthalmoplegia and multiple sclerosis. She has a somewhat silly, wide-eyed facial expression, in addition to obvious malalignment of the eyeballs. There is no dementia. This facial appearance is similar to that of an adolescent of 15 years of age with presumed multiple sclerosis. The characteristic facial expression is seen in Fig. 8-46, B. She is not demented.

The facial appearance in Wilson's disease seems to depend to some extent on the type of the disease. As was discussed in Chapter 6, patients with the juvenile-onset, rapidly progressive "lenticular" form of Wilson's disease tend to have the fixed, silly smile that has been called the wil-

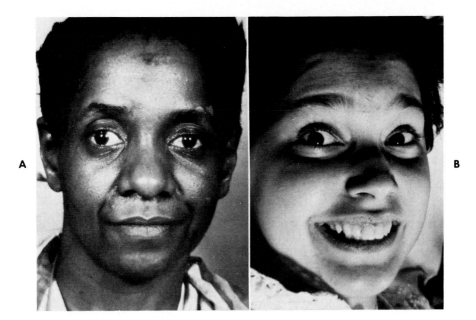

Fig. 8-46. Two patients with presumed multiple sclerosis. A, Forty-three-year-old woman with unconcerned, somewhat silly facial expression. Patient has a characteristic history of recurrences and remissions of neurophthalmologic deficits. Note exotropia related to an internuclearis ophthalmoplegia. B, Fifteen-year-old postpubescent girl in whom retrobulbar neuritis developed suddenly, several months before the time of this photograph. Full recovery ensued. Soon before this photograph was taken, she began to display silly and facetious behavior, and quadriparesis with sensory disturbances developed. Note characteristically silly and exaggerated facial appearance.

sonian risus. These patients have widespread histologic changes in the lenticular nucleus particularly. This striking facial involvement contrasts with the facial involvement of patients with the more slowly advancing, later-onset, "pseudosclerotic" form of Wilson's disease, which is characterized more by an expressionless or masked facies that is similar to the facial appearance in Parkinson's paralysis agitans (see Fig. 6-24). Transitional forms between the two types undoubtedly occur. Similarly, it is not uncommon to see a person with paralysis agitans who has a wide-open appearance or even, very rarely, a fixed smile. Fig. 8-47 shows several of Wilson's original patients. The photographs in Fig. 8-47, A and B, are "before" views of the well-advanced patients seen in Fig. 8-47, C and D.

*Seitelberger's infantile neuroaxonal dystrophy*, a rare degenerative disease of the central nervous system, has a fairly typical presentation. It is inherited as an autosomal recessive trait. Signs of peripheral neuropathy may predominate (Duncan and others, 1970). One patient with this

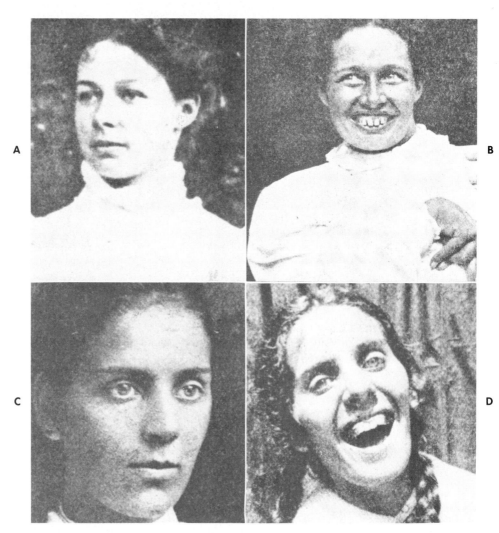

Fig. 8-47. Four photographs that originally appeared in S.A. Kinnier Wilson's article delineating hepatolenticular degeneration. A, Normal, attractive woman prior to commencement of neurologic symptoms. B, Same woman after disease was well developed. C, Another woman before beginning of symptoms. D, Same woman years after development of the disease. Note the dramatic differences between the normal facial appearances and the severely grimacing and demented expressions. The patient in B also shows evidence of athetotic dystonia of the upper extremities. The grimace in this form of Wilson's disease is often referred to as the wilsonian risus or smile and was originally pointed out in Wilson's classic description of the disorder. (From Wilson, S.: Brain 34:295, 1912.)

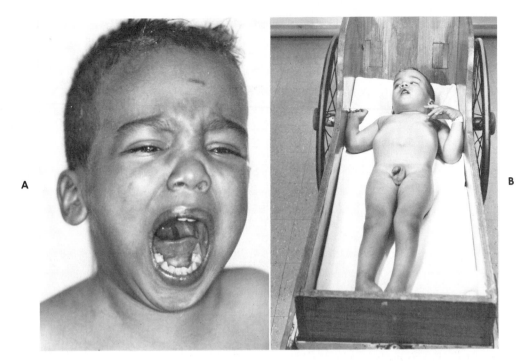

**Fig. 8-48.** Sixteen-month-old boy with infantile neuroaxonal dystrophy (INAD). **A,** Facial view showing extreme irritability and robust crying. There are no other obvious facial stigmata. (The mild scar on the forehead resulted from a fall several months before the photograph was taken.) **B,** Full-body view showing decorticate posturing characteristic of this child. INAD is a degenerative disease of the central and peripheral nervous system. The disorder has some characteristic clinical features, including a slowly progressing motor (usually pyramidal) system degeneration that originates in the spinal cord and progresses upward. There is associated dementia.

syndrome showed no characteristic facial stigmata other than those associated with being extremely agitated at all times (Fig. 8-48).

**Other peculiar facial expression syndromes.** There remains a large group of syndromes characterized by peculiar, not totally consistent abnormalities in facial expressions. The *Albers-Schönberg syndrome,* or infantile osteopetrosis, shows many unique facial and somatic features but few neurologic symptoms. Persons with this disorder are said to have an "agonized" facial expression, which is possibly explained in part by the osseous density of the bony orbits that typifies the disease. This causes pressure on the eyeball and the soft tissue of the orbit and results in mild proptosis, which, in combination with an associated enlarged cranium, produces the illusion of agony.

The whistling face syndrome, or craniocarpotarsal dysplasia of Freeman and Sheldon, which has been discussed before, is another of these syndromes, as are the Schwartz-Jampel and Marden-Walker syndromes. In all three syndromes, affected persons appear to be whistling.

Patients with the *Riley-Day syndrome* of familial dysautonomia have a number of somatic and neurologic abnormalities. It is reported that such patients have a "frightened" facial expression.

The face of a person with the Schwartz-Jampel symdrome, besides being set in a whistling posture, is also believed by many observers to appear "saddened." The patient in Figs. 7-23 and 7-25, *B*, who has the syndrome, does not, however, have such an appearance. Finally, patients with the *otopalatodigital (OPD) syndrome* are said to appear "pugilistic."

# References

Aarskog, D.: Pterygium syndrome, Birth Defects 7(6):232, 1971.

Aberfeld, D., Hinterbuchner, L., and Schneider, M.: Myotonia, dwarfism, diffuse bone disease and unusual ocular and facial abnormalities (a new syndrome), Brain 88:313, 1965.

Addy, D., and Hudson, F.: Diencephalic syndrome of infantile emaciation, Arch. Dis. Child 47:338, 1972.

Adie, W.: Argyll Robertson pupils, true and false, Brit. Med. J. 2:136, 1931.

Albright, F., Burnett, C., Smith, P., and Parson, W.: Pseudohypoparathyroidism – an example of "Seabright-bantam syndrome": report of three cases, Endocrinology 30:922, 1942.

Albright, F., Forbes, A., and Henneman, P.: Pseudo-pseudohypoparathyroidism, Trans. Assoc. Am. Phys. 65:337, 1952.

Alexander, G., and Norman, R.: Sturge-Weber syndrome, Baltimore, 1960, The Williams and Wilkins Co.

Allen, R., Dyken, P., and Lansky, L.: Degenerative diseases of the central nervous system. In Swaiman, K., and Wright, F.: The practice of pediatric neurology, St. Louis, 1975, The C. V. Mosby Co., pp. 714-774.

Alter, M., and Kennedy, W.: The Marinesco-Sjögren syndrome: hereditary cerebello-lental degeneration with mental retardation, Minn. Med. 51:901-906, 1968.

AMA drug evaluations, ed. 3, Littleton, Mass., 1977, Publishing Sciences Group, Inc.

Angelman, H.: "Puppet" children: a report on three cases, Dev. Med. Child. Neurol. 7:681, 1965.

Angle, C., McIntire, M., and Moore, R.: Cloverleaf skull Kleeblattschädel deformity syndrome, Am. J. Dis. Child. 114:198-202, 1967.

Apert, E.: De l'acrocephalosyndactyli, Bull. Soc. Med. Hosp. (Paris) 23:1310, 1906.

Apert, E.: New observations on acrocephalosyndactyly, Bull. Soc. Med. Hosp. (Paris) 47: 1672, 1923.

Arey, L.: Developmental anatomy, Philadelphia, 1974, W. B. Saunders Co.

Aubry, M.: Varieté singuliere d'alopecie congenitale; alopecie suturale, Ann. Dermatol. Syphiligr. (Paris) 4:899, 1893.

Austin, J., and others: Studies in globoid (Krabbe) leukodystrophy (GLD). V. Controlled enzymatic studies in ten human cases, Arch. Neurol. 23:502, 1970.

Banker, B., Robertson, J., and Victor, M.: Spongy degeneration of the central nervous system in infancy, Neurology (Minneap) 14:981, 1964.

Batten, F., and Gibbs, H.: Myotonia atrophica, Brain 32:187-205, 1909.

Bearn, A.: Wilson's disease. In Stanbury, J., Wyngaarden, J., and Fredrickson, D., editors: The metabolic basis of inherited disease, ed. 3, New York, 1972, McGraw-Hill Book Co.

Becker, K., and others: Klinefelter's syndrome: clinical and laboratory findings in 50 patients, Arch. Intern. Med., 118:314-321, 1966.

Beighton, P.: The Ehlers-Danlos syndrome, London, 1970, William Heinemann Medical Books, Ltd.

Berardinelli, W.: An undiagnosed endocrinometabolic syndrome: a report of two cases, J. Clin. Endocrinol. Metab. 14:193, 1954.

Berg, J., Delhanty, J., Faunch, J., and Ridler, M.: Partial deletion of short arm of a chromosome of the 4 and 5 group (Denver) in an adult male, J. Ment. Defic. Res. 9:219, 1965.

Bergsma, D., editor: The clinical delineation of birth defects. II. Malformation syndromes, Birth Defects 5(2): , 1969.

Bergsma, D., editor: International conference on morphogenesis and malformation of face and brain, New York, 1975, Alan R. Liss, Inc., National Foundation March of Dimes; Birth defects 11(7): , 1975.

Beuren, A.: Supravalvular aortic stenosis: a complex syndrome with and without mental retardation, Birth Defects 8(15):45, 1972.

Bisland, T.: The Laurence-Moon-Biedl syndrome, Am. J. Ophthalmol. 34:874, 1951.

Bjork, A.: Roentgencephalometric growth analysis. In Pruzansky, S., editor: Congenital anomalies of the face and associated structures, Springfield, 1961, Charles C Thomas, Publisher.

Black, J., and Bonharm-Carter, R.: Association between aortic stenosis and facies of severe infantile hypercalcemia, Lancet 2:745, 1963.

Bloom, D.: Cutaneous manifestations of systemic genetic diseases, N.Y. J. Med. 63:3070, 1963.

Boder, E., and Sedgwick, R.: Ataxia-telangiectasia: a familial syndrome of progressive cerebellar ataxia, oculocutaneous telangiectasia and frequent pulmonary infection, Pediatrics 21:526, 1958.

Bohm, E., and Strang, R.: Choroid plexus papillomas, J. Neurosurg. 18:493, 1961.

Book, J., and Hesselvik, L.: Acrocephalosyndactyly, Acta Paediatr. 42:359, 1953.

Book, J., Schut, T., and Reed, S.: A clinical and genetical study of microcephaly, Am. J. Ment. Defic. 57:637-660, 1953.

Bourneville, D.: Sclereuse tubereuse des circonvolutions cerebrales: idiste et epilepsie hemiplegique, Arch. Neurol. (Paris) 1:81, 1880.

Bowen, P., Lee, C., Zellweger, H., and Lindenberg, R.: A familial syndrome of multiple congenital defects, Johns Hopkins Med. J. 114:402, 1964.

Bower, B. and Jeavons, P.: The "happy puppet" syndrome, Arch. Dis. Child. 42:298-302, 1967.

Boyle, J., and others: Lesch-Nyhan syndrome: preventive control by prenatal diagnosis, Science 169:688, 1970.

Brachmann, W.: Ein Full von symmetrischer monoktylie durchul-nadefekt mit symmetrischer Flughantbildung in den fallenbogen savie andheren Abnormalitaten (Zwerghaftigkert, Halsrippen, Behaarung), J. Kinderheilkd 84:224, 1916.

Branch, C., and Dyken, P.: Choroid plexus papilloma and infantile spasms, Ann. Neurol. 5:302, 1979.

Branch, C., Swift, T., and Dyken, P.: Prolonged neonatal myasthenia gravis: electrophysiological studies, Ann. Neurol. 3:416, 1978.

Branch, C., Volcan, I., and Dyken, P.: Choroid plexus papilloma: a rare, treatable cause of infantile spasm syndrome, Proc. Child. Neurol. Soc. 6:17, 1977.

Burian, H., and Burns, C.: Ocular changes in myotonic dystrophy, Am. J. Ophthalmol. 63:22, 1967.

Caffey, J.: The whiplash shaken infant syndrome: manual shaking by the extremities with whiplash-induced intracranial and intraocular bleedings, linked with residual permanent brain damage and mental retardation, Pediatrics 54:396, 1974.

Cain, D., Griggs, D., Lackey, D., and Kagan, B.: Familial renal agenesis and total dysplasia, Am. J. Dis. Child. 128:377, 1974.

Campbell, B., and others: Waardenburg's syndrome. Arch. Dermatol. 86:718, 1962.

Carpenter, G.: Two sisters showing malformations of the skull and other congenital abnormalities, Rep. Soc. Study Dis. Child. (London) 1:110, 1901.

Carson, N., and Neill, D.: Metabolic abnormalities detected in a survey of mentally backward individuals in Northern Ireland. Arch. Dis. Child. 37:505, 1962.

Caughey, J., and Myrianthopoulos, N.: Dystrophia myotonica and related disorders, Springfield, Ill., 1963, Charles C Thomas, Publisher.

Chao, D.: Congenital neurocutaneous syndrome of childhood. III. Sturge-Weber diseases. J. Pediatr. 55:635-49, 1959.

Cockayne, E.: Dwarfism with retinal atrophy and deafness, Arch. Dis. Child. 11:1, 1936.

Cohen, M., Sr., and Cohen, M., Jr.: The oral manifestations of trisomy G (Down's syndrome), Baltimore, 1971, The Williams and Wilkins Co. Birth Defects 8(7):241-251, 1971.

Cohen, M., and Gorlin, R.: The Prader-Willi syndrome, Am. J. Dis. Child. 117:213, 1969.

Cohen, M., Jr., Sedano, H., Gorlin, R., and Jirasek, J.: Frontonasal dysplasia (median cleft face syndrome): comments on etiology and pathogenesis, Birth Defects 7(7):117, 1971.

Collins, E.: Case with symmetrical congenital notches in the outer part of each lower lid and defective development of the malar bones, Trans. Ophthalmol. Soc. U.K. 20:190, 1900.

Condron, C., and others: The supernumerary isochromosome 18 syndrome (+18 pi), Birth Defects 10(10):36, 1974.

Crawfurd, M.: Multiple congenital anomaly associated with an extra autosome, Lancet 2:22, 1961.

Crawfurd, M.: Multiple congenital anomaly associated with an extra autosome, Lancet 2:22, 1961.

Crome, L.: The association of phenylketonuria with leucodystrophy, J. Neurol. Neurosurg. Psychiatry 25:149, 1962.

Crome, L.: Microgyria, J. Pathol. 64:479-495, 1952.

Crome, L., and Sylvester, P.: Hydranencephaly (hydrencephaly), Arch. Dis. Child. 33:235, 1958.

Cross, H., McKusick, V., and Breen, W.: A new oculocerebral syndrome with hypopigmentation, J. Pediatr. 70:398, 1967.

Crowe, F., Schull, W., and Neal, J.: A clinical, pathological and genetic study of multiple neurofibromatosis, Springfield, Ill., 1956, Charles C Thomas, Publisher.

Cushing, H.: The basophil adenomas of the pituitary body and their clinical manifestations (pituitary basophilism), Bull. Johns Hopkins Hosp. 50:137, 1932.

Dandy, W.: The diagnosis and treatment of hydrocephalus due to occlusions of the foramina of Magendie and Luschka, Surg. Gynecol. Obstet. 32:112, 1921.

Danks, D., Tipett, P., Adams, C., and Campbell, P.: Cerebrohepatorenal syndrome of Zellweger, J. Pediatr. 86:382, 1975.

Darwin, C.: The variation of animals and plants

under domestication, London, 1875, John Murray Ltd.

Daum, S.,LeBlau, J., and Minuit, P.: Dysplasie telencephaliqne avec excroissance de l'os frontal, Sem. Hop. Paris 34:1893, 1958.

de Grouchy, J.: Chromosome 18: a topoligic approach, J. Pediatr. 66:414-431, 1965.

de Grouchy, J.: The 18p– and 18r syndromes, Birth Defects 5(5):74, 1969.

de Grouchy, J., Royer, P. Salmon, C., and Lamy, M.: Deletion partielle des bras longs du chromosome 18, Ruthol. Biol. 12:579, 1964.

Dejong, R.: Multiple sclerosis: history, definition and general considerations. In Viuken, P., and Bruyn, G.: Handbook of clinical neurology, vol. 9, Amsterdam, 1970, North Holland Publishing Co.

Dekaban, A.: Tables of cranial and orbital measurements, cranial volume, and derived indexes in males and females from 7 days to 20 years of age, Ann. Neurol. 2 (6):485-491, 1977.

de Lange, C.: Sur un type nonveau de degeneration (typus Amstelodausensis), Arch. Med. Enf. 36:713, 1933.

DeMyer, W.: The median cleft face syndrome: differential diagnosis of cranium bifidum occultum, hypertelorism, and median cleft nose, lip and palate, Neurology 17:961, 1967.

DeMyer, W.: Median facial malformations and their implications for brain malformations. In Bergsma, D., editor: Morphogenesis and malformation of the face and brain, New York, 1975, Alan R. Liss, Inc.; Birth Defects 11(7): 155-181, 1975.

DeMyer, W.: Prenatal and developmental defects. In Barnett, A., and Einhorn, A., editors: Pediatrics, ed. 15, New York, 1972, Appleton-Century-Crofts.

DeMyer, W.: Technique of the neurological examination. New York, 1974, McGraw-Hill Book Co.

DeMyer, W., and Zeman, W.: Alobar holoprosencephaly (arhinencephaly) with median cleft lip and palate: clinical, nosologic and electroencephalographic considerations, Confin. Neurol. 23:, 1963.

DeMyer, W., Zeman, W., and Palmer, C.: The face predicts the brain: diagnostic significance of median facial anomalies in holoprosencephaly (arhinencephaly), Pediatrics 34: 256, 1964.

Dennison, W.: The Pierre Robin syndrome, Pediatrics 36:336-41, 1965.

Dickerson, W.: Characteristic roentgenographic changes associated with tuberous sclerosis, Arch. Neurol. Psychiatr. (Chicago) 53:199, 1945.

Dieker, H., and others: The lissencephaly syndrome, Baltimore, 1969, The Williams and Wilkins Co.; Birth Defects 5(2):53-64, 1969.

DiGeorge, A., Olmsted, R., and Harley, R.: Waardenburg's syndrome, J. Pediatr. 57:649, 1960.

Dimitri, V.: Rev. Assoc. Med. Argent. 36:1029, 1923.

Dodge, H., Wood, M., and Kennedy, R.: Craniofacial dysostosis: Crouzon's disease, Pediatrics 23:98, 1959.

Dodge, P., Gamstrop, I., Byers, R., and Russell, P.: Myotonic dystrophy in infancy and childhood, Pediatrics 35:3-19, 1965.

Donohue, W.: Dysendocrinism, J. Pediatr. 32: 739, 1948.

Donohue, W. and Uchida, I.: Leprechaunism, J. Pediatr. 45:505, 1954.

Down, J.: Observations on an ethnic classification of idiots, London Hosp. Clin. Lec. Rep. 3: 259, 1866.

Dudding, B., Gorlin, R., and Langer, L.: The oto-palato-digital syndrome; a new symptom-complex consisting of deafness, dwarfism, cleft palate, characteristic facies and a generalized bone dysplasia, Am. J. Dis. Child. 113: 214, 1967.

Dukes, T., Green, J., and Dyken, P.: Half and half seizures: A rare type of neonatal seizure, Proc. Child. Neurol. Soc. 6:24, 1977.

Duncan, C., Strub, R., McGarry, P., and Duncan, D.: Peripheral nerve biopsy as an aid to diagnosis in infantile neuroaxonal dystrophy, Neurology 20:1024, 1970.

Dunn, H.: The Prader-Labhart-Willi syndrome: review of the literature and report of nine cases, Acta Paediatr. Scand. 186(Suppl.):1, 1968.

Dyken, P.: Ataxia in childhood, Postgrad. Med. 50(2), 93, 1971.

Dyken, P.: The changing syndromes of dystrophia myotonica, Neurology 19:292, 1969.

Dyken, P.: Extraocular myotonia in families of dystrophia myotonica, Neurology 16:738, 1966.

Dyken, P.: Half and half seizures, Dev. Med. Child Neurol. 11:94-95, 1969.

Dyken, P.: Headaches in children, Amer. J. Fam. Physic. 11:105, 1975.

Dyken, P.: Identification of two neonatal dystrophia myotonica syndromes, Proc. C.N.S. 4:11, 1975.

Dyken, P.: Marfan's syndrome and dystrophia myotonica, N. Engl. J. Med. 274:915, 1966.

Dyken, P.: Retinal changes in neuronal ceroid-lipofuscinosis, Arch. Ophthalmol. 94:687, 1976.

Dyken, P., and Buchanan, D.: Early onset dystrophia myotonica, Proc. Inst. Med. Chic. 25: 301, 1965.

Dyken, P., and Cully, W.: Another population of phenylketonuria? studies on atypical phenylketonurics, Dev. Med. Child Neurol. 11:718, 1969.

Dyken, P., Dukes, T., Hartlage, P., and Muller, J.: Infiltrating brain stem glioma and Von Recklinghausen's disease, Proc. C.N.S. 6:25, 1977.

Dyken, P., and Haar, F.: Congenital left hemiparesis, hemiatrophy and hemiathetosis: inherited as an autosomal dominant, Proc. C.N.S. 4:14, 1975.

Dyken, P., and Harper, P.: Congenital dystrophia myotonica, Neurology 23:465, 1973.

Dyken, P., and Kolar, O.: Dancing eyes, dancing feet: infantile polymyoclonia, Brain 91:305, 1968.

Dyken, P., Langstrom, D., and Harrington, G.: Pictorial atlas of ten neurocutaneous diseases, Pediatr. Basics, 6:10, 1972.

Dyken, P., Miller, M., Swift, A., and Waldo, K.: Facial features of pediatric neurological syndromes: a programmed approach to the differentiation of the normal and the abnormal face, Proc. C.N.S. 6:25, 1977.

Dyken, P., and Trefz, J.: Comparison of blood and brain and the ultrastructural classification of neuronal ceroid lipofuscinosis, Proc. C.N.S. 8:55, 1979.

Dyken, P., and Zeman, W.: A clinical, pathological, and genetic study of an unusual form of Tay-Sachs disease with macular degeneration in the family, J. Neurol. Neurosurg. Psychiatry, 27:29-37, 1964.

Edwards, J., Norman, R., and Roberts, J.: Sex linked hydrocephalus: report of a family with 15 affected members, Arch. Dis. Child. 36:481, 1961.

Engel, E., and Forbes, A.: Cytogenetic and clinical findings in 48 patients with congenitally defective or absent ovaries, Medicine 44:135, 1965.

Epstein, C., Martin, G., Schultz, A., and Motulsky, A.: Werner's syndrome; a review of its symptomatology, natural history, pathologic features, genetics and relationship to the natural aging process, Medicine 45:177, 1966.

Epstein, C., and others: Hereditary dysplasia of bone with kyphoscoliosis, contractures and abnormally shaped ears, J. Pediatr. 73:379, 1968.

Estrada, M., Dyken, P., Gurbani, S., and Huff, T.: Chronic form of adrenoleukodystrophy, Clin. Res. 26:821A, 1979.

Falk, R., and others: Partial trisomy of chromosome 11: a case report, Am. J. Ment. defic. 77: 383, 1973.

Fanconi, G., and others: Chronische Hypercalcaemie kombinert mit Osteosklerosis, Hyperazotaemis, Mundenvuchs and kongenitalen Missbildungen, Helv. Paediatr. Acta 7:314, 1952.

Farmer, T.: Pediatric neurology, New York, 1968, Hoeber Medical Division, Harper and Row, Publishers, Inc.

Fazen, L., Elmore, J., and Nadler, H.: Mandibulo-facial dysostosis (Treacher-Collins syndrome), Am. J. Dis. Child. 113:405-410, 1967.

Ferguson-Smith, M.: Karyotype-phenotype correlations in gonadal dysgenesis and their bearing on the pathogenesis of malformations, J. Med. Genet. 2:142, 1965.

Feingold, M.: The Face and syndrome identification. In Bergsma, D., editor: Morphogenesis and malformation of face and brain, New York, 1975, Alan R. Liss, Inc.; Birth Defects 11(7):213-215, 1975.

Feingold, M.: Normal values for selected physical parameters: an aid to syndrome delineation, Birth Defects 10(13): 1974.

Feingold, M., O'Connor, J., Berkman, M., and Darling, D.: Kleeblattschädel syndrome, Am. J. Dis. Child. 118:589-594, 1969.

Fienman, N., and Yakovac, W.: Neurofibromatosis in childhood, J. Pediatr. 76:339, 1970.

Fitch, N., Pinsky, L., and Lachance, R.: A form of bird-headed dwarfism with features of premature senility, Am. J. Dis. Child. 120:260, 1970.

Flippen, J.: Cranio-facial dysostosis of Crouzon, Pediatrics 5:90, 1950.

Forland, M.: Cleidocranial dysostosis: a review of the syndrome and report of a sporadic case with hereditary transmission, Am. J. Med. 33: 792, 1962.

Franceschetti, A., and Klein, D.: The mandibulo-facial dysostosis: a new hereditary syndrome, Acta Ophthalmol (Kbh) 27:143, 1949.

Frasier, S., and Kogut, M.: Adolescent acromegaly: studies of growth hormone and insulin metabolism, J. Pediatr. 71:832, 1967.

Freeman, M., and others: The Roberts syndrome, Clin. Genet. 5:1, 1974.

Fulton, W., and Dyken, P.: Neurological syndromes of systemic lupus erythematosus, Neurology 14:317, 1964.

Gardner, F.: No leper's clapper: Robert the Bruce, 1274-1329, Surg. Gynecol. Obstet. 94: 373, 1952.

Garland, H., and Moorhouse, D.: An extremely rare recessive hereditary syndrome including cerebellar ataxia, oligophrenia, cataracts and other features, J. Neurol. Neurosurg. Psychiatry 16:110, 1953.

Gazit, E., Goodman, R., Katznelson, B., and Rotem, Y.: The wrinkly skin syndrome: a new heritable disorder of connective tissue, Clin. Genet. 4:186, 1973.

Gerritsen, T., Vaughn, J., and Waisman, H.: The identification of homocystine in the urine, Biochem. Biophys. Res. Commun. 9:493, 1962.

Gibson, J.: Congenital hydrocephalus due to atsesia of the foramen of Magendie, J. Neuropathol. Exp. Neurol. 14:244, 1955.

Gilbert, W., Jr., Smith, J., and Nyhan, W.: The Sjögren-Larsson syndrome, Arch. Ophthalmol. 80:308, 1968.

Gilchrist, K., Gilbert, E., Shahidi, N., and Opitz, J.: The evaluation of infants with the Zellweger (cerebro-hepato-renal) syndrome, Clin. Genet. 7:413, 1975.

Gilford, H.: Ateleiosis: a disuse characterized by conspicuous delay of growth and development, Med. Chirurg. Trans. 85:305, 1902.

Goldenhar, M.: Associations malformations de l'oeil at de l'oreille, J. Genet. Hum. 1:243, 1952.

Goltz, R., Hult, A., Goldfarb, M., and Gorlin, R.: Cutix laxa: a manifestation of generalized elastolysis, Arch. Dermatol. 92:373, 1965.

Goltz, R., Peterson, W., Gorlin, R., and Ravits, H.: Focal dermal hypoplasia, Arch. Dermatol. 86:708-17, 1962.

Gomez, M., Groover, R., and Mellinger, J.: Tumors of the brain and spinal cord. In Swaiman, K., and Wright, F.: The practice of pediatric neurology, St. Louis, 1975, The C. V. Mosby Co.

Goodman, R., and Gorlin, R.: The face in genetic disorders, ed. 2, St. Louis, 1977, The C. V. Mosby Co.

Gordon, H.: Craniostenosis, Br. Med. J. 2:792, 1959.

Gorlin, R., Anderson, R., and Blaw, M.: Multiple lentigenes syndrome, Am. J. Dis. Child. 117:652, 1969.

Gorlin, R., and Cohen, M.: Frontometaphyseal dysplasia: a new syndrome, Am. J. Dis. Child. 118:487-494, 1969.

Gorlin, R., Meshin, L., and St. Geme, J.: Oculodentodigital dysplasia, J. Pediatr. 63:69, 1963.

Gorlin, R., and Psaume, J.: Orodigoto-facial dysostosis—a new syndrome, J. Pediatr. 61:520, 1962.

Gorlin, R., and others: Multiple mucosal neuromas, pheochromocytoma, medullary carcinoma of the thyroid: a syndrome, Cancer 22:293, 1968.

Grabb, W.: The first and second branchial arch syndrome, Plast. Reconstr. Surg. 36:485-508, 1965.

Graves, R.: Clinical lectures, Ind. Med. and Surg. J. 7:516, 1835.

Greig, D.: Hypertelorism, Edinburgh Med. J. 31:560, 1924.

Greig, D.: Oxycephaly, Edinburgh Med. J. 33:189, 1926.

Gurbani, S., Dyken, P., and Estrada, M.: Tay-Sachs disease and detection of the carrier state in a large black family, Ann. Neurol. 6:184, 1975.

Guyton, A. Textbook of medical physiology, ed. 4, Philadelphia, 1971, W. B. Saunders Co.

Haar, F., and Dyken, P.: Hereditary nonprogressive athetotic hemiplegia: a new syndrome, Neurology 27(9):849, 1977.

Haines, R., and Mohiuddin, A.: Handbook of human embryology, Baltimore, 1965, The Williams and Wilkins Co.

Hall, B.: Aglossia-adactylia, Birth Defects 7(11):233, 1971.

Hallermann, W.: Vogelgesicht and Cataracta congenita. Klin. Monatsbl. Augenheilkd. 113:315, 1948.

Hallervorden, J., and Spatz, H.: Eigenartige Erkrankuna im extrapyramidalen System mit besonderer Beteihigung des Globus pallidus und der Substantia nigra, Z. Ges. Neurol. Psychiatr. 79:254, 1922.

Hanson, J., and Smith, D.: U-shaped palatal defect in the Robin anomalad: developmental and clinical relevance, J. Pediatr. 87:30, 1975.

Hanson, P., and Rowland, L.: Moebius syndrome and facioscapulohumeral muscular dystrophy, Arch. Neurol. 24:31-39, 1971.

Harper, P.: Sturge-Weber syndrome with Klippel-Trénaunay-Weber syndrome, Birth Defects 7(8):314, 1971.

Harper, P., and Dyken, P.: Early onset dystrophia myotonica: evidence supporting a maternal environmental factor, Lancet 2:53, 1972.

Harper, R., Orti, E., and Baker, R.: Bird-headed dwarfs (Seckel's syndrome), J. Pediatr. 70:799, 1967.

Harper, P., Rivas, M., Bias, W., Hutchinson, J., Dyken, P., and McKusick, V.: Genetic linkage confirmed between the locus for myotonic dystrophy and the ABH-secretion and Lutheran blood group loci, Am. J. Hum. Genet. 24:310, 1972.

Hart, M., Malamud, N., and Ellis, W.: The Dandy-Walker syndrome, a clinicopathological study based on 28 cases, Neurology 22:771, 1972.

Hartwell, S., Pickrell, K., and Quinn, G.: Congenital anhidrotic ectodermal dysplasia, Clin. Pediatr. 4:383-86:1965.

Hecht, F., and others: Leukaemia and lymphocytes in ataxia-telangiectasia, Lancet 2:1193, 1966.

Henderson, J.: The congenital facial diplegia syndrome: clinical features, pathology and aetiology, Brain 62:381-403, 1939.

Herrlin, K., and Hillborg, P.: Neurological signs in a juvenile form of Gaucher's disease, Acta Paediatr. 51:137, 1962.

Hess, R., Kaveggia, L., and Opitz, J.: The N syndrome, a new multiple congenital anomaly—mental retardation syndrome, Clin. Genet. 6:237, 1974.

Holden, K., and Dekaban, A.: Neurological involvement in nevus unis lateris and nevus linearis sebaceus, Neurology 22:879, 1972.

Hoefnagel, D., and Penry, J.: Partial facial paralysis in young children, New Engl. J. Med. 262:1126, 1960.

Holmes, G.: An attempt to classify cerebellar disease; with a note on Marie's hereditary cerebellar ataxia, Brain 30:545, 1907.

Holmes, L., and others: Mental retardation: an atlas of diseases with associated physical abnormalities, New York, 1972, Macmillan, Inc.

Holtermüller, K., and Wiedemann, H.: Kleeblattschädel syndrome, Med. Monatsschr. 14:439, 1960.

Horowitz, S., Morishima, A., and Vinkka, H.: The position of the external ear in Turner's syndrome, Clin. Genet. 9:333, 1976.

Horrocks, P.: Trans. Ophthalmol. Soc. U.K. 3:106, 1883.

Horta-Barbosa, L., and others: Some characteristics of SSPE measles virus (34718), Proc. Soc. Exp. Biol. Med. 134:17, 1970.

Hsia, Y., Bratu, M., and Herbordt, H.: Genetics of the Meckel syndrome (dysencephalia splanchnocystica), Pediatrics 48:237, 1971.

Hunter, C.: A rare disease in two brothers, Proc. R. Soc. Med. 10:104, 1917.

Hurler, G.: Ueber einen Typ Muliples Abartangen, vorwiegend am Skelettsystem, Z. Kinderheilkd. 24:220, 1919.

Hutchinson, J.: Congenital absence of hair and mammary glands, Med. Chir. Trans. 69:473, 1886.

Huttenlocher, P., and others: Osteo-chondromuscular dystrophy: a disorder manifested by multiple skeletal deformities, myotonia and dystrophic changes in muscle, Pediatrics 44:945, 1969.

Insley, J.: Syndrome associated with a deficiency of part of the long arm of chromosome No. 18, Arch. Dis. Child. 42:140-146, 1967.

Jabbour, J., Duenas, D., Gilmartin, R., and Gottlieb, M.: Pediatric neurology handbook, ed. 2, Flushing, N.Y., 1976, Medical Examination Publishing Co., Inc.

Jabbour, J., and others: Subacute sclerosing panencephalitis: a multidisciplinary study of eight cases, J.A.M.A. 207:2248, 1969.

Jabbour, J. and Taybi, H.: Craniotelencephalic dysplasia, Am. J. Dis. Child. 108:627, 1964.

Jarcho, S., and Levin, P.: Hereditary malformation of the vertebral Bodies, Bull. Johns Hopkins Hosp. 62:216, 1938.

Jervis, G.: Phenylpyruvic oligophrenia: inductory study of 50 cases of mental deficiency associated with excretion of phenylpyruvic acid, Arch. Neurol. Psychiatry 38:944, 1937.

Johnson, V., Mulder, R., and Hosen, R.: The Wolf-Hirschhorn (4p−) syndrome, Clin. Genet. 10:104, 1976.

Jones, K., and Cohen, M.: The Crouzon syndrome, J. Med. Genet. 10:398, 1973.

Jones, W.: Cherubism: a thumb nail sketch of its diagnosis and a conservative method of treatment, Oral Surg. 20:648, 1965.

Kahn, A., and Fulmer, J.: Acrocephalosyndactylism, New Engl. J. Med. 252:379, 1955.

Kalischer, S.: Berl. Klin. Wochenschr. 4:1059, 1897.

Kalliala, E., and Taskinen, P.: Cleidocranial dysostosis, report of six typical cases and one atypical case, Oral Surg. 15:808, 1962.

Kay, L., and Haskell, R.: Color atlas of orofacial diseases, Chicago, 1971, Year Book Medical Publishers, Inc.

Kearns, T., and Sayre, G.: Retinitis pigmentosa, external ophthalmoplegia and complete heart block, Arch. Ophthalmol. 60:280, 1958.

Kenyon, A.: Hyperpituitarism. In Cecil, R., and Loeb, R., editors: Textbook of medicine, Philadelphia, 1956, W. B. Saunders Co.

Kirkham, T., and Werner, E.: The ophthalmic manifestations of Rothmund's syndrome, Can. J. Ophthalmol. 10:1, 1975.

Kissel, P., and Schmitt, J.: Les formes viscerales des phikomatoses. In Michaux and Feld, editors: Les phakomatoses cerebrales, 1963, SPEI.

Klippel, M., and Feil, A.: Anomalie de la colonne vertebrale par absence des vertebres cervicales; cage thoracogne remontant jusqu'à la base du crane, Bull. Mem. Soc. Anat. 87:185, 1912.

Kloepfer, H., Platon, R., and Hansche, W.: Manifestations of a recessive gene for microcephaly in a population isolate, J. Genet. Hum. 13:52, 1964.

Krabbe, K.: A new familial infantile form of diffuse sclerosis, Brain 39:74, 1916.

Kunstadter, R.: Melkersson's syndrome: a case report of multiple recurrences of Bell's palsy and episodic facial edema, Am. J. Dis. Child. 110:559, 1965.

Kurlander, G., DeMyer, W., and Campbell, J.: Roentgenology of the median cleft face syndrome, Radiology 88:473-78, 1967.

Kushnick, T., and Matsushita, G.: Partial deletion of long arms of chromosome 18, Pediatrics 42:194-97, 1968.

Laband, P., Habib, G., and Humphreys, G.: Hereditary gingival fibromatosis: report of an affected family with associated splenomegaly and skeletal and soft tissue abnormalities, Oral Surg. 17:339, 1964.

Laestadius, N., Aase, J., and Smith, D.: Normal inner canthal and outer orbital dimensions, J. Pediatr. 74:465-468, 1969.

Lagos, J., and Gomez, M.: Tuberous sclerosis: reappraisal of a clinical entity, Mayo Clin. Proc. 42: 26, 1967.

Landouzy, L., and Dejerine, J.: De la myopathie atrophique progressive, Rev. Med. Franc. 5:81, 253, 1885.

Laron, Z.: The syndrome of familial dwarfism and high plasma immunoreactive human growth hormone, Birth Defects 10(4):231, 1974.

Larsen, L., Schottstaedt, L., and Bost, F.: Multiple congenital dislocations associated with characteristic facial abnormality, J. Pediatr. 37:574, 1950.

Lejeune, J., Ganthier, M., and Turpin, R.: Etude des chromosomes somatiques de neuf enfants mongoliens, C. R. Acad. Sci. (Paris) 248:1721, 1959.

Lejeune, J., and others: Trois cas de deletion partielle du bras coutc'n chromosome 5. C. R. Acad. Sci. (Paris) 257:3098, 1963.

Lemli, L., and Smith, D.: The XO syndrome: a study of the differential phenotype in 25 patients, J. Pediatr. 63:577, 1965.

Lenz, W.: Resessiv-geschlects-gebunden M: Prophthalmie mit nultiplen Miosbildungen, Z. Kinderheilkd. 77:384, 1955.

Leroy, J., and Crocker, A.: Clinical definition of the Hurler-Hunter phenotypes – a review of 50 patients, Am. J. Dis. Child. 112:518, 1966.

Lesch, M., and Nyhan, W.: Familial disorder of uric acid metabolism and central nervous system function, Am. J. Med. 36:561, 1964.

Lichtenstein, L.: Histiocytosis-X eosinophilic granuloma of bone, Letterer-Siwe disease, and Schüller-Christian disease: further observation of pathological and clinical importance, J. Bone Joint Surg.[Am.] 46:76, 1964.

Lloyd, K., and Dennis, M.: Cowden's disease: a possible new symptom complex with multiple system involvement, Ann. Intern. Med. 58:136, 1963.

Lorber, J.: Hydranencephaly with normal development, Dev. Med. Child. Neurol. 7:628, 1965.

Louis-Barr, M.: Sur un syndrome progressif comprenant des telangiectasis capillaires cutanées et conjonctivales à disposition naevoide et des troubles cerebelleux, Confin. Neurol. 4:32, 1941.

Lowe, C., Terrey, M., and MacLachlan, E.: Organic-aciduria, decreased renal ammonia production, hydrophthalmos and mental retardation, Am. J. Dis. Child. 83:164, 1952.

Lowry, R., and Guichon, V.: Congenital contractural arachnadactyly: a syndrome simulating Marfan's syndrome, Can. Med. Assoc. J. 107: 531, 1972.

MacGillivray, R.: Cutis verticis gyrata and mental retardation, Scott. Med. J. 12:450, 1967.

MacGregor, F.: Transformation and identity: the face and plastic surgery, New York, 1974, Quadrangle/The New York Times Book Co.

Mackenzie, N., and Emery, J.: Deformities of the cervical cord in children with neurospinal dysraphism, Dev. Med. Child. Neurol. 25 (Suppl.):58, 1972.

Mann, T., and Russell, A.: Study of a microcephalic midget of extreme type, Proc. R. Soc. Med. 52:1024, 1959.

Manning, J., and Adour, K.: Facial paralysis in children, Pediatrics 49:102, 1972.

Marden, P., and Walker, W.: A new generalized connective tissue syndrome, Am. J. Dis. Child. 112:225, 1966.

Marfan, A.: Un cas de deformation congenitale des quatre membres plus pronouncée aux extremities characterisée par l'allongement des os avec un certain degre d'amincissement, Bull. Mem. Soc. Med. Hop. Paris 13:220, 1896.

Marie, P., and Sainton, P.: Observation d'-hydrocephalie hereditaire (père et fils), par vie de development du crave et du cerveau, Bull. Mem. Soc. Med. Hop. Paris 14:706, 1897.

Marinesco, G., Draganesco, S., and Vasiliu, D.: Nouvelle maladie familiale caracterisé par une cataracte congenitale et un arret du developpement somato-neuro-phychique, Encephale 26:97, 1931.

Marshall, R., and Smith, D.: Frontodigital syndrome: a dominantly inherited disorder with normal intelligence, J. Pediatr. 77:129, 1970.

McArthur, R., and Edwards, J.: DeLange syndrome: report of 20 cases, Can. Med. Assoc. J. 96:1185-98, 1967.

McDonald, J., and Kelley, W.: Lesch-Nyhan syndrome, altered kinetic properties of mutant enzyme, Science 171:689, 1971.

McKusick, V.: Heritable disorders of connective tissue, ed. 4, St. Louis, 1972, The C. V. Mosby Co.

McKusick, V.: Mendelian inheritance in man, Baltimore, 1975, Johns Hopkins University Press.

Meislin, A., and Rothfield, N.: Systemic lupus erythematosus, Pediatrics 42:1, 37, 1968.

Melnick, J., and Needles, C.: An undiagnosed bone dysplasia: a two family study of four generations and three generations, Am. J. Roentgenol. Radium Ther. Nucl. Med. 97:39, 1966.

Mende, I.: Uber eine Familie hereditar-degeneratives Taubstummes mit mongoloidem Einschlay und teilweisen Leukismus der Hunt und Hoare, Arch. Kinderheilkd. 79:214, 1926.

Meredith, H.: Change in a dimension of the frontal bone during childhood and adolescence, Anat. Rec. 134:769, 1959.

Merritt, H., and Moore, M.: The Argyll Robertson pupil: an anatomic-physiologic explanation of the phenomenon with a survey of its occurrence in neurosyphilis, Arch. Neurol. Psychiatr. 30:357, 1933.

Milhorat, T.: Pediatric neurosurgery, Philadelphia, 1978, F. A. Davis Co.

Moebius, P.: Uber angeborene doppolseitige Abducens-Facialis-Lahmany, Munch. med. Wochenschn. 35:91, 1888.

Moore A.: Observations on facial growth and its clinical significance, Am. J. Orthod. 45:399, 1959.

Moosa, A., and Dubowitz, V.: Peripheral neuropathy in Cockayne's syndrome, Arch. Dis. Child. 45:674, 1970.

Morris, J., and MacGillivray, R.: The mental capacity in achondroplasia, J. Ment. Sci. 99: 547, 1953.

Moser, H., Prensky, A., Wolfe, H., and Rosman, N.: Farber's lipogranulomatosis: report of a case and demonstration of an excess of free ceramide and ganglioside, Am. J. Med. 47:869, 1969.

Moynahan, E.: Multiple symmetrical moles with psychic and somatic infantilism and genital hypoplasia: first male case of a new syndrome, Proc. R. Soc. Med. 55:959, 1962.

Muller, J., and Zeman, W.: Degenerescence systematisee optico-cochleo-dentelee, Acta Neuropath. (Berlin) 5:26, 1965.

Murray, J.: On three peculiar cases of molluscum fibrosum in children of one family (neurofibromatosis), Med. Chir. Trans. 38: 235, 1873.

Muzj, E.: Orofacial anthropometrics, Hempstead, N.Y., 1970, Index Publishers Corp.

Myrianthopoulos, N.: Huntington's chorea: review, J. Med. Genet., 3:298, 1966.

Nellhaus, G.: Head circumference from birth to eighteen years: practical composite international and interracial graphs, Pediatrics 41: 106-111, 1968.

Nevin, H., Burrows, D., Allen, G., and Kernohan, D.: Aglossia-aductylia syndrome, J. Med. Genet. 12:89, 1975.

Newton, F., Rosenberg, R., Lampert, P. and O'-Brien, J.: Neurological involvement in Urbach-Wiethe's disease (lipoid proteinosis): a clinical, ultrastructural and chemical study, Neurology 21:1205, 1971.

Noonan, J., and Ehmke, D.: Associated noncardiac malformations in children with congenital heart disease, J. Pediatr. 63:468, 1963.

Opitz, J., and Howe, J.: The Meckel syndrome (dysencephalia splanchnocystica — the Gruber syndrome), Birth Defects 5(2):167, 1969.

Opitz, J., Johnson R., McCreadie, S., and Smith, D.: The C syndrome of multiple congenital anomalies, Baltimore, 1969, Williams and Wilkins Co.; Birth Defects 5(2):161-166, 1969.

Paddison, R., Moossy, J., Derbes, V., and Kloepfer, W.: Cockayne's syndrome: a report of five cases with biochemical, chromosomal, dermatologic, genetic and neuropathologic observations, Dermatol. Trop. 2:195, 1963.

Parkins, F., and Barbers, G.: Abnormalities of development of the palate and soft tissues of the mouth. In Nelson, W., Vaughan, V., and McKay, R.: editors: Textbook of pediatrics, ed. 9, Philadelphia, 1969, W. B. Saunders Co.

Parry, C., editor: Collections from the unpublished medical writings of the late Caleb Hillier Parry, London, 1825, Underwoods.

Patau, K., and others: Multiple congenital anomaly caused by an extra autosome, Lancet 1: 790, 1960.

Patten, B.: Human embryology, ed. 3, New York, 1968, McGraw-Hill Book Co.

Patten, B.: The normal development of the facial region. In Pruzansky, S., editor: Congenital anomalies of the face and associated structures, Springfield, Ill., 1961, Charles C Thomas, Publisher.

Peskova, H., and Stockar, B.: Hemiatrophia facies progressiva: Romberg's disease, Acta Chir. Plast. 3:276, 1961.

Peush, B.: Arnold-Chiari malformations: morphogenesis, Arch. Neurol. 12:527, 1956.

Pincus, J. Subacute necrotizing encephalomyelopathy (Leigh's disease): a consideration of clinical features and etiology, Dev. Med. Child. Neurol. 14:87, 1972.

Pitner, S., Edwards, J., and McCormick, W.: Observations on the pathology of the Moebius syndrome, J. Neurol. Neurosurg. Psychiatry 28:362, 1965.

Poser, C., and van Bogaert, L.: Natural history and evolution of the concept of Schilder's diffuse sclerosis, Acta Neurol. Scand. 31:285, 1958.

Prader, A., Labbart, A., and Willi, H.: Ein Syndrome von Adipositas, Kleinwuchs, Kryptochismus und Oligophrenie nach mystonieartigen Zustand im Neugeboren-enalter, Schweiz Med. Wochenschr. 86:1260, 1956.

Prensky, A.: Metechromatic leukodystrophy. In Swaiman, K., and Wright, F., editors: The practice of pediatric neurology, St. Louis, 1975, The C.V. Mosby Co., p. 412.

Preus, M., and Fraser, F.: The cerebro-oculo-facio-skeletal syndrome, Clin. Genet. 5:294, 1974.

Pries, C., and others: The EEC syndrome, Am. J. Dis. Child. 127:840, 1974.

Pryor, H.: Objective measurement of interpupillary distance, Pediatrics 44:973-977, 1969.

Pryor, H., and Thelander, H.: Abnormally small head size and intellect in children, J. Pediatr. 73:593-598, 1968.

Puretic, S., Puretic, B., Fiser-Herman, M., and Adamcic, M.: A unique form of mesenchymal dysplasia, Br. J. Perinatal. 74:8, 1962.

Rabe, E.: Subdural effusions in children, Pediatr. Clin. N. Am. 14:831, 1967.

Reed, W., and others: Xeroderma pigmentosum: clinical and laboratory investigation of its basic defect, J.A.M.A. 207:2073, 1969.

Remnick, H.: Embryology of the face and oral cavity, Rutherford, N. J., 1970, Fairleigh Dickinson University Press.

Renwick, J., Bundey, S., Ferguson-Smith, M., and Izatl, M.: Confirmation of linkage of the loci for myotonic dystrophy and ABH secretion, J. Med. Genet. 8:407, 1971.

Richter, R.: Infantile subacute necrotizing encephalopathy with predilection for the brain stem, J. Neuropathol. Exp. Neurol. 16:281, 1957.

Riley, H., Jr., and Smith, W.: Macrocephaly, pseudopapilledema and multiple hemangiomata: a previously undescribed heredofamilial syndrome, Pediatrics 26:293, 1960.

Rimoin, D., and Edgerton, M.: Genetic and clinical heterogeneity in the oral-facial-digital syndromes, J. Pediatr. 71:94, 1967.

Rimoin, D., Merimee, T., and McKusick, V.: Growth hormone deficiency in man; an isolated recessively inherited defect, Science 152:1635, 1966.

Robinson, M., Silverman, F., and Smith, H.: A newly recognized dwarfing syndrome, Am. J. Dis. Child. 117:645, 1969.

Rogers, B.: Embryology of the face and introduction to craniofacial anomalies. In Converse, J. editor: Reconstructive plastic surgery, Philadelphia, 1977, W. B. Saunders Co.

Rogers, B.: Microtia, "lap," "cup," and protruding ears: four directly related congenital deformities? In Longacre, J, editor: Craniofacial anomalies, Philadelphia, 1968, J.B. Lippincott Co.

Romberg, M.: Klinische Ergebnisse, Berlin, 1846, A. Forstner.

Rossman, R.: The ectodermal dysplasias, Cutis 4:1246-48, 1968.

Rubinstein, J., and Taybi, H.: Broad thumbs and toes and facial abnormalities, Am. J. Dis. Child. 105:588, 1963.

Russell, A.: A diencephalic syndrome of emaciation in infancy and childhood, Arch. Dis. Child 26:274, 1951.

Sachs, B.: On arrested cerebral development with special reference to its cortical pathology, J. Nerv. Ment. Dis. 14:541, 1887.

Sanfilippo, S., Podosin, R., Langer, L., and Good, A.: Mental retardation associated with acid mucopolysacchariduria (heparitin sulfate type), J. Pediatr. 63:837, 1963.

Schaumberg, H., Richardson, E., and Johnson, P.: Schilder's disease, sex-linked recessive transmission with specific adrenal changes, Arch. Neurol. 27:458, 1972.

Schneider, P. and Kennedy, E.: Sphingomyelinase in normal human spleens and in spleens from subjects with Niemann-Pick disease, J. Lipid Res. 8:202, 1967.

Schwartz, O., and Jampel, R.: Congenital blepharophimosis associated with a unique generalized myopathy, Arch. Ophthalmol. 68:52, 1962.

Seckel, H.: Bird-headed dwarfs, Springfield, Ill., 1960, Charles C Thomas, Publisher.

Sedano, H., Cohen, M., Jirasek, J., and Gorlin, R.: Frontonasal dysplasia, J. Pediatr. 76:906-913, 1970.

Sedgwick, R., and Boder, E.: Ataxia-telangiectasia. In Vinken, P., and Bruyn, G.: Handbook of clinical neurology, vol. 14, Amsterdam, 1972, North Holland Publishing Co.

Senior, B., and Gellis, S.: The syndromes of total lipodystrophy and partial lipodystrophy, Pediatrics 33:593, 1964.

Seuanez, H., Mane-Gãrzon, F., and Kolski, R.: Cardio-cutaneous syndrome (the "LEOPARD" syndrome): review of the literature and a new family, Clin. Genet. 9:266, 1976.

Shiller, J.: Craniofacial dysostosis of Crouzon: a case report and pedigree with emphasis on heredity, Pediatrics 23:107, 1959.

Shy, G., and Magee, K.: A new congenital nonprogressive myopathy, Brain 79:610, 1956.

Sjögren, T.: Hereditary congenital spinocerebellar ataxia combined with congenital cataract and oligophrenia, Acta Psychiatr. Scand. 46 (Suppl.):286, 1917.

Sjögren, T., and Larsson, T.: Oligophrenia in combination with congenital ichthyosis and spastic disorders, Acta Psychiatr. Scand. (Suppl.):113:1, 1957.

Smith, D.: Autosomal abnormalities, Am. J. Obstet. Gynecol. 90:1055, 1964.

Smith, D.: Recognizable patterns of human malformation, Philadelphia, 1970, W. B. Saunders Co.

Snyder, C.: Syndrome of gingival hyperplasia, hirsutism and convulsions, J. Pediatrics 67:499, 1965.

Solitare, G.: The cri du chat syndrome: neuropathologic observations, J. Ment. Defic. Res. 11:267, 1967.

Solomons, G., Zellweger, H., Jahnke, P. and Opitz, E.: Four common eye signs in mongolism, Am. J. Dis. Child. 110:46-50, 1965.

Sotos, J., Dodge, P., Muirhead, D., Crawford, J., and Talbot, N.: Cerebral gigantism in childhood, N. Engl. J. Med. 271:109, 1964.

Sperber, G.: Craniofacial embryology, Baltimore, 1973, The Williams and Wilkins Co.

Steinert, H.: Dystrophia musculorum progressiva retiahens, Kasnistisches und Kritisches zur Le'hre von den hereditaren Krenkheiten, Mitt. Grenzgeb. Med. Chir. Lena. 81:105, 1909.

Stickler, G., and others: Hereditary progressive arthro-ophthalmopathy, Proc. Mayo Clin. 40: 433, 1965.

Streiff, E.: Dysmorphie mandibulofaciale (tete d'oiseau) et alterations oculaires, Ophthalmologica 120:79, 1950)

Sturge, W.: Trans, Clin. Soc. Lond. 12:162, 1879.

Sugar, A., Bigger, J., Podos, S.: Hallermann-Streiff-Francois syndrome, J. Pediatr. Ophthalmol. 8(4):234, 1971.

Sugarman, G., and Reed, W.: Two unusual neurocutaneous disorders with facial cutaneous signs, Arch. Neurol. 21:242, 1969.

Suzuki, K., and Suzuki, Y.: Globoid cell leucodystrophy (Krabbe's disease): deficiency of galactocerebroside beta-galactosidase, Proc. Natl. Acad. Sci. U.S.A. 66:302, 1970.

Swaiman, K.: Other lipid diseases. In Swaiman, K., and Wright, E., editors: The practice of pediatric neurology, St. Louis, 1975, The C.V. Mosby Co., p. 421.

Swift, T., Ignacio, O., and Dyken, P.: Neonatal dystrophia myotonica: electrophysiological studies, Am. J. Dis. Child. 129:734, 1975.

Szanto, J., and Gallyas, F.: Study of iron metabolism in neuropsychiatric patients: Hallervorden-Spatz disease, Arch. Neurol. 14:438-42, 1966.

Tanner, J.: Growth at adolescence, Oxford, 1962, Blackwell Scientific Publications.

Tay, W.: Symmetrical changes in the region of the yellow spot in each eye of an infant, Trans. Ophthalmol. Soc. U.K. 1:55, 1881.

Taybi, H.: Diastrophic dwarfism. Radiology 80:1, 1963.

Taybi, H.: Generalized skeletal dysplasia with multiple anomalies. Am. J. Roentgenol. Radium Ther. Nucl. Med. 88:450, 1962.

Taylor, R.: Heredofamilial mononeuritis multiplex with branchial predilection, Brain 83:113, 1960.

Temtamy, S.: Carpenter's syndrome: acrocephalopolysyndactyly: an autosomal recessive syndrome, J. Pediatr. 69:111, 1966.

Temtamy, S., and McKusick, V.: Synopsis of hand malformation with particular emphasis on genetic factors, Birth Defects 5(3):125, 1969.

Tessier, P.: Anatomical classification of facial, craniofacial and laterofacial cleft, J. Maxillofac. Surg. 4:69, 1976.

Thurnam, J.: Two cases in which the skin, hair and teeth were very imperfectly develop. Proc. R. Med. Chir. Soc. 31:71, 1848.

Tuomaala, P., and Haapanen, E.: Three siblings with similar anomalies in the eyes, bones and skin, Acta Ophthalmol. (Kbh.) 46:365, 1968.

Turner, H.: A syndrome of infantilism, congenital webbed neck and cubitus valgus, Endocrinology 23:566, 1938.

Tyler, F., and Stephens, F.: Studies in disorders of muscle. II. Clinical manifestations and inheritance of facioscapulohumeral dystrophy in a large family, Ann. Intern. Med. 32:640, 1950.

Urbach, E., and Wiethe, C.: Lipodosis cutis et mucosae, Virchows Arch. [Pathol. Anat.] 273, 285, 1929.

Van Der Hoeve, J.: Eye symptoms in tuberous sclerosis of the brain, Trans. Ophthalmol. Soc. U.K. 40:329, 1920.

Von Reuss, A.: Zuckeraussoheiduny im Sanglingsalter, Wien. Med. Wochenschr. 58:799-803, 1908.

Waardenburg, P.: A new syndrome combining developmental anomalies of the eyelids, eyebrows and nose root with pigmentary defects of the iris, head, and hair and with congenital deafness, Am. J. Hum. Genet. 3:195, 1951.

Wagenmann, A.: Multiple Neurome des Auges und der Funge, Ber. Dtsch. Ophthalmol. Ges. 43:282, 1922.

Walsh, F.: Clinical neurophthalmology, ed. 2, Baltimore, 1957, The Williams and Wilkins Co.

Walshe, J.: The physiology of copper in man and its relationship to Wilson's Disease, Brain 90: 149, 1967.

Walshe, J., and Cumings, J., editors: Wilson's disease, some current concepts (symposium on Wilson's disease), Oxford, 1961, Blackwell Scientific Publications.

Warburg, M.: Anophthalmos complicated by mental retardation and cleft palate, Acta Ophthalmol. 38:394-404, 1960.

Warkany, J., and others: Congenital malformations in autosomal trisomy syndromes, Am. J. Dis. Child. 112:502, 1966.

Weber, F.: J. Neurol. Psychopath. 3:134, 1922.

Wells, C., and Shy, G.: Progressive familial choreoathetosis with cutaneous telangiectasia, J. Neurol. Neurosurg. Psychiatry 20:98, 1957.

Werner, S., Coleman, J., and Franzen, L.: Ultrasonographic evidence of consistent orbital involvement in Graves' disease, N. Engl. J. Med. 290:1447, 1974.

Wilkins, R., and Brody, I.: Tuberous Sclerosis, Arch. Neurol. 22:475-477, 1970.

Williams J., Barratt-Boyes, B., and Lowe, J.: Supravalvular aortic stenosis, Circulation 24: 1311, 1961.

Wilson, S.: Progressive lenticular degeneration: familial nervous disease associated with cirrhosis of the liver, Brain 34:295, 1912.

Winter, G., and Simpkiss, M.: Hypertrichosis with hereditary gingival hyperplasia, Arch. Dis. Child. 49:394, 1974.

Witkop, C.: Heterogeneity in gingival fibromatosis, Birth Defects 7(7):210, 1971.

Wolman, M., Sterk, V., Gatt, S., and Frenkel, M.: Primary familial xanthomatosis with involvement and calcification of the adrenals, Pediatrics 28:742, 1961.

Woolf, C., Woolf, R., and Broadbent, T.: Genetic and nongenetic variables related to cleft lip and palate, Plast Reconstr. Surg. 32:65, 1963.

Wright, F., Benton, J., and Bornhofen, T.: Congenital structural defects. In Swaiman, K., and Wright, E., editors: The practice of pediatric neurology, St. Louis, 1975, The C. V. Mosby Co.

Wyburn-Mason, R.: Arterio-venous aneurysm of mid-brain and retina, facial naevi and mental changes. Brain 66:163, 1943.

Zaleski, W., Houston, C., Pozsonyi, L., and Ying, K.: The XXXXY chromosome anomaly: report of three new cases and review of 30 cases from the literature, Can. Med. Assoc. J. 94:1143, 1966.

Zehender, W.: Eine Missgehurt mit hautaber-vachsenen Augen oder Kryptophthalmus, Klin. Monatsbi. Angenheilkd. 10:225, 1872.

Zellweger, H., and Ionasescu, V.: Early onset of myotonic dystrophy in infants, Am. J. Dis. Child. 125:601, 1973.

Zellweger, H., Ionasescu, V., Simpson, J. and Burmeister, L.: The problem of trisomy 22, Clin. Pediatr. 15:601, 1976.

Zeman, W., Donahue, S., Dyken, P., and Green, J.: The neuronal ceroid lipofuscinoses (Batten-Vogt syndrome). In Vinken, P., and Bruyn, G., editors: Handbook of clinical neurology, vol. 10, Amsterdam, 1970, North Holland Publishing Co., pp. 522-617.

Zeman, W., and Dyken, P.: Dystonia musculorum deformans. In Vinken, P., and Bruyn, G., editors: Handbook of clinical neurology, vol. 6, Amsterdam, 1968, North Holland Publishing Co., pp. 517-543.

Zeman, W., and Dyken, P.: Dystonia musculorum deformans: clinical, genetic and pathoanatomical studies, Psychiatry Neurol. Neurochir. 70:77, 1967.

Zeman, W., and Dyken, P.: Neuronal ceroid-lipofuscinosis (Batten's disease): relationship to amaurotic familial idiocy? Pediatrics 44:570, 1969.

Zundel, W., and Tyler, F.: The muscular dystrophies, N. Engl. J. Med. 273:537, 1965.

# Index

## A

Abnormal eye movements, 68-70
Abnormalities
of buccal surface and gums, 92
syndromes characterized by, 333-337
of central middle face, 263-273
of cheeks, 88
of chin, 90
syndromes characterized by, 325-326
of conjunctiva, syndromes characterized by, 223-229
of cornea and lens, syndromes characterized by, 210-218
craniofacial
in achondroplasia, 138
caused by subdural effusions, 153
cranioplastic, 153
of ears, syndromes characterized by, 285-294
of external lower face, 83-91
of eye distances, 73
of eyelid, 70-72
syndromes characterized by, 229-243
facial
subdivisions for describing, 14
in tuberous sclerosis, 282
in facial expression, 397-422
of first branchial arch, 91
gingival, 92
of hair, syndromes characterized by, 166-172
of head posture, syndromes characterized by, 344-349
of iris, 65
and pupil, syndromes characterized by, 202-210
of jaws, syndromes characterized by, 328-333
of lens, syndromes characterized by, 218-223
of lips, 89
lower facial segment, 82-101
middle facial segment, 58-81
of middle nose, 77
of mouth, 28-29, 88-90
neck, 82-101, 98-101
neurogenic, 153
of ocular alignment, syndromes characterized by, 254-262
in orbital slant, syndromes characterized by, 243-254
of palpebral fissures, 79
associated with phenytoin ingestion, 333-335
in position of head, 97-98

Abnormalities—cont'd
involving posture and protrusion of tongue, 96
of proximal nose, 76-77
pupillary, 62-66
involving size and protrusion of eyes, 60-62
of teeth, 93
syndromes characterized by, 337-338
of tongue, 93-97, 338-344
topographic, 96-97
topographic, 91
in total facial contour and size, syndromes characterized by, 360-376
Achondroplasia, 138-140
craniofacial abnormalities in, 138
macrocephaly in, 138
mental retardation in, 140
somatic features of, 138-140
Acne vulgaris, 76
Acrobrachycephalies, 107-117
without pronounced digital deformity, 114-116
Acrocephalopolysyndactyly, 110
Acrocephalosyndactyly
type I, 108
type II, 110
type III, 111
type IV, 111
type V, 112
type VI, 114
Acrocephaly, 108
Acromegaly, 328, 329
Addisonian bronzing, 388-391
Addison's disease, 388
Adenoma sebaceum, 75, 76
of Balzer, 279
of Pringle, 279
in tuberous sclerosis, 278-279
Adie's syndrome, 204, 205
Adrenoleukodystrophy, 389, 411-414, 416
Adrenomyeloneuropathy, 389
Adult face, 30
Aging, facial syndrome, 382-385
Aging process and face, 31
Aglossia, 96
Albers-Schonberg syndrome, 421
Albinism
oculocutaneous, 385-386, 387
partial, 172
Albright's hereditary osteodystrophy, 169, 364
Albright's polyostotic fibrous dysplasia, 175
Alcohol syndrome, fetal, 241
Alexander's disease, 149, 411

Alopecia and baldness, 166-169
Alopecia areata, 169
Alper's disease, 411
Amaurotic familial idiocies, 148, 411
Anencephaly, 135, 156-158
Aneurysms, 231
  galenic, hydrocephalus caused by, 133
Angiofibroma, 76
  in tuberous sclerosis, 282
Angiofibromatosis in patients with tuberous sclerosis, 281
Angioneurotic edema, 94
Angioosteohypertrophy of Klipper-Trenaunay-Weber, 313
Anisocoria, 63, 203
Ankyloglossum superius syndrome, 403
Anomalies, congenital, of intracranial vessels, 231
Anophthalmia, 62, 71, 195
Anoxia, perinatal cerebral, 322
Antecollis, 98
Anticonvulsant administration, chronic, 333-335
Antimongoloid slanting, 79, 247-254
Apert's syndrome, 108-110, 252
  facial appearance of patient with, 116
Aqueductal stenosis, 130-133
  acquired, 133
Arachnodactyly, congenital contractural, syndrome of, 361-362
Arcus senilis, 66
Argentosis, 388
Argininosuccinicaciduria, 169
Argyll Robertson pupil, 64, 204
Arnold-Chiari syndrome, 130-131, 134-135
Arteriovenous malformation, deep, 133
A-shaped tilt, 79
Astrocytomas, 190
Ataxia, myoclonic, with multiple cranial nerve palsies, 258-259
Ataxia-plus, myoclonic, syndrome, 259
Ataxia-telangiectasia, 76, 223-227, 416-418
  major abnormalities of, 225
Atrophy
  hemifacial, 201, 395, 396
  and hypoplasia of tongue, 95-96
  spinal muscular, progressive, 342-343, 344
  of tongue, 96
Aural points, 17

**B**

Bacterial meningitides as cause of subdural effusion, 155-156
Baldness
  and alopecia, 166-169
  frontal, 167
Balzer, adenoma sebaceum of, 279
Banded tongue, 96
Beckwith-Wiedemann syndrome, 341-342, 343
Bell's palsy, 300-301
Bell's phenomenon, 235

Beta-glucuronidase deficiency, 215
Bielschowsky-Jansky syndrome, 410, 411, 412
Birthmarks, 91, 92
  and hemihyperplasia of lower face, syndromes characterized by, 311-316
  and other skin blemishes, 73-76
Bones
  eosinophilic granuloma of, 336-337
  major, of newborn skull, 10-11
Bony orbits, lateral, and zygomata, 77-79
Bourneville's disease, 277-282
Bra in masses, 231
Brachial plexus palsy, 287
Brachmann-DeLange syndrome, 372
Brachial plexus neuritis
  familial, 270
    recurrent, 247
Brachial plexus palsy, 287
Brachycephaly, 118
Brachycollis, 100
  and pterygium colli, syndromes characterized by, 353-358
Brachyfacial and fat facial syndromes, 364-372
Brachyfacial person, 18
Brain
  herniation of, 231
  smooth, 160
Branchial arch, 5-9, 11, 13
  first
    abnormalities of, 91
    syndromes, 247-254, 298-299, 332-333
Broad thumbs syndrome, 248-250
Bronzing, addisonian, 388-391
Brow line, 14
Brushfield spots, 65-66
Buccal surface and gums, 92-93
  abnormalities of, syndromes characterized by, 333-337
Buphthalmos, 60-61, 191-195

**C**

C syndrome, 247
"Café-au-lait spots," 189-190
Calcifications, "railroad track," 194-195
Calcifying epitheliomas, 180
Caloric nystagmus, 70
Canavan's disease, 149, 411
Canthal lines, 17
Canthus, displaced, 22-24
Canthus-iris relationships, 23
Carbon monoxide poisoning, 345
Carnitine myopathy, 326
Carotid cavernous arteriovenous fistula, 227, 228
Carpenter's syndrome, 110
  facial appearance of patient with, 116
Cataract, congenital, syndromes, 218
Cat's eye syndrome, 201, 247, 252, 273, 274, 350, 371-372
Cebocephaly, 265
Central lower face; *see* Lower face, central

Central middle face; *see* Middle face, central
Cephalus, extreme, 108
Cerebral dysgenesis, 162
Cerebral gigantism, 350
    and abnormal jaws, syndromes characterized
        by, 328-333
Cerebrohepatorenal syndrome, 364, 365
Cerebrooculofacioskeletal syndrome, 243
Cerebrosidoses, 145
Cerebrotendinous xanthomatosis, 243, 244
Ceroid-lipofuscinosis, neuronal, 169-170, 260-
        262, 410, 411, 412
Cheeks
    abnormalities of, 88
    and mouth, 27-29, 83-84
Cherubism, 328-332
Child abuse and neglect, 154-155, 162
Chin
    abnormalities of, 90
        syndromes characterized by, 325-326
    and jaws, 29, 90-91
        abnormalities of, 91
    triangular, syndromes of, 326-327
Chondrodysplasia punctata, 247
Chondrodystrophy; *see* Achondroplasia
Chorea
    benign familial, 322
    Huntington's, 322, 415
    Sydenham's, 322
Choroid plexus papilloma, 135
Chotzen's syndrome, 111
Chromosome abnormalities, holoprosencephaly
        associated with, 267
Cleft lip and palate, 83-84
    syndromes characterized by, 296-299
Cleidocranial dysostosis, 123
Cleidocranial dysplasia, 350
Cloverleaf dysostosis, 123
Cloverleaf skull anomalad, 252
Coarse facial syndromes, 372-376
Cockayne's syndrome, 161, 200, 378-382
    facial features of, 378
    neurologic symptoms and signs of, 378
    variant of, 380-381
Collagen disease, 231
Coloboma, iridal, syndromes characterized by,
        201
Congenital toxoplasmosis, 68
Conjunctiva, syndromes characterized by abnor-
        malities of, 223-229
Conjunctival telangiectasis, 76, 225
Conjunctival vessels, dilated, syndromes involv-
        ing, 227-229
Conradi's syndrome, 247
Corectasis, 63
Cornea and lens, syndromes characterized by
        abnormalities of, 210-218
Corneal clouding syndromes, 213-215
Corneal reflection sign, 21, 22-24, 66-68
Coronal suture, premature closure of, 116
Coup de sabre, 175-176, 276-277

Cover-uncover test, 67
Cowden's syndrome, 391-393
Cranial base, 8
Cranial lines, vertical, 16
Cranial nerve palsies, multiple, myoclonic
        ataxia with, 258-259
Cranial neurocutaneopathies, 172-180
Cranial points, upper, 17
Cranial poliosis and white forelocks, 170-172
Cranial shagreen patch, 173
Cranial skin, congenital absence of, 169
Cranial sutures, syndromes characterized by
        premature closures of, 104-122
Cranial and upper facial segment, 19-20
    syndromes of, 102-180
Craniocarpotarsal dysplasia, 320
Craniodysostoses, 298
Cranioface, segments of, 8-9
Craniofacial abnormalities
    in achondroplasia, 138
    caused by subdural effusions, 153
Craniofacial dysostosis, 119
Craniofacial leukoderma, 170, 175, 206, 284,
        406
    of Sugarman-Reed, 284-285
Cranioplastic abnormalities, 153
Craniosynostoses, 104
Craniotelencephalic dysplasia, 128, 270
Cranium
    embryologic formation of, 11
    and face, embryogenesis of, 5-13
Cretinism, 339-342
Cri-du-chat syndrome, 273, 274, 371-372
Cross' syndrome, 201, 215, 335, 386
Crouzon's syndrome, 119-122
    milder forms of, 120
    somatic findings in, 119
Cryptophthalmos syndrome, 197
"Cushingoid syndrome," 370
Cushing's syndrome, 370
Cutaneous pigmentary lesions, diffuse, syn-
        dromes characterized by, 385
Cutaneous and subcutaneous involvement, gen-
        eralized, disorders with, 395-397
Cutis laxa, 393
Cyclopia, 265
Cyclopic monster, 195
Cytogenic disorders, 349-350

**D**

Dandy-Walker syndrome, 130, 133-135
Darier's syndrome, 393
de Grouchy's syndrome, 267, 350
Deformities, osseous, 117
DeLange-Brachmann syndrome, 323
DeLange's syndrome, 166, 169, 171, 273-276,
        360, 372
Dementia syndromes, 407-414
Dementia-emaciation syndrome, 170, 381
DeMorsier's syndrome, 201
DeSanctis-Cacchione syndrome, 393-394

Devic's neuromyelitis optica, 285, 286
Diabetes mellitus, 231, 300
Diastrophic dwarfism, 299
Diencephalic syndrome, 378, 379
Diparesis, facial, 87-88
   or facial palsy, syndromes characterized by,
      299-311
Diplegia, facial, 87-88
Disproportion, fiber-type, congenital, 326
Dolichofacial person, 18
Dolichoscaphocephalies, 104-106
Dolichostenocollis, syndromes characterized by,
      349-353
Dolichostenofacial person, 18
Dolichostenofacial syndromes, 360-364
Dolicocollis, 99
Donohue's syndrome, 170, 382
Down's syndrome, 207-208, 245-247, 322-323,
      339
   phenotypical, 247
   true, 247
Down-turned mouths, 89
Dreschfield-Taylor-Erickson syndrome, 247
Duane's retraction syndrome, 308
Dwarfism
   diastrophic, 299
   Montreal-type, 384-385
   nanocephalic, 159
   pituitary, 384
   Seckel's bird-headed, 159-160
Dysgenesis, cerebral, 162
Dyskinesia
   senile orofacial, 322
   tardive, 322
Dysmigration, 204-206
Dysmigration syndrome, 175
Dysostosis
   cleidocranial, 123
   cloverleaf, 123
   craniofacial, 119
   mandibulofacial, 333
   otomandibular, 196
Dysplasia
   cleidocranial, 350
   craniocarpotarsal, 252, 320, 421
   craniotelencephalic, 128, 270
   ectodermal, 169, 337-338
   fibrous, 175
      Albright's polyostotic, 175
   frontonasal, 128, 273
   oculodento-osseus, 201
   septo-optic, 201
Dystonia musculorum deformans, 243, 322,
      344-348
Dystonias, symptomatic, 345
Dystopia canthorum, 22-24, 60, 72
Dystrophia myotonia, 232, 234, 235, 405
Dystrophia myotonica, 167, 179, 301-307, 338,
      349, 350, 399, 401
   congenital, 264, 291
   distal, congenital, with prognathism, 329-332

Dystrophia myotonica—cont'd
   early-onset form of, 304
   facial stigmata in, 302-324
Dystrophy
   infantile neuroaxonal, 421
   muscular, facioscapulohumeral, 349
   osteochondromuscular, 318-320, 321
   Settelberger's infantile neuroaxonal, 419-421

E

Ears, 79-81
   abnormalities of, 80
      syndromes characterized by, 285-294
   external, embryologic formation of, 12
   frontal facial viewing of, 79
   jug, 81
   large and floppy, syndromes of, 290-291
   lobules of, large, 81
   low-set, syndromes of, 285-290
   normal, 25-26
   protruding, 81
   set of, 26
   syndromes of, 291-294
Eaton-Lambert syndrome, 232
Ectoderm, 5
Ectodermal dysplasia, 169, 337-338
Edema, angioneurotic, 94
Edwards' syndrome, 252
EEC syndrome, 298
Ehlers-Danlos syndrome, 393
Elastolysis, generalized, 393
Elfin-facies syndrome, 215
Emaciation, facial, syndromes, 378-382
Embryo, human, frontal aspect of, 6
Embryogenesis of face and cranium, 5-13
Embryologic formation
   of cranium, 11
   of external ear, 12
   of eye, 11-12
   of lower face, 12-13
   of middle face, 11-12, 59
   of nose, 12
Embryonic face, adult analogues of, 7
Embryonic parts, facial derivatives of, 7
Empyema, subdural, 156
Encephalitis periaxialis diffusa, 389
Encephaloceles, 126
Encephalomyelopathy, subacute necrotizing,
      257
   hypoxic, 165-166
   Leigh's, 238
   TORCH, 161-162
"Encephalotrigeminal hemangiomatosis," 191
Endoderm, 5
End-position nystagmus, 70
Enophthalmos, 62, 71
Eosinophilic granuloma of bone, 336-337
Epicanthal fold, 22, 71-72
Epitheliomas, calcifying, 180
Erythematosus, lupus, 333
Esotropia, 68

Esotropia—cont'd
  progressive, syndromes of, 256
Ethmocephaly, 265
Exophthalmos, 60-61, 182-185
  and proptosis, distinction between, 61
Exotropia, 68
  other degenerative diseases associated with,
      262
External lower face; see Lower face, external
Extrapyramidal facies, 415-421
Eyeball
  malalignment of, 66-68
  movements of, spontaneous, abnormal, 70
  syndromes of, dissociative, and multiple scle-
      rosis, 254-256
Eyelid
  abnormalities of, 70-72
    syndromes characterized by, 229-243
  development of, 12
  upper, drooping of, 70
Eyes, 59-72
  abnormalities involving size and protrusion
      of, 60-62
  distances between, abnormalities of, 73
  embryologic formation of, 11-12
  measurement of distances between, 21-22
  movements of, abnormal, 68-70
  myopic, 63
  normal, 20
    proportions of, 21
  pupillary abnormalities of, 62-66
  slanting of, 78-79
  structures of, 20-24

**F**

Fabry's disease, 148
Face
  abnormalities of; see Abnormalities, facial
  adult, 30
  and aging process, 31
  aging syndrome of, 382-385
  central lower; see Lower face, central
  contour and size of, total, abnormalities in,
      syndromes characterized by, 360-376
  and cranium, embryogenesis of, 5-13
  diparesis syndromes of, 401-403
  division of, 8-9
  emaciation syndrome of, 378-382
  embryonic, adult analogues of, 7
  external lower; see Lower face, external
  features of
    general, 29-30
    nomenclature in describing, 3-4
  growth of, 30-32
  internal lower; see Lower face, internal
  lower; see Lower face
  middle; see Middle face
  nerve lesions of, upper-motor, 85
  normal, 1-31
  total, syndromes of, 359-422
Facial and cranial segment, upper, 19-20

Facial and cranial segment, upper—cont'd
  syndromes of, 102-180
Facial derivatives of embryonic parts, 7
Facial diplegia and diparesis, 87-88
Facial expression
  abnormal, syndromes of, 397-422
  peculiar, syndromes characterized by, 414-422
  syndromes, other peculiar, 421-422
Facial gestalt, 3
Facial hirsutism, 91, 169-170
Facial immobility, syndromes characterized by,
      399-403
Facial lines; see Lines, facial
Facial observation, 2-5
  improving skills in, 4-5
  of mother, 2
  of physician, 2-3
  process of, 3
  systematized approach, 2
Facial palsy, 299-311
  complete or peripheral, 86
  and paresis, unilateral, 85-87
Facial paresis
  extrapyramidal, 86
  long-standing, unilateral, 87
Facial proportion, normal, 17-18
Facial segments; see Segments
Facies
  extrapyramidal, 415-421
  Potter, 385
Facioscapulohumeral muscular dystrophy, 309,
      349
Farber's lipogranulomatosis, 148
Fat facial and brachyfacial syndromes, 364-372
Fetal alcohol syndrome, 241
Fetal face syndrome, 372
Fever, 103
Fibrous dysplasia, 175
  Albright's polyostotic, 175
First-arch syndromes, 285-290
Fish mouths, 89
Fistula, arteriovenous, 186, 228
  acquired, 186
    cavernous-carotid, 186-187, 227, 228
  congenital, 186
Floppy-baby syndromes, 342-343
Fluid accumulations, traumatic subdural, 153
Fontanels, major, of newborn skull, 10-11
Frohlich's syndrome, 370
Frontal aspect of human embryo, 6
Frontal bossing syndromes, 126-129
Frontonasal dysplasia, 128, 273
Frontonasal process, 5-9, 11, 13
Frontonasal prominence, 8
Furrowed tongue, 96

**G**

Galactosemia, 218-220
Galenic aneurysm, hydrocephalus caused by,
      133
Gangliosidoses, 141

Gangliosidoses—cont'd
  GM$_1$, 145
  GM$_2$, 411
Gaucher's disease, 130, 145
Gaze, conjugate dissociation in, 255
Gerodermia osteodysplastica hereditaria, 385
Gestalt, facial, 3
Gigantism, cerebral, 350
  and abnormal jaws, syndromes characterized by, 328-333
Gingival abnormalities, 92
Gingival hyperplasia, 333-336
Giraffism, 99, 352-353
Glaucoma, 193-194
  congenital, 216
Glioma, pontine, 256-257, 258
β-Glucuronidase deficiency, 215
Goiter, acquired, 340
Goldenhar's syndrome, 229, 252, 253, 291
Goltz's syndrome, 201
Granuloma, eosinophilic, 336
Graves' disease, 182, 184
Grieg's syndrome, 272-273
Growth, facial, 30-32
Gums and buccal surface, 92-93
  abnormalities of, syndromes characterized by, 333-337

**H**

Hair, 29
  abnormalities of, syndromes characterized by, 166-172
  facial, excessive, 91, 169-170
Hairline, nasal line, 14
Half-and-half syndrome, 207-209, 395
Hallermann-Streiff syndromes, 169, 199-200, 215, 251-252, 333
Hallervorden-Spatz syndrome, 320-322, 323, 327, 333, 345
  facial features of, 322
Hand-Schuller-Christian syndrome, 336-337
Hanhart's syndrome, 403
Happy puppet syndrome, 96, 146-148, 343-344
Harada's syndrome, 206
Head
  abnormalities in position of, 97-98
  injuries of, acute, 231
  posture of, abnormal, syndromes characterized by, 344-349
  tilt of, 98
  water, 130
Heavy metal poisonings, 169
Hemangioma
  mixed, 399
    cavernous, Klippel-Trénaunay syndrome with, 397
    Riley-Smith syndrome with, 397
  pia-arachnoid, 193
  port wine, 191, 312
  scaphocephaly syndrome, midline, 105-106, 107, 108

Hematoma, subdural
  acute, 153
  chronic, 154
Hemifacial atrophy, 395, 396
Hemihyperplasia and birthmarks of lower face, syndromes characterized by, 311-316
Hemiplegia-hemihypoplasia-hemiathetosis syndrome, 348-349
  hereditary, 262
Hemochromatosis, 388
*Hemophilus influenzae*, 155
Hepatolenticular degeneration, 420
  Wilson's, 345
Herpes zoster infections, 285, 286
Hess, N syndrome of, 364
Heterochromia, 65
  syndromes, 206-210
Heterotropia, 68, 69
  nonprogressive, 262
Hirsutism, facial, 91, 169-170
Histiocytosis X, 231, 336-337
Holoprosencephalic anomalad, alobar, 297-298
Holoprosencephalies, 135, 195, 264-267, 296-298
  associated with chromosome abnormalities, 267
  semilobar, 266-267
Homocystinuria, 220-221, 362-363
  clinical picture of, 221
  facial features of, 221-223
Horizontal lines
  facial, 14-16
  major, 15
  mental, 14
  midfacial, 14
  oral, 14
  vertex, 14
Horizontal segments, major, 18-19
Horner's syndrome, 202-206, 229, 231
  acquired, 202
  congenital, 204-206
  sympathetic disturbance in, 202
Hunter mucopolysaccharidoses, 169
Hunter-Hurler megalencephaly, 141
Hunter's syndrome, 273, 275, 372-375
Huntington's chorea, 322, 415
Hurler mucopolysaccharidoses, 169
Hurler-Hunter varieties of mucopolysaccharidoses, 291, 292
Hurler's syndrome, 213, 215, 341, 372-375
Hurler-Scheie syndrome, 215
Hutchinson-Gilford progeria, 169
Hutchinson-Gilford syndrome, 382-384
  variant of, 384
Hyaline neuropathy, megalencephaly associated with, 149
Hyalinosis cutis et mucosae, 394-395
Hydranencephaly, 135-137
  and hydrocephalus, distinction between, 137
  transillumination as sign for, 137
  true nature of, 135
Hydrocephalies, 130-138

Hydrocephalies—cont'd
   congenital malformation syndromes causing, 130
   caused by galenic aneurysm, 133
   and hydranencephaly, distinction between, 137
Hypercalcemia, infantile, 215, 217
Hyperpigmentation syndromes, diffuse, 386-390
Hyperplasia
   gingival, 333-336
   midface, 73, 74
Hypertelorism, 73, 263
   median cleft face syndrome with, 128
   ocular, 22
   syndromes, 270
Hyperthyroidism, 182-185
Hypertrichosis universalis congenita, 170
Hypertropia, 68
Hypoglossia-hypodactylia syndrome, 403
Hypoparathyroidism, idiopathic, 169
Hypopigmentation syndromes, diffuse, 385-386, 387
Hypoplasia
   and atrophy of tongue, 95-96
   focal dermal, 201
   midface, 73, 74
   otoculomandibular, 196
Hypotelorism, 73, 263
   syndromes, 267-270
Hypothyroidism, 243
   acquired infantile, with goiter, 325-326
   congenital, 339, 340
   nongoitrous, 339
Hypotrichosis, 169
Hypotropia, 68
Hypoxia, perinatal cerebral, 345
Hypoxic encephalopathy, 165-166

I
Idiocies, amaurotic
   familial, 411
   juvenile, 260-262
Idiopathic hypoparathyroidism, 169
Immobile face syndromes, 403
Infantile neuroaxonal dystrophy, 421
Infantile osteopetrosis, 421
Intercanthal line, 14, 15
Internal lower face; see Lower face, internal
Internuclearis ophthalmoplegia, 418, 419
Intracranial vessels, congenital anomalies of, 231
Iris
   abnormalities of, 65
   colobomas of, 210
   color changes in, 66
   development of, 12
   and pupil, abnormalities of, syndromes characterized by, 202-210
Iris-canthus relationships, 23

J
Jadassohn, nevus of, 178
Jakob-Creutzfelt disease, 407
Jaws
   abnormal, and cerebral gigantism, syndromes characterized by, 328-333
   angle points of, 14, 17
   angled, 91
   and chin, 29, 90-91
      abnormalities of, 91
Jug ear, 81
Juvenile amaurotic idiocy, neuronal ceroidlipofuscinosis, 260-262

K
Kayser-Fleischer ring, 66, 212, 213
Kearns-Sayre syndrome, 238-240
Kernicterus, 322
Kleeblättschadel syndrome, 123
Klinefelter's syndrome, 349, 351, 364
Klippel-Feil anomalad, 323, 353-355, 356
Klippel-Trénaunay syndrome, 313-314, 398
   with cavernous hemangioma, 397
Klüver-Bucy syndrome, 169
Krabbe's disease, 145, 411
Krabbe's globoid cell leukodystrophy, 184-185
Kuru, 407

L
Labial line, canthal, 17
Laron's type dwarfism, 384
Laron's type panhypopituitarism, 384
Larsen's syndrome, 270-271, 272, 299
Lateral canthal lines, 17
Laurence-Moon-Biedl syndrome, 370
Lawrence-Berardinelli syndrome, 382
Leather patch, 173
Leigh's disease, 257
Leigh's subacute necrotizing encephalomyelopathy, 238
Lejeune syndrome, 252
Lens
   development of, 12
   syndromes characterized by abnormalities of, 218-223
Lenticular syndromes, 220-223
Lentigines, multiple, 394
Lentiginosis, central facial, 394, 395
Lenz, microphthalmia syndrome of, 197-198, 215
Leopard syndrome, 394
Leprechaunism, 382
Leprosy, 239, 309-311, 395, 396
   causes of, 309
   lepromatous, 169
Lesch-Nyhan syndrome, 316
   facial features of, 318
   syndromes similar to, 318
Lesions
   acute oculomotor, 231

Lesions—cont'd
  nerve
    lower-motor, 86
    shock type, 85
    upper-motor facial, 85
Letterer-Siwe syndrome, 336-337
Leukemia, 231
Leukoderma
  and adenoma sebaceum, tuberous sclerosis with, 397
  congenital, 282-285
  craniofacial, 170, 175, 206, 284, 406
    congenital, 317
    of Sugarman-Reed, 284-285
Leukodystrophy, 149, 388-389
  Krabbe's globoid cell, 184-185
  metachromatic, 145, 389, 411
Linear scleroderma, 176
Lines
  brow, 14
  canthal, 17
  cranial, vertical, 16
  facial, 13-18
    horizontal, 14-16
    oblique, 17
    vertical, 16-17
  horizontal, major, 14, 15
  intercanthal, 14, 15
  mental, upper, 14
  nasal, hairline, 14
  oblique, major, 18
  pupillary, vertical, 17
  vertical
    major, 16
    midfacial, 16-17
Lipidoses, 141
  sulfatide, 145
Lipodystrophy
  congenital, 382
  facial, 399
Lipogranulomatosis, Farber's, 148
Lipoid proteinosis, 394-395
Lips
  abnormalities of, 89
  abnormally large, 89-90
  cleft, 83-84, 296-299
  mutilated and abnormally positioned, syndromes characterized by, 316-322
  upper
    tenting of, 87-88
    thin, 89
Lissencephalic syndrome, 160-161, 170
Lobulated tongue, 97
Louis-Barr, ataxia-telangiectasia of, 226
Lower face
  central, 83-84
    syndromes of, 296
  embryologic formation of, 12-13
  external, 28, 83-91
  internal, 92-97
  peripheral, 90-91

Lower face—cont'd
  peripheral—cont'd
    syndromes of, 325-333
Lower facial segment, 27-29
  and neck
    abnormalities of, 82-101
    syndromes of, 295-358
Lower-motor nerve lesions, 86
Lowe's oculocerebrorenal syndrome, 201, 218
Lupus erythematosus, 76, 333

M
Macrocephaly
  in achondroplasia, 138
  simple, syndromes characterized by, 130-156
  from subdural accumulations, 149-156
Macroglossia, 93-94
  acquired, 94
  and other tongue abnormalities, syndromes characterized by, 338-344
Macrophthalmia, 60-61
  and pseudomacrophthalmia, distinction between, 61
Macrostomia or microstomia, syndromes characterized by, 322-325
Mandible, primitive, 13
Mandibulofacial dysostosis, 333
Maple syrup urine disease, 149
Marden-Walker syndrome, 320, 403, 421
Marfanian habitus, 221
Marfan's syndrome, 221, 223, 350, 360-364
  clinical features of, 360-361
  facial features of, 360-361
  variants of, 362
Marinesco-Sjogren syndrome, 200-201, 215, 218-220
Maroteaux-Lamy syndrome, 215
Maxilla, primitive, 13
Measles, 407
Meckel's syndrome, 270, 299
Medial canthal lines, 17
Median cleft face syndrome, 273
  with hypertelorism, 128
Megalencephaly, 141-149
  Hunter-Hurler, 141
  associated with hyaline neuropathy, 149
  syndromes characterized by, 141
Megalocornea, 61, 215, 217
  syndromes of, 215-218
Melkersson-Rosthenal syndrome, 300, 309-311, 341, 342
Melnick and Needles, osteodysplasty of, 350
Meningitides, bacterial, as cause of subdural effusion, 155
Menkes' kinky hair syndrome, 169
Mental line
  horizontal, 14
  upper, 14
Mental point, 14
Mental retardation syndromes, 403-407
Mesenchyma, 5

Mesoderm, 5
Metachromatic leukodystrophy, 145, 411, 389
Methionine breakdown, 221
Microcephaly
  causes of, 161-162
  primary, 158-161
  secondary, 161-166
  syndromes characterized by, 156-166
Micrognathia, 90
Microphthalmia, 62, 71, 195-201
  Lenz's type of, 197-198, 215
Microstomia or macrostomia, syndromes char-
    acterized by, 322-325
Middle face
  central, syndromes of, 182-277
  cutaneous lesions of, 75
  embryologic formation of, 11-12
  lateral
    skin blemish syndromes of, 282-285
    syndromes of, 277-294
Middle facial segment, 20-27
  abnormalities of, 58-81
  embryologic origin, 59
  syndromes of, 181-294
Midface hypoplasia and hyperplasia, 73, 74
Midface proper, 26-27
  and nasal base, 72-76
Midfacial line
  horizontal, 14
  vertical, 16-17
Midline hemangioma-scaphocephaly syndrome,
    105-106
Miosis, 63
Mitochondrial myopathies, 238
Mitten hands, 108
MMM syndrome, 268, 323-325
Moebius' sign, 183
Moebius' syndrome, 235, 307-309, 399, 403
  diagnosis of, 308
Mohr's syndrome, 111-112
Mongoloid slanting, 77-79
Mongoloid syndromes, 245-247
Monilethrix, 169
Monosomy 21 and 21 q− syndrome, 252
Montreal-type dwarfism, 384-385
Morquio's syndrome, 215
Mouth
  abnormalities of, 28-29, 88-90
  and cheeks, 27-29, 83-84
  corners of, 14
  down-turned, 89
  fish, 89
  internal, 29, 92
  primitive, 13
  puckered, 88
Mucolipidoses, 339-341, 376
Mucopolysaccharidoses, 141, 213, 215, 275, 339-
    341, 372
  excessive facial hair in, 169-170
  facial features of, 375-376, 377
  Hunter forms of, 215, 374

Mucopolysaccharidoses—cont'd
  Hurler-Hunter varieties of, 291, 292
  Sanfilippo's, 172
Multiple mucosal neuroma syndrome, 350
Multiple pterygium syndrome, 299
Multiple sclerosis, 418, 419
  and other dissociative eyeball syndromes,
    254-256
  symptoms and signs of, 255
Multisegmental involvement, syndromes of,
    360-397
Mumps, 300
Murray-Puretic syndrome, 335-336
Muscular atrophy, spinal, progressive, 342-343,
    344
Muscular dystrophy, 349
  facioscapulohumeral, 234, 237, 309, 349, 403
  myotonic, 232, 234, 235, 262
Myasthenia gravis, 232-233, 399
  congenital, 232
  late, 238
Myasthenoid syndrome, 232
Mydriasis, 63
Myoclonic ataxia with multiple cranial nerve
    palsies, 258-259
Myoclonic ataxia-plus, 405
  syndrome of, 259
Myoclonus, 407, 408, 409
Myopathy
  carnitine, 326
  mitochondrial, 238
  nemaline, 241, 326, 349, 403
Myotonic dystrophy, 301-307
  distal, congenital, with prognathism, 329-332
  muscular, 232, 234, 235, 262
Myotonic eye sign, 236

N

N syndrome, 170, 270, 350-351, 382
  of Hess, 364
Nanocephalic dwarfism, 159
Nasal base
  and bridge, variations in, 25
  and midface proper, 72-76
Nasal bridge and tip, 76-77
Nasal line hairline, 14
Nasal placodes, 12
Nasolabial fold, 87
Neck
  abnormalities of, 82-101
  excessively short and broad, 101
  extremely long, 98
  and lower facial segment, syndromes of, 295-
    358
  syndromes of, 344-358
  torter, congenital absence of, 98
  webbed, 101
Nemaline myopathy, 231, 326, 349, 403
Nerve lesions
  lower-motor, 86
  release type, 85

Nerve lesions — cont'd
  shock type, 85
  upper-motor facial, 85
Neural crest, 5
Neuritis, familial brachial plexus, 270
Neurocutaneopathies, cranial, 172-180
Neuroectoderm, 5
Neurofibromatosis, 175, 187-190, 314-315
Neurogenic abnormalities, 153
Neuromuscular disorders, 349
Neuromyelitis optica, Devic's, 285, 286
Neuronal ceroid-lipofuscinosis, 169-170, 260-262, 410, 411, 412
Nevus (nevi)
  craniofacial, Sturge-Weber syndrome with, 397
  of Jadassohn, 178
  organoid, 178
  port wine, 312, 313
  telangiectatic, 225, 227
Nevus flammeus, 400
  midline, 228
  port wine, 192
Newborn skull, major bones, sutures, and fontanels of, 10-11
Niemann-Pick disease, 145
Nomenclature in describing facial features, 3-4
Nonchromosomal dysplastic syndromes, 350
Noonan's syndrome, 252, 270, 271, 358
Normal face, 1-31
Nose, 24-25
  distal, abnormalities of, 77
  embryologic formation of, 12
  middle, abnormalities of, 77
  of normal face, 24
  proximal, abnormalities of, 76-77
  saddle, 77
  of sarcoidosis, 77
  variations in, 25
Notochord, 5
Nystagmus, 68-69
  caloric, 70
  end-position, 70
  opticokinetic, 68-69
  rotational, 70

O

Oblique facial lines, 17
  major, 18
Observation, facial; see Facial observation
Ocular alignment
  abnormal, syndromes characterized by, 254-262
  test of, 66-67
Ocular hypertelorism, 22, 270
Ocular protrusion and abnormal size, syndromes characterized by, 182-201
Oculocutaneous albinism, 385-386, 387
Oculomotor palsy, 203-204
ODO syndrome, 201
OFD II syndrome, 298

OPD syndrome, 252, 293, 298-299, 422
Ophthalmoplegia
  acute, 229-231
  internuclear, 255
Ophthalmoplegia-plus syndrome, 238
Opitz trigonocephaly syndrome, 247
Opticocochleodentatic degeneration, 162, 262, 413
Opticokinetic nystagmus, 68-69
Oral cavity
  small, 93
  syndromes of, 333-344
Oral line, horizontal, 14
Orbital slant, abnormalities in, syndromes characterized by, 243-254
Oromandibular-limb hypogenesis syndrome, 403
Osseous deformities, 117
Osteochondromuscular dystrophy, 318-320, 321
Osteodysplasty of Melnick and Needles, 350
Osteodystrophy, hereditary, Albright's, 169, 364
Osteopetrosis, infantile, 421
Otic placodes, 12
Otopalatodigital syndrome, 293, 298-299, 422
Oxycephaly, 108
Oxyturricephaly, 119

P

Palate, cleft, 83-84, 296-299
  and cleft lip, 83-84
Palpebral fissures, abnormalities of, 79
Palsy
  Bell's, 300-301
  brachial plexus, 287
  facial, 299-311
    complete or peripheral, 86
    or facial diparesis, syndromes characterized by, 299-311
    and paresis, unilateral, 85-87
  oculomotor, 203-204
Panencephalitis, subacute sclerosing, 335, 389, 407, 411
Papilloma, choroid plexus, 135
Paralysis, idiopathic, 300-301
Paresis, facial
  extrapyramidal, 86
  and facial palsy, unilateral, 85-87
  long-standing unilateral, 87
Parietal points, 19-20
Parkinson's disease, 415, 416
Parry-Romberg syndrome, 175, 201, 276-277, 395, 396
Pelizaeus-Merzbacher disease, 262, 263, 411
Pfeiffer's syndrome, 114
Phenylketonuria, 172, 386
  alobar, 266-267, 268
  maternal, 166
Phenytoin treatment, 169
  abnormalities associated with, 333-335
Pierré Robin anomalad, 299
Pituitary dwarfism, 384

Pituitary dysfunctions, 231
Pituitary gigantism, acromegaly, 328, 329
Placodes
  aural, 17
  cranial, upper, 17
  jaw angle, 14, 17
  mental, 14
  nasal, 12
  otic, 12
  parietal, 19-20
  vertex, 14
Poisonings, heavy metal, 169
Poland's anomaly, 307, 308
Poliosis, cranial, and white forelocks, 170-172
Pontine glioma, 256-257, 258
Port wine hemangioma, 312
Port wine nevus, 312, 313
  flammeus, 172-173
Port wine stain, 191-193, 285, 288
Potter facies, 385
Potter's syndrome, 293, 385
Prader-Willi syndrome, 367-370
  etiology of, 369
  facial features of, 369
  neonatal and infantile features in, 369
Pringle, adenoma sebaceum of, 279
Proboscis, 77, 265
Progeria, 172, 382-384
  Hutchinson-Gilford, 169
Prognathism, 90
  congenital, myotonic distal dystrophy with, 329-332
  syndromes of, 328-332
Proptosis, 60-61, 185-190
  and exophthalmos, distinction between, 61
Proteinosis, lipoid, 394-395
Protruding ears, 81
Pseudohypoparathyroidism, 364-367
Pseudomacroglossia, 94
Pseudomacrophthalmia, 60-61
  and macrophthalmia, distinction between, 61
Pseudomicrophthalmia, 62
Pseudomucopolysaccharidosis, 377
Pseudo-pseudohypoparathyroidism, 364-367
Pseudoptosis, 70-71, 229
Pseudoxanthoma elasticum, 393
Pterygium colli, 100, 101
  and brachycollis, syndromes characterized by, 353-358
Ptosis, 70
  syndromes of, 229-241
Puckered mouth, 88
Pupils
  abnormalities of, 62-66
  Argyll Robertson, 64, 204
  asymmetry of, 63-64
  and iris, syndromes characterized by abnormalities of, 202-210
  irregularly shaped, 64
  lines of, vertical, 17
  reaction of, to light, 62

Pupils—cont'd
  resting, size and shape of, 63
  size of, 62-63
  wilsonian, 64-65

Q
Q sign, 96

R
"Railroad track" calcifications, 194-195
Ramsay Hunt's syndrome, 294
Release type nerve lesions, 85
Reticuloendothelioses, 336-337
Retina, development of, 11-12
Retrocollis, 98
Riley-Day syndrome, 422
Riley-Smith syndrome with mixed hemangioma, 397
Roberts' syndrome, 299
Rotational nystagmus, 70
Rothmund-Thomson syndrome, 384
Rubinstein-Taybi syndrome, 114, 248-250, 323

S
Saddle nose, 77
Saethre-Chotzen syndrome, 111
Sandhoff's disease, 141
Sanfilippo mucopolysaccharidoses, 169, 172, 215, 375-376
Sanfilippo's syndromes, 215, 375-376
Sarcoidosis, 231, 300
  nose in, 77
Scaphocephaly, 104
Scarred tongue, 97
Scheie's syndrome, 215
Schilder's disease, 389
Schwartz-Jampel syndrome, 241, 243, 318-320, 321, 403, 421, 422
  facial features of, 320
Scleroderma, 399
  linear, 176
Sclerosis
  multiple; see Multiple sclerosis
  tuberous, 170, 173-176, 277-282, 315-316, 317, 333, 334, 395, 397
    adenoma sebaceum in, 278-279
    angiofibromas in, 282
    angiofibromatosis in patients with, 281
    clinical features of, 278
    facial abnormalities in, 282
    with leukoderma and adenoma sebaceum, 397
  seizures in, 278
Seckel's bird-headed dwarfism, 159-160
Segments
  facial, 18-29
  horizontal, major, 18-19
  lower facial, 27-29
    abnormalities of, 82-101
  middle facial, 20-27
    abnormalities of, 58-81

Segments — cont'd
  middle facial — cont'd
    embryologic origin of, 59
    upper facial and cranial, 19-20
Settelberger's infantile neuroaxonal dystrophy,
    419-421
Shagreen patches, 279
Shock type nerve lesions, 85
Silver-Russell syndrome, 327
Sinus thrombosis
  cavernous, 186, 187
  lateral, 185-186
  superior sagittal, 185
Sjögren-Larsson syndrome, 393
Skin, 30
  cranial, congenital absence of, 169
Skin blemish syndromes
  diffuse 390-395
  of lateral middle face, 282-285
Skin blemishes and birthmarks, 73-76
Skull, newborn, major bones, sutures, and fon-
    tanels of, 10-11
Smooth brain, 160
Sock feet, 108
Sotos' syndrome, 252, 290-291, 328, 330, 350
Sphingolipidoses, 141, 148
Sphingomyelinoses, 141, 145
Spielmeyer-Sjögren disease, 412
Sprengel's deformity, 353
Squamousal sutures, patent, 116
Squints, 67-68
Stenosis
  aqueductal, 130-133
    acquired, 133
  supravalvular aortic, 215, 217
Stickler's syndrome, 299
Stomodeum, 13
Strabismus, 67-68
Sturge-Weber syndrome, 172, 191-195, 218, 227,
    229, 285, 311-313, 341, 395, 400
  atypical, 288
  with craniofacial nevus, 397
Subcutaneous and cutaneous involvement, gen-
    eralized, 395-397
Subdural accumulations, macrocephaly result-
    ing from, 149-156
Subdural effusion
  bacterial meningitides as cause of, 155-156
  craniofacial abnormalities caused by, 153
  empyema following, 156
Subdural empyema, 156
Subdural fluid accumulations, traumatic, 153
Subdural hematoma
  acute, 153
  chronic, 154
Sugarman-Reed, craniofacial leukoderma of,
    284-285
Sugarman-Reed syndrome, 206
Sulfatide lipidoses, 145
Supernumerary isochrome 18 syndrome, 350-
    364

Supravalvular aortic stenosis, 215, 217
Sutures
  coronal, premature closure of, 116
  cranial, syndromes characterized by pre-
    mature closures of, 104-122
  disturbances of, syndromes characterized by,
    123-129
  major, of newborn skull, 10-11
  squamousal, patent, 116
  synostosis of, syndromes characterized by, 128
Sydenham's chorea, 322
"Symptomatic dystomias," 345
Syndactyly, 107
Syndrome(s)
  Adie's, 204, 205
  Albers-Schonberg, 421
  ankyloglossum superius, 403
  Apert's; see Apert's syndrome
  Arnold-Chiari, 130-131, 134-135
  Beckwith-Wiedemann, 341-342, 343
  Bielschowsky-Jansky, 410, 411, 412
  Brachmann-DeLange, 372
  brachyfacial and fat facial, 364-372
  broad thumbs, 248-250
  C, 247
  Carpenter's; see Carpenter's syndrome
  cat-cry, 273, 274, 371-372
  cat's eye, 201, 247, 252, 273, 274, 350, 371-372
  of central lower face, 296-325
  of central middle face, 182-277
  cerebrohepatorenal, 364, 365
  cerebrooculofacioskeletal, 243
  characterized by
    abnormalities
      of buccal surface and gums, 333-337
      of chin, 325-326
      of conjunctiva, 223-229
      of cornea and lens, 210-218
      of ears, 285-294
      of eyelids, 229-243
      of facial expression, 397-422
      of hair, 166-172
      of head posture, 344-349
      of iris and pupil, 202-210
      of jaws and cerebral gigantism, 328-333
      of lens, 218-223
      of ocular alignment, 254-262
      in orbital slant, 243-254
      of teeth, 337-338
      in total facial contour and size, 360-376
    brachycollis and pterygium colli, 353-358
    cleft lip and palate, 296-299
    coloboma iridal, 201
    dementia or mental retardation, 403-414
    diffuse cutaneous pigmentary lesions, 385
    dolichostenocollis, 349-353
    facial emaciation and aging, 376-385
    facial immobility, 399-403
    facial palsy or facial diparesis, 299-311
    hemihyperplasia and birthmarks of lower
      face, 311-316

Syndrome(s)—cont'd
  characterized by—cont'd
    hypotelorism, hypertelorism, and other abnormalities of central middle face, 263-273
    laterally extending skin blemishes, 277-285
    macroglossia and other tongue abnormalities, 338-344
    megalencephaly, 141
    microcephaly, 156-166
    microstomia or macrostomia, 322-325
    mutilated and abnormally positioned lips, 316-322
    ocular protrusion and abnormal size, 182-201
    peculiar facial expressions, 414-422
    premature closures of cranial sutures, 104-122
    simple macrocephaly, 130-156
    suture disturbances, 123-129
  Chotzen's, 111
  coarse facial, 372-376
  Cockayne's; see Cockayne's syndrome
  of congenital absence of cranial skin, 169
  congenital cataract, 218
  of congenital contractural arachnodactyly, 361-362
  congenital malformation causing hydrocephalus, 130
  conjunctival, 229
  involving conjunctival vessels dilated, 227-229
  Conradi's, 247
  corneal clouding, 213-215
  Cowden's, 391-393
  cri-du-chat, 273, 274, 371-372
  Cross', 201, 215, 335, 386
  Crouzon's; see Crouzon's syndrome
  cryptophthalmos, 197
  "cushingoid," 370
  Cushing's, 370
  Dandy-Walker, 130, 133-135
  Darier's, 393
  de Grouchy's, 267, 350
  DeLange-Brachmann, 323
  DeLange's, 166, 169, 171, 273-276, 366, 372
  dementia, 407-414
  dementia-emaciation, 170, 381
  DeMorsier's, 201
  DeSanctis-Cacchione, 393-394
  diencephalic, 378, 379
  diffuse hyperpigmentation, 386-390
  diffuse hypopigmentation, 385-386, 387
  diffuse skin blemish, 390-395
  Donohue's, 170, 382
  Down's; see Down's syndrome
  Dreschfield-Taylor-Erickson, 247
  Duane's retraction, 308
  dysmigration, 175
  ear, 291-294
  Eaton-Lambert, 232

Syndrome(s)—cont'd
  Edwards', 252
  EEC, 298
  Ehlers-Danlos, 393
  elfin-facies, 215
  eyelid, 241-243
  facial aging, 382-385
  facial diparesis, 401-403
  facial emaciation, 378-382
  fetal alcohol, 241
  fetal face, 372
  first-branchial-arch, 247-254, 285-290, 298-299, 332-333
  floppy-baby, 342-343
  Frohlich's, 370
  frontal bossing, 126-129
  Goldenhar's, 229, 252, 253, 291
  Goltz's, 201
  Greig's, 272-273
  half-and-half, 207-209, 395
  Hallermann-Streiff, 169, 199-200, 215, 251-252, 333
  Hallervorden-Spatz; see Hallervorden-Spatz syndrome
  Hand-Schuller-Christian, 336-337
  Hanhart's, 403
  happy puppet, 96, 146-148, 343-344
  Harada's, 206
  hemiplegia-hemihypoplasia-hemiathetosis, 348-349
  heterochromia, 206-210
  Horner's; see Horner's syndrome
  Hunter's, 273, 275, 372-375
  Hurler's, 213, 215, 341, 372-375
  Hurler-Scheie, 215
  Hutchinson-Gilford; see Hutchinson-Gilford syndrome
  hypertelorism, 270
  hypoglossia-hypodactylia, 403
  hypotelorism, 267-270
  immobile face, 403
  Kearns-Sayre, 238-240
  Kleeblättschadel, 123
  Klinefelter's, 349, 351, 364
  Klippel-Trénaunay; see Klippel-Trénaunay syndrome
  Klüver-Bucy, 169
  of large and floppy ears, 290-291
  Larsen's, 270-271, 272, 299
  of lateral middle face, 277-294
    skin blemish, 282-285
  Laurence-Moon-Biedl, 370
  Lawrence-Berardinelli, 382
  Lejeune, 252
  lenticular, 220-223
  Leopard, 394
  Lesch-Nyhan; see Lesch-Nyhan syndrome
  Letterer-Siwe, 336-337
  lissencephalic, 160-161, 170
  of lower facial segment and neck, 295-358
  Lowe's oculocerebrorenal, 201, 218

Syndrome(s)—cont'd
  of low-set ears, 285-290
  macrostomia, 323-325
  Marden-Walker, 320, 403, 421
  Marfan's; *see* Marfan's syndrome
  Marinesco-Sjogren, 200-201, 215, 218-220
  Maroteaux-Lamy, 215
  Meckel's, 270, 299
  median cleft face, 273
    with hypertelorism, 128
  megalocornea, 215-218
  Melkersson-Rosthenal, 300, 309-311, 341, 342
  Menkes' kinky hair, 169
  microphthalmia, of Lenz, 197-198
  of middle facial segment, 181-294
  midline hemangioma-scaphocephaly, 105-106
  MMM, 268, 323-325
  Moebius'; *see* Moebius' syndrome
  Mohr's, 111-112
  mongoloid, 245-247
  monosomy 21 and 21q−, 252
  Morquio's, 215
  mucopolysaccharide, 372
  multiple mucosal neuroma, 350
  multiple pterygium, 299
  of multisegmental involvement, 360-397
  Murray-Puretic, 335-336
  myasthenoid, 232
  myoclonic ataxia-plus, 259
  N, 170, 270, 350-351, 382
  of neck, 344-358
  nonchromosomal dysplastic, 350
  Noonan's, 252, 270, 271, 358
  oculocerebrorenal, of Lowe, 201, 218
  ODO, 201
  OFD II, 298
  OPD, 252, 293, 298-299, 422
  "ophthalmoplegia-plus," 238
  Opitz trigonocephaly, 247
  of oral cavity, 333-344
  oromandibular-limb hypogenesis, 403
  otopalatodigital, 293, 298-299, 422
  4 p−, 299
  5 p+, 247
  9 p−, 247
  9 p+, 252
  11 p+, 252, 299
  Parry-Romberg, 175, 201, 276-277, 395, 396
  of peripheral lower face, 325-333
  Pfeiffer's, 114
  +18 pi, 364
  Potter's, 293, 385
  Prader-Willi; *see* Prader-Willi syndrome
  prognathism, 328-332
  of progressive estropia, 256
  ptosis, 229-241
  10 q+, 252
  13 q−, 276
  18 q−, 267, 350
  19 q−, 299

Syndrome(s)—cont'd
  22 q+, 350
  Ramsay Hunt's, 294
  Riley-Day, 422
  Riley-Smith, with mixed hemangioma, 397
  Roberts', 299
  Rothmund-Thomson, 384
  Rubinstein-Taybi, 114, 248-250, 323
  Saethre-Chotzen, 111
  Sanfilippo's, 215, 375-376
  Scheie's, 215
  Schwartz-Jampel; *see* Schwartz-Jampel syndrome
  Silver-Russell, 327
  Sotos', 252, 290-291, 328, 330, 350
  Stickler's, 299
  Sturge-Weber; *see* Sturge-Weber syndrome
  Sugarman-Reed, 206
  supernumerary isochrome 18, 350, 364
  supravalvular aortic stenosis−elfin facies−
    idiopathic hypercalcemia, 323
  teardrop pigment, 285, 286
  of total face, 359-422
  Treacher Collins, 252, 291-294, 322, 333-334
  triangular chin, 326-327
  trisomy 8, 350
  trisomy 13, 195-196
  trisomy 18, 276, 350
  trisomy 22, 252
  Tuomaala-Haapanen, 386
  Turner's; *see* Turner's syndrome
  of upper facial and cranial segment, 102-180
  Urbach-Wiethe, 394-395
  Vogt-Koyanagi, 206
  Waardenburg's, 72, 170, 175, 206, 207, 241,
    242, 271-272, 283, 284
  Waterman's, 169, 334, 335
  Werner's, 384
  whistling face, 252, 320, 399, 403, 421
  Williams, 215
  wrinkly skin, 385
  Wyburn-Mason's, 227-229
  XXXXY, 252, 299
  XXY, 349, 351
  XYY, 332
  Zellweger's, 360, 364, 365
  Zimmermann-Laband, 335
Synostosis, suture, syndromes characterized by,
    128

**T**

Tangier disease, 148
Tay-Sachs disease, 141-144, 391, 411
Teardrop pigment syndrome, 285, 286
Teeth
  abnormalities of, 93
    syndromes characterized by, 337-338
  characteristics of, 29
Telangiectasia, 225
  ataxia-, 76

Telangiectasia — cont'd
  conjunctival, 76
Telangiectatic nevi, 227
Temperature, elevation in, 103
Tented tilt, 79
Tenting of upper lip, 87-88
Thomsen's myotonia congenita, 301
Thrombosis, sinus; see Sinus thrombosis
Thyroid and pituitary dysfunctions, 231
Tongue, 93-97
  abnormalities of, 94, 97
    macroglossia, syndromes characterized by, 338-344
    involving posture and protrusion, 96
    topographic, 96-97
  asymmetrical fibrous bands of, 97
  atrophy and hypoplasia of, 95-96
  banded, 96
  fasciculations of, 95
  furrowed, 96
  lobulated, 97
  scarred, 97
  smallness of, 96
  unilateral atrophic involvement of, 95-96
Topographic abnormalities, 81
TORCH encephalopathies, 161-162
Torter, neck, congenital absence of, 98
Torticollis, 97
Torticollis dystonia, 100
Toxoplasma gondii, 165
Toxoplasmosis, congenital, 68, 165
Transillumination as sign for hydranencephaly, 137
Treacher Collins' syndrome, 252, 291-294, 323, 333-334
Trichinosis, 232
Trisomy, 207, 245-247
Trisomy 8 syndrome, 350
Trisomy 13, 267, 298, 299
  syndrome, 195-196
Trisomy 18, 252
  partial, 210
  syndrome, 276, 350
Trisomy 21, 78, 166, 270, 322-323, 339
Trisomy 22, 201, 247
  syndrome, 252
Tuberous sclerosis; see Sclerosis, tuberous
Tuomaala-Haapanen syndrome, 386
Turner's syndrome, 172, 242, 252, 270, 323, 355-358, 367, 385
  abnormalities in, 356-357
  facial features in 357-358
  male, 358
  types of, 255-256
Turricephaly, 108, 117-122

U

Upper facial and cranial segment, 19-20
  syndromes of, 102-180

Upper-motor facial nerve lesions, 85
Urbach-Wiethe syndrome, 394-395

V

V-shaped tilt, 79-80
Vascular malformations, congenital, 93
Vertex line, horizontal, 14
Vertex point, 14
Vertical lines
  cranial, 16
  facial, 16-17
  major, 16
  midfacial, 16-17
  pupillary, 17
Vitiligo, 170, 206
Vogt-Koyanagi syndrome, 206
von Graefe's sign, 183
von Hippel's disease, 193-195
von Recklinghausen's disease, 187-190, 194, 314-315, 391, 392, 405-406

W

Waardenburg's syndrome, 72, 170, 175, 206, 207, 241, 242, 271-272, 283, 284
Water head, 130
Waterman's syndrome, 169, 334, 335
Webbed neck, 101
Werdnig-Hoffmann disease, 342-343, 344
Werner's syndrome, 384
Whistling face syndrome, 252, 320, 399, 403, 421
White forelocks and cranial poliosis, 170-172
Williams' syndrome, 215
Wilsonian pupil, 64-65
Wilson's disease
  facial appearance in, 213, 418-419, 420
  hepatic form of, 212
  lenticular form of, 212
  "pseudosclerotic" form of, 211, 419
Wilson's hepatolenticular degeneration, 210-213, 214, 322, 345
Wolman's xanthomatosis with adrenal involvement, 148
Wrinkly skin syndrome, 385
Wyburn-Mason's syndrome, 227-229

X

Xanthomatosis
  cerebrotendinous, 243, 244
  Wolman's, with adrenal involvement, 148
Xeroderma pigmentosum, 393-394
XXXXY syndrome, 252, 299
XXY syndrome, 349, 351
XYY syndrome, 332

Z

Zellweger's syndrome, 360, 364, 365
Zimmermann-Laband syndrome, 335
Zygomata and lateral bony orbits, 77-79